# NEUROPROTECTION IN CRITICAL CARE AND PERIOPERATIVE MEDICINE

**Edited by**

David L. Reich, MD
*President and COO*
*The Mount Sinai Hospital*
*Horace W. Goldsmith Professor of Anesthesiology*
*Icahn School of Medicine at Mount Sinai*

Stephan A. Mayer, MD
*William T. Gossett Endowed Chair*
*Chair, Department of Neurology*
*Co-Director, Neuroscience Institute*
*Henry Ford Health System*

Suzan Uysal, PhD
*Associate Professor of Anesthesiology, Psychiatry and*
*Rehabilitation Medicine*
*Icahn School of Medicine at Mount Sinai*

OXFORD
UNIVERSITY PRESS

# OXFORD
UNIVERSITY PRESS

Oxford University Press is a department of the University of Oxford. It furthers
the University's objective of excellence in research, scholarship, and education
by publishing worldwide. Oxford is a registered trade mark of Oxford University
Press in the UK and certain other countries.

Published in the United States of America by Oxford University Press
198 Madison Avenue, New York, NY 10016, United States of America.

© Oxford University Press 2018

Library of Congress Cataloging-in-Publication Data
Names: Reich, David L. (David Louis), 1960– editor. | Mayer, Stephan A., editor. |
Uysal, Suzan, 1960– editor.
Title: Neuroprotection in critical care and perioperative medicine /
edited by David L. Reich, Stephan Mayer, Suzan Uysal.
Description: New York, NY : Oxford University Press, [2018] |
Includes bibliographical references.
Identifiers: LCCN 2017040791 | ISBN 9780190280253 (pbk.)
Subjects: | MESH: Neuroprotection | Perioperative Period | Critical Care
Classification: LCC RC341 | NLM WL 102 | DDC 616.8—dc23
LC record available at https://lccn.loc.gov/2017040791

9 8 7 6 5 4 3 2 1

Printed by WebCom, Inc., Canada

# Neuroprotection in Critical Care and Perioperative Medicine

To our families and loved ones.

# About the Cover

Entitled, "What's left behind?", these images are multiple axial slices of the same healthy human brain. They capture the eyes, cortex, and other neuroanatomy, including the optic nerve (bottom left panel) in high resolution. These images were acquired using ultra-high field (7 Tesla field strength) magnetic resonance imaging (MRI). Although the images were acquired as magnitude images, often displayed in grayscale, each panel was processed with a different colormap. The colormaps were chosen for their overall visual qualities, and each was initially developed to highlight different features of an image.

Cover artwork provided courtesy of:
Rebecca Feldman, PhD
Postdoctoral Fellow
Translational and Molecular Imaging Institute and Department of Radiology
Icahn School of Medicine at Mount Sinai
New York, New York

# Contents

# Contributors

**Christopher S. Ahuja, MD**
Division of Neurosurgery, Department of Surgery
Institute of Medical Science
University of Toronto
Toronto, Ontario

**Aws Alawi, MD**
Columbia University College of Physicians and Surgeons
New York, New York

**Zirka H. Anastasian, MD**
Assistant Professor of Anesthesiology
Columbia University Medical Center
New York, New York

**John G. Augoustides, MD, FASE, FAHA**
Professor, Cardiovascular and Thoracic Section
Department of Anesthesiology and Critical Care
Perelman School of Medicine
University of Pennsylvania
Philadelphia, Pennsylvania

**Karsten Bartels, MD**
Assistant Professor of Anesthesiology and Surgery
Cardiothoracic Anesthesiology and Critical Care Medicine
University of Colorado
Aurora, Colorado

**Jess W. Brallier, MD**
Assistant Professor, Department of Anesthesiology, Perioperative and Pain Medicine
Icahn School of Medicine at Mount Sinai
New York, New York

**Marco Carbonara, MD**
Neurointensive Care Unit, Fondazione IRCCS Ca' Granda Ospedale Maggiore Policlinico
Milan, Italy

**Eugene Chang, MD**
Professor, Department of Obstetrics and Gynecology
Medical University of South Carolina
Charleston, South Carolina

**Neeraj Chaudhary, MD, MRCS, FRCR**
Assistant Professor, Departments of Radiology and Neurosurgery
University of Michigan
Ann Arbor, Michigan

**Jan Claassen, MD, PhD**
Columbia University College of Physicians and Surgeons
New York, New York

**Neha S. Dangayach, MD**
Assistant Professor
Departments of Neurosurgery and Neurology
Institute of Critical Care Medicine
Icahn School of Medicine at Mount Sinai
Mount Sinai Health System
New York, New York

**Ramon Diaz-Arrastia, MD, PhD**
Department of Neurology
University of Pennsylvania Perelman School of Medicine
Philadelphia, Pennsylvania

**W. Dalton Dietrich, PhD**
The Miami Project to Cure Paralysis
Department of Neurosurgery,
Neurology and Biomedical
Engineering
University of Miami Miller School of
Medicine
Miami, Florida

**Lauren E. Dunn, MD**
Stroke Division, Department of
Neurology
Columbia University Medical Center
New York, New York

**Michael Fehlings, MD, PhD, FRCSC,
FACS, FRSC, FCAHS**
Professor of Neurosurgery
Vice Chair Research
Department of Surgery
Halbert Chair in Neural Repair and
Regeneration
Co-Chairman Spinal Program
University of Toronto
Head Spinal Program
Senior Scientist McEwen Centre for
Regenerative Medicine
Toronto Western Hospital
University Health Network
Toronto, Ontario

**Jared W. Feinman, MD**
Assistant Professor, Cardiovascular
and Thoracic Section
Department of Anesthesiology and
Critical Care
Perelman School of Medicine
University of Pennsylvania
Philadelphia, Pennsylvania

**Charles L. Francoeur, MD, FRCPC**
Critical Care Division, Department of
Anesthesiology and Critical Care
CHU de Québec-Université Laval
Québec, Canada

**Jonathan S. Gal, MD**
Assistant Professor, Department of
Anesthesiology, Perioperative and
Pain Medicine
Icahn School of Medicine at Mount Sinai
New York, New York

**Nishant Ganesh Kumar, MD**
Department of Surgery, Section of
Plastic Surgery
University of Michigan Health System
Ann Arbor, Michigan

**Joseph J. Gemmete, MD,
FACR, FSIR**
Professor, Departments of Radiology,
Neurosurgery, and Otolaryngology
University of Michigan
Ann Arbor, Michigan

**Julius Griauzde, MD**
Neurointerventional Radiology Fellow,
Departments of Radiology
University of Michigan
Ann Arbor, Michigan

**Lucy He, MD**
Resident Physician, Department of
Neurological Surgery
Vanderbilt University Medical Center
Nashville, Tennessee

**Eric J. Heyer, MD, PhD**
Professor Emeritus of Anesthesiology
and Neurology
Columbia University Medical Center
New York, New York

**Travis R. Ladner, MD**
Resident Physician, Department of
Neurological Surgery
Icahn School of Medicine at
Mount Sinai
New York, New York

**Ronald M. Lazar, PhD,
FAHA, FAAN**
Evelyn F. McKnight Endowed Chair in
Learning and Memory
Director, Evelyn F. McKnight Brain
Institute at UAB
Director, Division of
Neuropsychology
Department of Neurology
The University of Alabama at
Birmingham
Birmingham, Alabama

**David S. Liebeskind, MD, FAAN, FAHA, FANA**
Professor of Neurology and
    Director, Neurovascular Imaging
    Research Core
Director, UCLA Cerebral Blood Flow
    Laboratory
Associate Neurology Director, UCLA
    Stroke Center
UCLA Department of Neurology
Los Angeles, California

**G. Burkhard Mackensen, MD, PhD, FASE**
Professor of Anesthesiology, Chief,
    Division of Cardiothoracic
    Anesthesiology
UW Medicine Research &
    Education Endowed Professor in
    Anesthesiology
Adjunct Professor of Medicine,
    Department of Anesthesiology &
    Pain Medicine
UW Medicine Regional Heart Center
University of Washington
Seattle, Washington

**Carlos Marquez de la Plata, PhD**
Director of Rehabilitation Research,
    Pate Rehabilitation
Clinical Assistant Professor,
    Department of Psychiatry
University of Texas Southwestern
    Medical Center
Dallas, Texas

**Stephan A. Mayer, MD**
William T. Gossett Endowed Chair,
    Department of Neurology
Co-Director, Neuroscience Institute
Henry Ford Health System
Detroit, Michigan

**Diana Mayor, MD**
Division of Neurosurgery, Toronto
    Western Hospital, University Health
    Network
Krembil Research Institute, University
    Health Network
Toronto, Ontario

**J Mocco, MD, MS**
Professor and Vice Chair for
    Education
Department of Neurological Surgery
Icahn School of Medicine at
    Mount Sinai
New York, New York

**Aditya S. Pandey, MD**
Associate Professor, Departments of
    Neurosurgery and Radiology
University of Michigan
Ann Arbor, Michigan

**Axel Petzold, MD, PhD**
UCL Institute of Neurology, Molecular
    Neuroscience
Queen Square, London

**Joseph H. Pitcher, MD**
Pulmonary and Critical Care Fellow
Maine Medical Center, Department of
    Critical Care Services
Portland, Maine

**Jonathan J. Ratcliff, MD, MPH**
Assistant Professor of Emergency
    Medicine and Neurology
Emergency Neurosciences and
    Neuroscience Critical Care,
    Emory University School of
    Medicine
Marcus Stroke and Neuroscience
    Center, Grady Memorial Hospital
Department of Emergency
    Medicine, Division of Emergency
    Neurosciences
Department of Neurology, Division of
    Neurocritical Care
Emory University
Atlanta, Georgia

**David L. Reich, MD**
President and COO
The Mount Sinai Hospital
Horace W. Goldsmith Professor of
    Anesthesiology
Icahn School of Medicine at
    Mount Sinai
New York, New York

**Michael Reznik, MD**
Neurocritical Care Fellow
Columbia University Medical Center
  and Weill Cornell Medicine
Department of Neurology
New York, New York

**David B. Seder, MD, FCCP,
  FCCM, FNCS**
Interim Department Chief and Director
  of Neurocritical Care
Maine Medical Center Critical Care
  Services
Associate Professor of Medicine, Tufts
  University School of Medicine
Portland, Maine

**Magdy Selim, MD, PhD**
Professor of Neurology, Harvard
  Medical School
Chief, Stroke Division, Department of
  Neurology
Beth Israel Deaconess Medical Center
Boston, Massachusetts

**Tarek Sharshar, MD, PhD**
General Intensive Care Medicine
Assistance Publique Hôpitaux de Paris,
  Raymond Poincaré Hospital
University of Versailles
Garches, France
Laboratory of Human Histopathology
  and Animal Models
Institut Pasteur
Paris, France

**Nino Stocchetti, MD**
Department of Physiopathology and
  Transplantation, Milan University
Neurointensive Care Unit, Fondazione
  IRCCS Ca' Granda Ospedale
  Maggiore Policlinico
Milan, Italy

**Michael Tymianski, MD, PhD**
Division of Neurosurgery, Toronto
  Western Hospital, University
  Health Network
Department of Surgery, University
  of Toronto
Krembil Research Institute,
  University Health Network
Toronto, Ontario

**Suzan Uysal, PhD**
Associate Professor of Anesthesiology,
  Psychiatry and Rehabilitation
  Medicine
Icahn School of Medicine at
  Mount Sinai
New York, New York

**Matthew A. Warner, MD**
Assistant Professor of Anesthesiology
Division of Critical Care Medicine
Department of Anesthesiology
  and Perioperative Medicine
Mayo Clinic
Rochester, Minnesota

**Joshua Z. Willey, MD, MS**
Assistant Professor of Neurology
Stroke Division, Department of
  Neurology
Columbia University Medical Center
New York, New York

**David W. Wright, MD, FACEP**
Associate Professor
Vice Chair for Innovation and
  Discovery
Director, Emergency Neurosciences
Director, Injury Prevention Research
  Center, at Emory
Department of Emergency Medicine
Emory University School of Medicine
Atlanta, Georgia

**Guohua Xi, MD**
Professor, Department of
  Neurosurgery
University of Michigan
Ann Arbor, Michigan

# PART I
## PROTECTION STRATEGIES

# 1 Physiologic Modulators of Neural Injury After Brain and Spinal Cord Injury

W. Dalton Dietrich

## INTRODUCTION

Central nervous system (CNS) injuries such as traumatic brain injury (TBI), stroke, subarachnoid hemorrhage (SAH), and spinal cord injury (SCI) are worldwide clinical problems that produce long-term disability and mortality. To address these neurological conditions, much basic and clinical research has been devoted to understanding the pathophysiology of these injuries and testing therapeutic interventions.

After the primary CNS injury, there is a spectrum of secondary injury processes that may complicate the pathobiology and worsen outcomes.[1] Early management of physiological targets with evidence-based pre-hospital and emergency care therefore represents a critically important phase of care. There are several core physiological targets and management strategies that are essential for successful treatment of the severely injured patient in the pre-hospital setting and in the neuro-intensive care unit.[2] Goals and standards of care have been established for the pre-hospital triage, stabilization, and transport phases to limit life-threatening events that may aggravate secondary injury mechanisms.

Three physiological factors have emerged from the scientific literature as important targets for protecting injured neural tissue from secondary injury and promoting good outcomes and long-term recovery in patients with acute neurological injury. These are oxygen, glucose, and core temperature. The measurement and management of blood gases, blood pressure, and core temperature has been shown to be important when attempting to reduce secondary injury mechanisms. This chapter summarizes these physiological modulators of secondary neural injury and the management and treatment strategies that require critical consideration in terms of their potential impact on long-term outcome.

## OXYGEN TARGETS

Cerebral hypoxia has been shown to worsen outcome in animal models of brain and spinal cord injury.[3] Hemorrhagic shock and other pathological conditions that result in hypotension or decreased perfusion, such as intracranial or intrathecal hypertension, can reduce oxygen ($O_2$) delivery to the brain or spinal cord.[4] Cerebral hypoxic conditions and adequacy of oxygen supply to the brain therefore play a critical role in modulating secondary injury cascades.[5] Specific means to increase tissue oxygenation to normalize metabolism and promote the survival of neural tissue are therefore standards of care in the clinical setting.[6]

Hypotension is thought to worsen secondary brain injury.[7] Intraoperative hypotension is common in patients with isolated TBI undergoing emergency craniotomy, as well as in patients with multiorgan trauma. The early correction of hypotension, defined as systolic blood pressure of less than 90 mm Hg, is recommended.[8]

In animal models of TBI, an induced secondary hypoxic insult increases overall contusion volume and aggravates the long-term behavioral consequences associated with the primary insult.[9] In animal models of stroke and cardiac arrest, secondary hypoxia increases neuronal vulnerability, leading to greater infarct volumes and white matter pathology.[10] Hypoxia aggravates several secondary injury mechanisms, including excitotoxic processes and blood–brain barrier (BBB) disruption, which can enhance the infiltration of circulating blood cells and thereby increase inflammatory and secondary injury mechanisms.[5]

Tracheal intubation and normobaric oxygen therapy are commonly used to increase brain tissue oxygen partial pressure ($PbtO_2$).[11] Pre-hospital tracheal intubation is an effective strategy to normalize levels of oxygen in severely injured patients and improve outcomes; however, in some clinical settings (e.g., severe TBI), outcomes have varied. Sobuwa and colleagues reported that patients who underwent basic airway management had better outcomes than those who were intubated, whereas another study reported higher mortality with intubation.[12–13] This inconsistency may reflect that other factors, such as underlying patient conditions, surgeon experience, and use of sedative/neuromuscular blocking drugs, may also contribute to outcomes.[2,11]

Experimental and clinical studies indicate that the specific level of $O_2$ may be a critical factor in determining the benefits of normobaric oxygen therapy.[14] Excessive normobaric oxygen has been shown to have deleterious effects in experimental studies of TBI. Normobaric oxygen treatment has been reported to increase lesion volume and have no positive effect on behavioral measures in an animal model of moderate TBI.[15] The protective effects of hyperbaric resuscitation therapy for TBI are also controversial, with both beneficial and detrimental effects reported.[7,16] In a polytrauma TBI model, improved hippocampal neuronal survival was observed following hyperoxic resuscitation compared to normoxic resuscitation.[17] Another polytrauma model study using controlled cortical impact-induced TBI followed by 30 minutes of hemorrhagic shock induced by blood withdrawal found that hyperoxic resuscitation using 100% $O_2$ was associated with greater survival, no difference in cerebral cortical pathology, and worse neurological outcome.[4]

Hyperoxic resuscitation, however, has also been reported to increase oxidative stress, metabolic impairment, neuronal death, and poor neurological outcome under specific conditions. Some retrospective studies have led to similar conclusions regarding hyperoxic treatment following cardiac arrest, whereas others have failed to detect any harm caused by hyperoxia. Clinical investigations have found that high levels of oxygen are associated with worse prognosis after severe TBI.[14,18] A retrospective analysis of patients with severe TBI who were monitored with cerebral microdialysis and glutamate analysis found that incremental normobaric $O_2$ levels were associated with increased cerebral excitotoxicity.[14] These findings call into question the therapeutic value of supernormal oxygen tension in this patient population and highlight the importance of normal $PaO_2$ levels for optimal neural tissue survival and function.[2] Future resuscitation studies should include examination of titrated levels of inspired ventricular $O_2$ to determine benefits and risks in specific patient populations.

## GLYCEMIC CONTROL

Hyperglycemia is a common problem in a variety of conditions and is associated with poor outcomes (Table 1.1).[19-20] In the context of ischemic stroke, higher blood levels of glucose are associated with greater stroke severity and functional impairment.[21] In the context of TBI, elevated blood levels of glucose have been shown to correlate with poorer outcomes and may impair cerebrovascular reactivity.[22] After SCI, hyperglycemia on hospital admission has been found to be a significant risk predictor of poor functional outcome.[19]

Several mechanisms have been proposed as an explanation for the detrimental effects of hyperglycemia, including increased anaerobic metabolism, apoptotic cell death, and BBB breakdown.[23] It is not clear, however, whether the associations between hyperglycemia and adverse outcomes are due to direct deleterious effects produced by hyperglycemia or whether the degree of hyperglycemia simply represents a marker of brain injury severity. Thus, the management of blood glucose levels after brain injury is a subject of growing debate.[24] Several glucose-lowering therapies have resulted in an increased rate of hypoglycemic episodes, and varying recommendations regarding post-injury hyperglycemia management have been advanced. Currently, less strict degrees of glycemic control (120–180 mg/dL) are believed to be optimal in most ICU populations.[25-26]

In patients with acute ischemic stroke, hyperglycemia has been observed in more than one-third of patients on hospital admission, is significantly more common in patients with severe strokes, and is an independent predictor of poor functional outcome.[27] A randomized clinical trial comparing intensive intravenous insulin treatment versus subcutaneous insulin in patients with acute ischemic stroke, however, found that while intensive insulin treatment was more effective in restoring

**Table 1.1** Conditions that Can Lead to Low or High Dialysate Glucose

| High Dialysate Glucose | Low Dialysate Glucose |
|---|---|
| *Hyperemia* due to increased blood flow and thereby increased glucose delivery | *Ischemia* caused by insufficient blood flow causing decrease levels of tissue glucose |
| *Hyperglycemia* due to increased blood glucose that increases the dialysate glucose | *Hypoglycemia* due to decreased blood glucose that decreases the dialysate glucose |
| *Hypometabolism*: this will cause a decrease of glucose uptake into the cells and thereby lead to high extracellular glucose available to the microdialysis catheter | *Hypermetabolism*: this will cause an increase of glucose uptake into the cells and thereby lead to low extracellular glucose available to the microdialysis catheter |

Adapted from Rostami E. Glucose and the injured brain-monitored in the neurointensive care unit. *Front Neurol.* 2014;5:91.

normoglycemia, it was associated with greater infarct growth.[28] A Cochrane review concluded that there is no reliable evidence for glucose control in acute ischemic stroke.[27] More investigation is required to determine the most appropriate and safest strategies to minimize the potential detrimental effects of hyperglycemia after stroke.

Most experimental studies investigating the effects of hyperglycemia on TBI have administered relatively large doses of glucose sufficient to induce hyperglycemia.[29] In a model of closed head injury, the infusion of a large volume of dextrose led to increased mortality, increased cerebral edema, and worse neurological outcome.[30] In contrast, the induction of hyperglycemia 20 minutes after a controlled cortical impact injury had no effect on contusion volume or neuronal loss in the hippocampus.[31] In studies using lower doses of glucose, the effects on local cerebral metabolic rates of glucose and neuronal injury were attenuated.[32] Taken together, these preclinical findings indicate that glucose administration after TBI may not be detrimental and that glucose treatment may actively produce neuroprotective effects. Additional studies using varying doses of glucose in multiple models of TBI are needed to clarify this important issue.

## THERAPEUTIC HYPOTHERMIA AND TARGETED TEMPERATURE CONTROL

Hypothermia has a long history as a strategy for neuroprotection.[33] Early studies conducted in experimental models of global cerebral ischemia showed that relatively small variations in brain temperature during or following the insult critically determined the vulnerability of specific neuronal groups and BBB consequences.[34] Subsequent studies have reported that moderate hypothermia significantly improves histopathological and behavioral outcomes, while mild elevations in temperature that occur in severely injured patients aggravate outcomes. Multi-institutional studies have also reported that small alterations in temperature significantly affect many pathophysiological secondary injury mechanisms associated with acute and more chronic injury.[35] Currently, therapeutic hypothermia and targeted temperature management (TTM) protocols are major themes in the critical care literature addressing a variety of conditions (Table 1.2).[36-44] Importantly, therapeutic hypothermia has been suggested to be the most potent neuroprotective strategy.[45]

## Mechanisms Underlying Physiological and Temperature Effects

As previously described, the pathophysiology of brain and spinal cord injury involves multiple potential mechanisms, each of which may have a significant impact on neuronal dysfunction and/or cell death.[39,46] These mechanisms include cerebral ischemia and hypoxia, excitotoxicity, inflammation, oxidative stress, metabolic dysfunction, seizures, brain edema, and intracranial pressure (ICP) elevation.[36] Injury complexity must therefore be taken into consideration in the search for new treatments that can be successfully translated to the clinical setting. Additionally, the temporal profile of injury cascades is important as we consider treatment limitations for targeting specific physiological variables or pharmacotherapy. To this end, experimental investigations and clinical studies have revealed multiple secondary injury processes that are sensitive to small variations in brain temperature during or following a brain insult.

| Clinical Scenario | Efficacy | Evidence | Protocol |
|---|---|---|---|
| Cardiac arrest (VT or VF) | Effective | 2 small RCTs and multiple cohort studies | Temperature target 32–34°C for 12–24 h[63–65] |
| Neonatal hypoxic ischemic encephalopathy (HIE) | Effective | RCTs | Moderate to severe HIE, should be treated within 6 h of delivery to 32–34°C for 72 h, at slow rewarming rate[62,66] |
| Increased ICP | Effective | RCTs and cohort studies | 32–36°C (tailored according to ICP level)[78,80–81] |
| Cardiac arrest (PEA or asystole) | Possible | Case series | Target temperature 32–34°C for 12–24 h[47–50] |
| Hypoxic encephalopathy in hanging injury cases | Feasible | Case series | Target temperature 32–34°C >48 h[51–52] |
| Ischemic stroke | Feasible | Small RCTs, ongoing trials | 35°C for awake patients, 32–35°C for ventilated comatose patients[71–73,99] |
| Intracerebral hemorrhage | Unknown | Case series | Fever control[100] |
| Subarachnoid hemorrhage | Unknown | Case series | Fever control[100] |
| Traumatic brain injury | Unknown | RCTs with conflicting research findings, ongoing trials | Target temperature 32–34°C for > 48 h[44,79,82,86,94] |

*ICP*, intracranial pressure; *PEA*, pulseless electrical activity; *RCT*, randomized controlled trial; *VF*, ventricular fibrillation; *VT*, ventricular tachycardia.

Adapted from Andresen M, et al. Therapeutic hypothermia for acute brain injuries. *Scand J Trauma Resusc Emerg Med.* 2015;23:42.

Temperature-sensitive processes include excitotoxicity, free radical generation, programmed cell death, and neuroinflammation.[39,46–49] Using in vivo microdialysis, early cerebral ischemia studies reported that extracellular levels of glutamate and indicators of free radical formation were significantly reduced with post-injury hypothermia compared to normothermia.[49] Cellular and molecular experiments have also shown that hypothermia alters apoptotic mechanisms and may affect programmed cell death signaling cascades. In addition to neuronal benefits, hypothermia reduces vascular permeability abnormalities and glial responses that occur after brain and spinal cord injury.[50–51] Hypothermia also reduces a variety of inflammatory cellular responses to injury and levels of pro-inflammatory cytokines within the injured tissues. Recently, hypothermia has been reported to reduce inflammasome activation, a critical step in the innate immune response to brain injury.[52] Finally, several studies have emphasized the importance of post-injury temperature in reparative processes that may contribute to recovery mechanisms, such as neurogenesis, angiogenesis, and synapse/circuit formation.[47] Together, these findings support the use of therapeutic hypothermia on the basis of beneficial alterations to mechanisms of neuronal injury and reparative processes.

## Therapeutic Hypothermia in Cerebral Ischemia and Stroke

It is well established that brain temperature is a critical factor in determining the pathological consequences of global cerebral ischemia.[35] Today, therapeutic hypothermia is used to treat out-of-hospital cardiac arrest patients and neonates with hypoxic encephalopathy, following multicenter randomized trials that reported long-term benefits.[38,53–56]

The beneficial effects of hypothermia in focal cerebral ischemia have also been established in preclinical studies. In multiple animal models of focal ischemia, hypothermia results in reduced infarct volumes and improved functional outcomes.[57–58] The efficacy of protection varies with the model of ischemia (e.g., temporary vs. permanent); duration of ischemia; and timing, duration, and depth of cooling. Hypothermia has proved to be especially protective in models using transient middle cerebral artery occlusion (MCAo), where cooling during the reperfusion phase consistently reduces infarct volumes.

Several early-phase clinical trials have tested therapeutic hypothermia for neuroprotection after ischemic stroke.[59–62] These studies have demonstrated the ability to safely cool patients with specific methodologies while establishing proactive shivering protocols without the need for tracheal intubation. The Intravenous Thrombolysis Plus Hypothermia for Acute Treatment of Ischemic Stroke (ICTuS-L) study, which compared the combination of thrombolysis and therapeutic hypothermia versus thrombolysis alone, reported encouraging results in terms of both feasibility and safety.[63]

Several large randomized clinical trials addressing the efficacy of therapeutic hypothermia in ischemic stroke are in progress.[57] The ICTuS 2/3 trial is projected to enroll 1,600 patients. The EuroHYP-1 is an open randomized phase III clinical trial with projected enrollment of 1,500 patients. It is hoped that these and future studies will provide additional support for hypothermia as a treatment strategy for acute ischemic stroke.

## Therapeutic Hypothermia in Traumatic Brain Injury

Clifton and colleagues first reported that mild hypothermia following a lateral fluid percussion brain injury improved motor recovery.[37] Since then, therapeutic hypothermia has been extensively tested in multiple models of TBI of focal and diffuse injury.[49,64] These studies have shown that early posttraumatic hypothermia using systemic cooling strategies reduces contusion volumes and protects against patterns of selective neuronal vulnerability. Posttraumatic hypothermia also attenuates diffuse axonal injury and blood-brain barrier damage.[65] In addition to improving histopathological outcomes, posttraumatic hypothermia has beneficial effects on clinically relevant behavioral outcome measures, including sensorimotor assessment and cognitive function.[49] Many studies have reported that posttraumatic hypothermia results in improved hippocampal-dependent cognitive function, as assessed by the

Morris water maze navigation test and fear conditioning paradigms. Although most publications have reported the beneficial effects in experimental studies of posttraumatic hypothermia, some have emphasized limitations of the strategy using mild hypothermia in models of severe cortical contusive injury.

An important variable in determining the efficacy of any clinical intervention is the therapeutic window. One shortcoming of many potentially useful neuroprotective strategies has been the lack of a well-defined treatment window for improving long-term outcomes. Markgraf and colleagues evaluated the therapeutic window of hypothermia after cortical impact injury on brain edema and functional outcomes.[66] Early cooling improved outcome, whereas a delay of hypothermia initiation 90 minutes post-injury failed to reduce edema formation or improve behavioral outcome. It should be noted, however, that a relatively restricted 3-hour duration of hypothermia was tested in this experimental study. Based on the current knowledge regarding the progressive nature of many pathological mechanisms, a long duration of treatment initiated within several hours after injury may be optimal to improve long-term outcome.

The efficacy of therapeutic hypothermia after TBI is also affected by the rate of rewarming following the cooling phase.[67] In the experimental setting, posttraumatic hypothermia followed by slow rewarming provides maximal protection in terms of axonal damage, microvascular damage and dysfunction, and contusional expansion. Hypothermia followed by rapid rewarming inhibits these protective effects and, in many cases, exacerbates the traumatically induced pathology and its functional consequences. Clinical evidence also suggests that the benefits of posttraumatic hypothermia are optimized with slow rewarming, thus reducing the potential for rebound vasodilation and elevated ICP.

Single-institution clinical studies have reported beneficial effects of hypothermia on ameliorating ICP elevations and neurological outcomes following TBI.[68–70] Encouraging findings have been presented by several groups showing that posttraumatic hypothermia improved patient survival and functional outcome following severe TBI.[71]

Unfortunately, when therapeutic hypothermia was tested in several multicenter TBI trials targeting adult or pediatric populations, no benefit on neurological outcome was observed.[72] Multiple multicenter studies found either no difference or worse mortality rates in the hypothermia group compared to a normothermia group.[43,73–75] A significant variation in critical care across sites was reported for the National Brain Injury Study Hypothermia (NABIS:H) trial that was considered to be a confounding variable. Large multicenter clinical trials in pediatric TBI patients also found no significant benefit for therapeutic hypothermia.[72,76] Other investigators have continued to conduct clinical trials of therapeutic hypothermia for severe TBI.[77–78] The Eurotherm 3235 Trial examined the effects of titrated therapeutic hypothermia (32–35°C) on ICP and neurological outcome.[79] This trial, which enrolled 387 patients at 47 centers in 18 countries, has recently reported that therapeutic hypothermia, while successfully reducing ICP, did not improve functional recovery. This trial may have failed to improve neurological outcome because hypothermia was initiated well after the acute injury and may not have influenced the early posttraumatic secondary injury mechanisms that are known to be critical for long-term outcome.

Clifton and colleagues reported a post hoc analysis of data from the NABIS:H multicenter trials indicating beneficial effects of therapeutic hypothermia in a subset of patients with severe TBI.[37] Early hypothermia was associated with improved outcomes in patients requiring surgical decompression for focal insults, but no such association was observed in patients with diffuse injury. These observations led to the hypothesis that early cooling prior to decompression surgery may benefit patient outcomes by reducing the detrimental effects of reperfusion injury that can occur after cortical decompression. Studies reported by Yokobori and colleagues showed that mild hypothermia prior to decompression surgery significantly reduced overall histological injury and improved biomarker indicators of tissue damage.[80] These novel findings emphasize the concept that specific therapeutic interventions may be most appropriate for selective types of severe TBI and that early hypothermic treatment may be most beneficial in conditions where reperfusion injury or elevated ICP are dominant secondary injury mechanisms.

Several meta-analyses of the literature examining hypothermia therapy have been conducted. Li and Yang showed that moderate hypothermia treatment reduced mortality and unfavorable clinical neurological outcomes.[81] In a more recent systematic review of therapeutic hypothermia, Crossley and colleagues examined 18 studies that provided mortality data.[82] They concluded that there is evidence to suggest that therapeutic hypothermia may be beneficial but that the majority of trials have been of low quality with unclear allocation concealment. There is, therefore, a need for more high-quality randomized controlled trials for therapeutic hypothermia after TBI.[83]

While moderate reductions in temperature during controlled cooling trials may be protective, it is known that inadvertent hypothermia in the acute injury setting is associated with increased mortality.[7] Because the severity of brain damage due to the traumatic impact accounts for the majority of early mortality after TBI, inadvertent hypothermia is thought to be a consequence of damage to key temperature regulatory areas in the brain.[84]

### Therapeutic Hypothermia in Spinal Cord Injury

Preclinical and clinical data support the use of therapeutic hypothermia and TTM after SCI.[85-87] Experimental studies have shown that cooling after moderate SCI results in reduced overall contusion volume and improved motor recovery. In contrast, an induced period of *hyperthermia* after SCI has been shown to result in worse functional recovery compared to normothermic SCI. These experimental observations have led to clinical studies that have assessed the safety and efficacy of therapeutic hypothermia in patients with severe cervical SCI. To date, the clinical use of early cooling after severe SCI appears to be safe and may improve long-term outcomes.[85] A multicenter randomized phase II trial is planned to critically assess this experimental treatment in SCI patients.

### Therapeutic Hypothermia in Subarachnoid Hemorrhage

The occurrence of delayed cerebral ischemia in SAH is a major contributor to morbidity and mortality.[88-89] In contrast to cardiac arrest, stroke, and TBI, limited studies have assessed the effects of therapeutic hypothermia in SAH.[90] In these studies, a hypothermia-related reduction in ICP has been commonly reported.[91] In a clinical study of low-grade SAH where early and prolonged therapeutic hypothermia was tested, patients experienced a reduced degree of vasospasm and lower rates of delayed cerebral infarction.[92] Randomized controlled trials in SAH patients with delayed cerebral ischemia are needed to clarify whether this is a reasonable therapeutic approach.

## Hyperthermia and Fever Control

Experimental and clinical studies have documented the deleterious effects of mild hyperthermia in multiple animal models of brain injury (including cerebral ischemia and trauma) and clinical outcomes.[87,93] Elevations in intra- or post-injury temperature aggravate histopathology and behavioral deficits, as well as increase mortality. After cerebral ischemia, hyperthermia has been reported to accelerate the appearance of selective neuronal pathology and increase infarct volume.[87] With TBI, an induced period of hyperthermia (39°C) 24 hours after the traumatic insult was reported to increase mortality, increase contusion volume, and worsen patterns of BBB permeability and inflammatory cell infiltration.[87,94] Similar findings have been reported after spinal cord injury, where posttraumatic hyperthermia increased contusion volume and long-term motor deficits.[87]

In the clinical arena, many brain-injured patients demonstrate periods of hyperthermia.[95] These periods of hyperthermia have been correlated with longer ICU stays and worse outcomes. TTM strategies that inhibit or limit periods of reactive hyperthermia may therefore improve outcomes in severely injured patients.[96] In TBI, fever control management has also been associated with a reduction in mortality.[73,97] A recent multicenter clinical trial performed in cardiac arrest patients found that TTM was associated with improved outcomes.[38] Patients cooled to either 33°C or 36°C had better clinical outcomes than historical controls in whom temperature was not critically managed, although there was no significant difference in outcomes between the 33°C and 36°C groups. In summary, current clinical data support the need for hyperthermia prevention by TTM and fever control in various forms of brain injury.

Mild TBI (mTBI) and concussion are common problems, especially in athletes and military personnel, and can lead to chronic neurological symptoms. Recently, the question of whether brain temperature elevations following mTBI influence outcome has been addressed.[98] This topic is highly relevant since active individuals prone to head injuries may experience elevated core temperatures during strenuous activities, especially in warm environments. Sakurai and colleagues reported that rats that underwent mild fluid percussion brain injury under mild hyperthermia (39°C) had significantly more histopathological damage compared to animals that underwent normothermic mTBI.[99] Mildly hyperthermic animals showed evidence of a mild cortical contusion with cortical neuronal loss adjacent to underlying white matter tracts. In contrast, only limited evidence for histopathological damage was observed in normothermic mTBI animals. To determine if these morphological changes correlated with functional deficits, Titus and colleagues, using a similar experimental paradigm, reported that animals in the hyperthermic mTBI condition had behavioral deficits, whereas animals in the normothermic mTBI condition displayed normal behavior.[100] These findings indicate the importance of brain temperature on the histopathological and functional consequences of mTBI and concussion. The data suggest that mild elevations in temperature could exacerbate mTBI, concussion pathology and neurological deficits, and that preventive strategies such as targeted temperature therapy may be beneficial.

## CONCLUSION

Several physiological factors during the early post-injury phase play a major role in influencing the severity and long-term consequences of brain and spinal cord injury. These physiological variables include blood pressure, oxygen tension, hyperglycemia, and body temperature, all of which can affect secondary injury mechanisms and exacerbate neural tissue damage. Continuous monitoring of these physiological variables in the days following an injury, with appropriate interventions, can improve outcomes and may prevent complications. Physiological monitoring and use of evidence-based medical practices with neuroprotective and reparative strategies will provide the best approach for long-term improvement in patients.

## REFERENCES

1. Chesnut RM, Marshall LF, Klauber MR, et al. The role of secondary brain injury in determining outcome from severe head injury. *J Trauma.* 1993;34(2):216–22.

2. Wijayatilake DS, Jigajinni SV, Sherren PB. Traumatic brain injury: physiological targets for clinical practice in the prehospital setting and on the Neuro-ICU. *Curr Opin Anaesthesiol.* 2015;28(5):517–24.

3. Oddo M, Levine JM, MacKenzie L, et al. Brain hypoxia is associated with short-term outcome after severe traumatic brain injury independently of intracranial hypertension and low cerebral perfusion pressure. *Neurosurgery.* 2011;69(5):1037–45; discussion 1045.

4. Proctor JL, Scutella D, Pan Y, et al. Hyperoxic resuscitation improves survival but worsens neurologic outcome in a rat polytrauma model of traumatic brain injury plus hemorrhagic shock. *J Trauma Acute Care Surg.* 2015;79(4 Suppl 2):S101–9.

5. Hazelton JL, Balan I, Elmer GI, et al. Hyperoxic reperfusion after global cerebral ischemia promotes inflammation and long-term hippocampal neuronal death. *J Neurotrauma.* 2010;27(4):753–62.

6. Balan IS, Fiskum G, Hazelton J, Cotto-Cumbria C, Rosenthal RE. Oximetry-guided reoxygenation improves neurological outcome after experimental cardiac arrest. *Stroke.* 2006;37(12):3008–13.

7. Jeremitsky E, Omert L, Dunham CM, Protetch J, Rodriguez A. Harbingers of poor outcome the day after severe brain injury: hypothermia, hypoxia, and hypoperfusion. *J Trauma.* 2003;54(2):312–9.

8. Brain Trauma Foundation, American Association of Neurological Surgeons, Congress of Neurological Surgeons, et al. Guidelines for the management of severe traumatic brain injury. I. Blood pressure and oxygenation. *J Neurotrauma.* 2007;24 Suppl 1:S7–13.

9. Yan EB, Satgunaseelan L, Paul E, et al. Post-traumatic hypoxia is associated with prolonged cerebral cytokine production, higher serum biomarker levels, and poor outcome in patients with severe traumatic brain injury. *J Neurotrauma.* 2014;31(7):618–29.

10. Jalal FY, Yang Y, Thompson JF, Roitbak T, Rosenberg GA. Hypoxia-induced neuroinflammatory white-matter injury reduced by minocycline in SHR/SP. *J Cereb Blood Flow Metab.* 2015;35(7):1145–53.

11. Bossers SM, Schwarte LA, Loer SA, Twisk JW, Boer C, Schober P. Experience in prehospital endotracheal intubation significantly influences mortality of patients with severe traumatic brain injury: a systematic review and meta-analysis. *PLoS One.* 2015;10(10):e0141034.

12. Karamanos E, Talving P, Skiada D, et al. Is prehospital endotracheal intubation associated with improved outcomes in isolated severe head injury? A matched cohort analysis. *Prehosp Disaster Med.* 2014;29(1):32–6.

13. Sobuwa S, Hartzenberg HB, Gedult H, Uys C. Outcomes following prehospital airway management in severe traumatic brain injury. *S Afr Med J.* 2013;103(9):644–6.

14. Quintard H, Patet C, Suys T, Marques-Vidal P, Oddo M. Normobaric hyperoxia is associated with increased cerebral excitotoxicity after severe traumatic brain injury. *Neurocrit Care.* 2015;22(2):243–50.

15. Talley Watts L, Long JA, Manga VH, Huang S, Shen Q, Duong TQ. Normobaric oxygen worsens outcome after a moderate traumatic brain injury. *J Cereb Blood Flow Metab.* 2015;35(7):1137–44.

16. Tolias CM, Reinert M, Seiler R, Gilman C, Scharf A, Bullock MR. Normobaric hyperoxia-induced improvement in cerebral metabolism and reduction in intracranial pressure in patients with severe head injury: a prospective historical cohort-matched study. *J Neurosurg.* 2004;101(3):435–44.

17. Blasiole B, Bayr H, Vagni VA, et al. Effect of hyperoxia on resuscitation of experimental combined traumatic brain injury and hemorrhagic shock in mice. *Anesthesiology.* 2013;118(3):649–63.

18. Rincon F, Kang J, Vibbert M, Urtecho J, Athar MK, Jallo J. Significance of arterial hyperoxia and relationship with case fatality in traumatic brain injury: a multicentre cohort study. *J Neurol Neurosurg Psychiatry.* 2014;85(7):799–805.

19. Kobayakawa K, Kumamura H, Saiwai H, et al. Acute hyperglycemia impairs functional improvement after spinal cord injury in mice and humans. *Sci Transl Med.* 2014;6(256):256ra137.

20. Jauch-Chara K, Oltmanns KM. Glycemic control after brain injury: boon and bane for the brain. *Neuroscience.* 2014;283:202–9.

21. Stead LG, Gilmore RM, Bellolio MF, et al. Hyperglycemia as an independent predictor of worse outcome in non-diabetic patients presenting with acute ischemic stroke. *Neurocrit Care.* 2009;10(2):181–6.

22. Donnelly J, Czosnyka M, Sudhan N, et al. Increased blood glucose is related to disturbed cerebrovascular pressure reactivity after traumatic brain injury. *Neurocrit Care.* 2015;22(1):20–5.

23. Godoy DA, Di Napoli M, Rabinstein AA. Treating hyperglycemia in neurocritical patients: benefits and perils. *Neurocrit Care.* 2010;13(3):425–38.

24. Cinotti R, Ichai C, Orban JC, et al. Effects of tight computerized glucose control on neurological outcome in severely brain injured patients: a multicenter sub-group analysis of the randomized-controlled open-label CGAO-REA study. *Crit Care.* 2014;18(5):498.

25. NICE-SUGAR Study Investigators for the Australian and New Zealand Intensive Care Society Clinical Trials Group and the Canadian Critical Care Trials Group, Finfer S, Chittock D, et al. Intensive versus conventional glucose control in critically ill patients with traumatic brain injury: long-term follow-up of a subgroup of patients from the NICE-SUGAR study. *Intensive Care Med.* 2015;41(6):1037–47.

26. Rostami E. Glucose and the injured brain-monitored in the neurointensive care unit. *Front Neurol.* 2014;5:91.

27. Bellolio MF, Gilmore RM, Ganti L. Insulin for glycaemic control in acute ischaemic stroke. *Cochrane Database Syst Rev.* 2014;1:CD005346.

28. Rosso C, Corvol JC, Pires C, et al. Intensive versus subcutaneous insulin in patients with hyperacute stroke: results from the randomized INSULINFARCT trial. *Stroke.* 2012;43(9):2343–9.

29. Shijo K, Ghavim S, Harris NG, Hovda DA, Sutton RL. Glucose administration after traumatic brain injury exerts some benefits and no adverse effects on behavioral and histological outcomes. *Brain Res.* 2015;1614:94–104.

30. Talmor D, Shapira Y, Artru AA, et al. 0.45% saline and 5% dextrose in water, but not 0.9% saline or 5% dextrose in 0.9% saline, worsen brain edema two hours after closed head trauma in rats. *Anesth Analg.* 1998;86(6):1225–9.

31. Cherian L, Hannay HJ, Vagner G, Goodman JC, Contant CF, Robertson CS. Hyperglycemia increases neurological damage and behavioral deficits from post-traumatic secondary ischemic insults. *J Neurotrauma.* 1998;15(5):307–21.

32. Moro N, Ghavim S, Harris NG, Hovda DA, Sutton RL. Glucose administration after traumatic brain injury improves cerebral metabolism and reduces secondary neuronal injury. *Brain Res.* 2013;1535:124–36.

33. Karnatovskaia LV, Wartenberg KE, Freeman WD. Therapeutic hypothermia for neuroprotection: history, mechanisms, risks, and clinical applications. *Neurohospitalist.* 2014;4(3):153–63.

34. Busto R, Dietrich WD, Globus MY, Valdes I, Scheinberg P, Ginsberg MD. Small differences in intraischemic brain temperature critically determine the extent of ischemic neuronal injury. *J Cereb Blood Flow Metab.* 1987;7(6):729–38.

35. Wang H, Wang B, Normoyle KP, et al. Brain temperature and its fundamental properties: a review for clinical neuroscientists. *Front Neurosci.* 2014;8:307.

36. Andresen M, Gazmuri JT, Marin A, Requeira T, Rovegno M. Therapeutic hypothermia for acute brain injuries. *Scand J Trauma Resusc Emerg Med.* 2015;23:42.

37. Clifton GL, Valadka A, Zygun D, et al. Very early hypothermia induction in patients with severe brain injury (the National Acute Brain Injury Study: Hypothermia II): a randomised trial. *Lancet Neurol.* 2011;10(2):131–9.

38. Nielsen N, Wetterslev J, Cronberg T, et al. Targeted temperature management at 33 degrees C versus 36 degrees C after cardiac arrest. *N Engl J Med.* 2013;369(23):2197–206.

39. Han Z, Liu X, Luo Y, Ji X. Therapeutic hypothermia for stroke: Where to go? *Exp Neurol.* 2015;272:67–77.

40. Hoedemaekers CW, Ezzahti M, Gerritsen A, van der Hoeven JG. Comparison of cooling methods to induce and maintain normo- and hypothermia in intensive care unit patients: a prospective intervention study. *Crit Care.* 2007;11(4):R91.

41. Kliegel A, Losert H, Sterz F, et al. Cold simple intravenous infusions preceding special endovascular cooling for faster induction of mild hypothermia after cardiac arrest: a feasibility study. *Resuscitation.* 2005;64(3):347–51.

42. Bernard SA, Smith K, Cameron P, et al. Induction of prehospital therapeutic hypothermia after resuscitation from nonventricular fibrillation cardiac arrest. *Crit Care Med.* 2012;40(3):747–53.

43. Borgquist O, Friberg H. Therapeutic hypothermia for comatose survivors after near-hanging-a retrospective analysis. *Resuscitation.* 2009;80(2):210–2.

44. Jehle D, Meyer M, Gemme S. Beneficial response to mild therapeutic hypothermia for comatose survivors of near-hanging. *Am J Emerg Med.* 2010;28(3):390 e1–3.

45. Lyden PD, Krieger D, Yenari M, Dietrich WD. Therapeutic hypothermia for acute stroke. *Int J Stroke.* 2006;1(1):9–19.

46. Yenari MA, Han HS. Neuroprotective mechanisms of hypothermia in brain ischaemia. *Nat Rev Neurosci.* 2012;13(4):267–78.

47. Yenari MA, Han HS. Influence of therapeutic hypothermia on regeneration after cerebral ischemia. *Front Neurol Neurosci.* 2013;32:122–8.

48. Dietrich WD. The importance of brain temperature in cerebral injury. *J Neurotrauma.* 1992;9 Suppl 2:S475–85.

49. Dietrich WD, Bramlett HM. The evidence for hypothermia as a neuroprotectant in traumatic brain injury. *Neurotherapeutics.* 2010;7(1):43–50.

50. Dietrich WD, Busto R, Halley M, Valdes I. The importance of brain temperature in alterations of the blood-brain barrier following cerebral ischemia. *J Neuropathol Exp Neurol.* 1990;49(5):486–97.

51. Jiang JY, Lyeth BG, Kapasi MZ, Jenkins LW, Povlishock JT. Moderate hypothermia reduces blood-brain barrier disruption following traumatic brain injury in the rat. *Acta Neuropathol.* 1992;84(5):495–500.

52. Tomura S, de Rivero Vaccari JP, Keane RW, Bramlett HM, Dietrich WD. Effects of therapeutic hypothermia on inflammasome signaling after traumatic brain injury. *J Cereb Blood Flow Metab.* 2012;32(10):1939–47.

53. Shankaran S, Laptook AR, Ehrenkranz RA, et al. Whole-body hypothermia for neonates with hypoxic-ischemic encephalopathy. *N Engl J Med.* 2005;353(15):1574–84.

54. Bernard SA, Gray TW, Buist MD, et al. Treatment of comatose survivors of out-of-hospital cardiac arrest with induced hypothermia. *N Engl J Med.* 2002;346(8):557–63.

55. Hypothermia After Cardiac Arrest Study Group. Mild therapeutic hypothermia to improve the neurologic outcome after cardiac arrest. *N Engl J Med.* 2002;346(8):549–56.

56. Shankaran S, Pappas A, McDonald SA, et al. Childhood outcomes after hypothermia for neonatal encephalopathy. *N Engl J Med.* 2012;366(22):2085–92.

57. Wu TC, Grotta JC. Hypothermia for acute ischaemic stroke. *Lancet Neurol.* 2013;12(3):275–84.

58. van der Worp HB, Sena ES, Donan GA, Howells DW, Macleod MR. Hypothermia in animal models of acute ischaemic stroke: a systematic review and meta-analysis. *Brain.* 2007;130(12):3063–74.

59. Lyden PD, Allgren RL, Ng K, et al. Intravascular Cooling in the Treatment of Stroke (ICTuS): early clinical experience. *J Stroke Cerebrovasc Dis.* 2005;14(3):107–14.

60. De Georgia MA, Krieger DW, Abou-Chebl A, et al. Cooling for Acute Ischemic Brain Damage (COOL AID): a feasibility trial of endovascular cooling. *Neurology.* 2004;63(2):312–7.

61. Schwab S, Georgiadis D, Berrouschot J, Schellings PD, Graffagnino C, Mayer SA. Feasibility and safety of moderate hypothermia after massive hemispheric infarction. *Stroke.* 2001;32(9):2033–5.

62. Els T, Oehm E, Voigt S, Klisch J, Hetzel A, Kassubek J. Safety and therapeutical benefit of hemicraniectomy combined with mild hypothermia in comparison with hemicraniectomy alone in patients with malignant ischemic stroke. *Cerebrovasc Dis.* 2006;21(1-2):79–85.

63. Hemmen TM, Raman R, Guluma KZ, et al. Intravenous thrombolysis plus hypothermia for acute treatment of ischemic stroke (ICTuS-L): final results. *Stroke.* 2010;41(10):2265–70.

64. Dietrich WD, Atkins CM, Bramlett HM. Protection in animal models of brain and spinal cord injury with mild to moderate hypothermia. *J Neurotrauma.* 2009;26(3):301–12.

65. Oda Y, Gao G, Wei EP, Povlishock JT. Combinational therapy using hypothermia and the immunophilin ligand FK506 to target altered pial arteriolar reactivity, axonal damage, and blood-brain barrier dysfunction after traumatic brain injury in rat. *J Cereb Blood Flow Metab.* 2011;31(4):1143–54.

66. Markgraf CG, Clifton GL, Moody MR. Treatment window for hypothermia in brain injury. *J Neurosurg.* 2001;95(6):979–83.

67. Povlishock JT, Wei EP. Posthypothermic rewarming considerations following traumatic brain injury. *J Neurotrauma.* 2009;26(3):333–40.

68. Sadaka F, Veremakis C. Therapeutic hypothermia for the management of intracranial hypertension in severe traumatic brain injury: a systematic review. *Brain Inj.* 2012;26(7-8):899–908.

69. Schreckinger M, Marion DW. Contemporary management of traumatic intracranial hypertension: is there a role for therapeutic hypothermia? *Neurocrit Care.* 2009;11(3):427–36.

70. Tokutomi T, Morimoto K, Miyagi T, Yamaguchi S, Ishikawa K, Shigemori M. Optimal temperature for the management of severe traumatic brain injury: effect of hypothermia on intracranial pressure, systemic and intracranial hemodynamics, and metabolism. *Neurosurgery.* 2003;52(1):102–11; discussion 111–2.

71. Marion DW, Penrod LE, Kelsey SF, Obrist WD, Kochanek PM, Palmer AM. Treatment of traumatic brain injury with moderate hypothermia. *N Engl J Med.* 1997;336(8):540–6.

72. Beca J, McSharry B, Erickson S, et al. Hypothermia for traumatic brain injury in children: a phase II randomized controlled trial. *Crit Care Med.* 2015;43(7):1458–66.

73. Maekawa T, Yamashita S, Nagao S, Hayashi N, Ohashi Y; Brain-Hypothermia Study Group. Prolonged mild therapeutic hypothermia versus fever control with tight hemodynamic monitoring and slow rewarming in patients with severe traumatic brain injury: a randomized controlled trial. *J Neurotrauma.* 2015;32(7):422–9.

74. Maekawa T. Therapeutic hypothermia for severe traumatic brain injury in Japan. 2015; Available from: http://clinicaltrials.gov/ct2/show/NCT00134472.

75. Clifton GL, Miller ER, Choi SC, et al. Lack of effect of induction of hypothermia after acute brain injury. *N Engl J Med.* 2001;344(8):556–63.

76. Hutchison JS, Ward RE, Lacroix J, et al. Hypothermia therapy after traumatic brain injury in children. *N Engl J Med.* 2008;358(23):2447–56.

77. Lei J, Gao G, Mao Q, et al. Rationale, methodology, and implementation of a nationwide multicenter randomized controlled trial of long-term mild hypothermia for severe traumatic brain injury (the LTH-1 trial). *Contemp Clin Trials.* 2015;40:9–14.

78. Nichol A, Gantner D, Presneill J, et al. Protocol for a multicentre randomised controlled trial of early and sustained prophylactic hypothermia in the management of traumatic brain injury. *Crit Care Resusc.* 2015;17(2):92–100.

79. Andrews PJ, Sinclair HL, Rodriguez A, et al. Hypothermia for intracranial hypertension after traumatic brain injury. *N Engl J Med,* 2015;373:2403–12.

80. Yokobori S, Gajavelli S, Mondello S, et al. Neuroprotective effect of preoperatively induced mild hypothermia as determined by biomarkers and histopathological estimation in a rat subdural hematoma decompression model. *J Neurosurg.* 2013;118(2):370–80.

81. Li P, Yang C. Moderate hypothermia treatment in adult patients with severe traumatic brain injury: a meta-analysis. *Brain Inj.* 2014;28(8):1036–41.

82. Crossley S, Reid J, McLatchie R, et al. A systematic review of therapeutic hypothermia for adult patients following traumatic brain injury. *Crit Care.* 2014;18(2):R75.

83. Sydenham E, Roberts I, Alderson P. Hypothermia for traumatic head injury. *Cochrane Database Syst Rev.* 2009;(1):CD001048.

84. Sharma D, Brown MJ, Curry P, Noda S, Chesnut RM, Vavilala MS. Prevalence and risk factors for intraoperative hypotension during craniotomy for traumatic brain injury. *J Neurosurg Anesthesiol.* 2012;24(3):178–84.

85. Dididze M, Green BA, Dietrich WD, Vanni S, Wang MY, Levi AD. Systemic hypothermia in acute cervical spinal cord injury: a case-controlled study. *Spinal Cord.* 2013;51(5):395–400.

86. Dietrich WD, Levi AD, Wang M, Green BA. Hypothermic treatment for acute spinal cord injury. *Neurotherapeutics.* 2011;8(2):229–39.

87. Dietrich WD, Bramlett HM. Hyperthermia and central nervous system injury. *Prog Brain Res.* 2007;162:201–17.

88. Steiner T, Juvela S, Unterberg A, et al. European Stroke Organization guidelines for the management of intracranial aneurysms and subarachnoid haemorrhage. *Cerebrovasc Dis.* 2013;35(2):93–112.

89. Kollmar R, Staykov D, Dorfler A, Schellinger PD, Schwab S, Bardutzky J. Hypothermia reduces perihemorrhagic edema after intracerebral hemorrhage. *Stroke.* 2010;41(8):1684–9.

90. Badjatia N, Fernandez L, Schmidt JM, et al. Impact of induced normothermia on outcome after subarachnoid hemorrhage: a case-control study. *Neurosurgery.* 2010;66(4):696–700; discussion 700–1.

91. Seule MA, Muroi C, Mink S, Yonekawa Y, Keller E. Therapeutic hypothermia in patients with aneurysmal subarachnoid hemorrhage, refractory intracranial hypertension, or cerebral vasospasm. *Neurosurgery.* 2009;64(1):86–92; discussion 92–3.

92. Kuramatsu JB, Kollmar R, Gerner ST, et al. Is hypothermia helpful in severe subarachnoid hemorrhage? An exploratory study on macro vascular spasm, delayed cerebral infarction and functional outcome after prolonged hypothermia. *Cerebrovasc Dis.* 2015;40(5-6):228–35.

93. Natale JE, Joseph JG, Helfaer MA, Shaffner DH. Early hyperthermia after traumatic brain injury in children: risk factors, influence on length of stay, and effect on short-term neurologic status. *Crit Care Med.* 2000;28(7):2608–15.

94. Dietrich WD, Alonso O, Halley M, Busto R. Delayed posttraumatic brain hyperthermia worsens outcome after fluid percussion brain injury: a light and electron microscopic study in rats. *Neurosurgery.* 1996;38(3):533–41; discussion 541.

95. Commichau C, Scarmeas N, Mayer SA. Risk factors for fever in the neurologic intensive care unit. *Neurology.* 2003;60(5):837–41.

96. Puccio AM, Fischer MR, Jankowitz BT, Yonas H, Darby JM, Okonkwo DO. Induced normothermia attenuates intracranial hypertension and reduces fever burden after severe traumatic brain injury. *Neurocrit Care.* 2009;11(1):82–7.

97. Hifumi T, Kuroda Y, Kawakita K, et al. Fever control management is preferable to mild therapeutic hypothermia in traumatic brain injury patients with Abbreviated Injury Scale 3-4: a multi-center, randomized controlled trial. *J Neurotrauma,* 2015;33:1047–53.

98. Kochanek PM, Jackson TC. It might be time to let cooler heads prevail after mild traumatic brain injury or concussion. *Exp Neurol.* 2015;267:13–17.

99. Sakurai A, Atkins CM, Alonso OF, Bramlett HM, Dietrich WD. Mild hyperthermia worsens the neuropathological damage associated with mild traumatic brain injury in rats. *J Neurotrauma.* 2012;29(2):313–21.

100. Titus DJ, Furones C, Atkins CM, Dietrich WD. Emergence of cognitive deficits after mild traumatic brain injury due to hyperthermia. *Exp Neurol.* 2015;263:254–62.

# 2 Pharmacologic Neuroprotection

## Nino Stocchetti and Marco Carbonara

## INTRODUCTION

Acute cerebral tissue damage due to traumatic or vascular injuries results in a cascade of biochemical events that amplifies the damage caused by the initial insult and contributes to long-term sequelae. This cascade develops over time and may be attenuated or limited by several pharmacologic interventions. Protection against such secondary injury mechanisms potentially would be of enormous benefit to individuals who sustain such injuries, their families, and society at large.

In the laboratory setting, animal models reproducing the pathophysiology of acute brain damage due to trauma, ischemia, and hemorrhage have been developed. Progressive secondary brain injury mechanisms have been identified, and targeted treatments have been tested. A variety of endpoints have been studied, from histological examination of tissue, to behavioral assessment of cerebral functions. Based on favorable experimental results, numerous promising compounds have been tested in clinical trials. This chapter will review the findings of clinical trials of pharmacologic neuroprotection in four specific pathologies: traumatic brain injury (TBI), subarachnoid hemorrhage (SAH), ischemic stroke, and hypoxic-ischemic encephalopathy in adults due to cardiac arrest.

## MOLECULAR MECHANISMS OF SECONDARY INJURY

Traumatic and vascular (hemorrhagic or ischemic) acute brain injuries are complex and different in many ways, but share some similar pathways and mechanisms of injury.[1] The initial injury can be amplified and exacerbated by further physiologic alterations activated after the insult, during an extended time window in which the brain remains vulnerable to secondary injury. Energy failure from insufficient oxygen and glucose delivery or mitochondrial dysfunction induces sustained depolarization of neurons and a massive release of glutamate. This excitatory amino acid activates a number of downstream signaling pathways promoting excessive intra- and extracellular liberation of ions, especially calcium. An increased intracellular concentration of calcium triggers phospholipase activation, further mitochondrial failure, and apoptosis. The ionic influx leads to cytotoxic cellular edema. Further propagation of depolarization waves triggered by excitotoxicity aggravates the ongoing cellular energy crisis that is occurring in surrounding tissue. Finally, ischemia and reperfusion amplify free radical production, which produces tissue acidosis and cell membrane disruption as ischemic tissue progresses to irreversible tissue infarction.

Cellular necrosis and apoptosis resulting from these processes early in the ischemic cascade start an inflammatory response that recruits leukocytes, activates Toll-like receptors, and promotes a pro-inflammatory phenotype of microglia. This microglial activation further produces pro-inflammatory cytokines and adhesion molecules. The mechanisms by which inflammation contributes to secondary brain injury are not completely understood but include free radical production and vascular alterations that often affect the permeability of the blood–brain barrier (BBB). This "sterile immune reaction" recruits central nervous system (CNS) resident and systemic inflammatory cells and may have protective as well as deleterious effects, often lasting weeks or months after injury.[2]

## PHARMACOLOGIC NEUROPROTECTION IN TRAUMATIC BRAIN INJURY

TBI affects millions of people worldwide every year.[3] The incidence is underestimated, however, because many cases of mild TBI go unrecognized and are not included in statistics. TBI is associated with high rates of mortality, morbidity, and life-long disability, with high personal, familial, and societal costs. Methods for treating the acute lesions of TBI and limiting secondary injury have therefore been sought for decades.

TBI is not a single entity, but rather encompasses a variety of primary cerebral lesions, including extracerebral hematomas, contusions, and traumatic axonal injury (TAI). The various primary pathologies are associated with different mechanisms of secondary injury. Hematomas rapidly compress the brain, causing tissue distortion, herniation, and vascular compression leading to ischemia. Contusions cause tissue necrosis, edema, damage to the BBB, and an inflammatory response. TAI results from rotational forces that damage white matter pathways within the cerebral hemispheres and brainstem. In clinical TBI, therefore, multiple lesions and multiple mechanisms of secondary injury often coexist.

Over the past 40 years, the pathophysiology of TBI has been experimentally investigated in multiple models and species.[4] Animal models of TBI include balloon expansion to replicate hematoma growth, weight-drop models for TAI, fluid percussion for contusions, and controlled cortical impact models. These experimental models provide the opportunity to investigate TBI pathophysiology under controlled conditions.

Mechanisms of secondary injury include vascular alterations, BBB damage, edema accumulation, complement activation, excitatory amino acid overload, and intracellular perturbations such as free radical activation, calcium influx, mitochondrial damage, and lipid peroxidation. These mechanisms have been studied as possible targets for treatment, and multiple molecules have been shown to have neuroprotective effects in numerous experimental studies.[5-9] Based on the promising evidence of pharmacologic neuroprotection in preclinical studies of TBI, numerous clinical trials have been conducted in patients with TBI.

## Barbiturates

Barbiturates were the first agents to be extensively tested as neuroprotectants in various pathologies, beginning with resuscitation from global temporary ischemia due to cardiac arrest. These drugs have multiple mechanisms of action, including reduction of the cerebral metabolic rate, suppression of pathological (and physiological) electrical activity, clearance of free radicals, vasoconstriction and edema reduction, and reduction of intracranial pressure (ICP). Due to this profile, the barbiturates qualified for therapeutic use in TBI.

In the 1980s, the main indication for barbiturates in the context of TBI was refractory high ICP. A more aggressive approach consisting of prophylactic induction of barbiturate coma was tested in a small randomized trial, but there was no outcome benefit and a greater incidence of arterial hypotension.[10] A 2012 literature review confirmed that barbiturate treatment is not associated with improved outcomes in acute TBI patients, but is associated with a greater incidence of hemodynamic side effects.[11]

## Modern Trials of Pharmacologic Neuroprotection for Traumatic Brain Injury

Major trials of pharmacologic neuroprotection published since the 1990s are summarized in Tables 2.1 and 2.2. Table 2.1 lists clinical trials of pharmacologic agents aimed at a single mechanism of neuroprotection (although some of the agents may act as neuroprotectants by multiple mechanisms). The major targets are excitotoxicity (Cerestat, Selfotel, repinotan, gacyclidine, traxoprodil, and amantadine), oxidative damage (pegorgotein, tirilazad, and citicoline), and inflammation (cyclosporin). None of these trials showed outcome benefit in TBI patients. Other failed drugs include calcium channel blockers (nimodipine) and bradykinin antagonists (Bradycor and Anatibant). Two retrospective studies have reported more favorable outcomes in TBI patients who were receiving β-blocker medications prior to injury, but a prospective randomized trial is lacking.

Table 2.2 lists trials of compounds that have been proposed for multiple targets. Progesterone has demonstrated anti-apoptotic, anti-inflammatory, and anti-oxidant properties. Dexanabinol, a synthetic cannabinoid, targets various pathophysiological mechanisms including glutamate excitotoxicity, free-radical damage, and inflammatory response. Erythropoietin has erythropoietic, anti-inflammatory, antiapoptotic, and anti-oxidant properties.

The large number of studies conducted in search of pharmacologic agents with neuroprotective properties for TBI indicates the extent of the investment made in this field. Some small-scale studies appear to have confirmed some of the benefits expected based on preclinical studies; however, no single large-scale randomized controlled trial (RCT) has demonstrated pharmacologic neuroprotection for TBI.[12] The discrepancy between the preclinical and clinical study findings has been surprising and requires explanation.

**Table 2.1** Major trials of pharmacological neuroprotection with agents directed toward a single mechanism in TBI

| Compound Study Name | Main Mechanism of Action | Patients Enrolled | Therapeutic Window | Reference |
|---|---|---|---|---|
| Nimodipine | Calcium channel blocker | 351 | 12 hours if comatose | 1992[78] |
| Pegorgotein | Reactive oxygen species scavenger | 463 | 8 hours | 1996[79] |
| Cerestat | Noncompetitive NMDA receptor antagonist | 340 | 8 hours | Unpublished, conducted in 1997 |
| Tirilazad mesylate | Antioxidant aminosteroid | 1,120 | 4 hours | 1998[80] |
| Bradycor (deltibant, CP-1027) | Bradykinin antagonist | 139 | 12 hours | 1999[81] |
| D-CPP-ene Sandoz | Glutamate antagonist | 920 | 12 hours | Unpublished, conducted in 1999 |
| Selfotel (CGS 19755) | NMDA receptor antagonist | 693 | 8 hours | 1999[82] |
| Repinotan (BAY x 37022001) | 5-HT1A agonist | 60 | 24 hours | 2001[83] |
| Gacyclidine | NMDA receptor antagonist | 51 | 2 hours | 2004[84] |
| Traxoprodil | NMDA receptor antagonist | 404 | 8 hours | 2005[85] |
| Anatibant | Inhibitor of kinin-kallikrein system | 25 | 12 hours | 2005[86] |
| β-Adrenergic blockade | Beta adrenergic receptor blocker | 420 | Pre exposure | 2007[87] |
| Cyclosporin | Immunosuppressive and antiapoptotic | 50 | 12 hours | 2009[88] |
| Recombinant factor VIIa (rFVIIa) | Restore coagulation in traumatic intracerebral hemorrhage | 97 | 6 h | 2008[89] |
| Cyclosporin a | Immunosuppressive and antiapoptotic | 50 | 12 hours | 2009[90] |
| β-Adrenergic blockade | Beta adrenergic receptor blocker | 2,601 | Pre exposure | 2010[91] |
| Amantadine | NMDA antagonist and indirect dopamine agonist | 184 | 4 to 16 weeks | 2012[92] |
| Citicoline | Precursor of membrane lipid | 1,213 | 24 hours | 2012[93] |

Table 2.2 Major trials of pharmacological neuroprotection with agents directed toward multiple mechanisms in TBI

| Compound Study Name | Multiple Mechanisms of Action | Patients Enrolled | Therapeutic Window | Publication Year |
|---|---|---|---|---|
| Triamcinolone | Anti inflammatory, anti edema | 396 | 4 hours | 1995[94] |
| CRASH | Corticosteroid | 10,008 | 8 hours | 2004[95] |
| Dexanabinol | Cannabinoid receptor agonist | 846 | 6 hours | 2006[96] |
| Magnesium sulfate | Calcium antagonist, smooth muscle relaxant | 488 | 8 hours | 2007[97] |
| Dual cannabinoid CB1 | Receptor agonist KN38-7271 | 97 | 6 hours | 2012[98] |
| Progesteron | Sex steroid hormone | 159 | 8 hours | 2012[99] |
| Progesteron | Sex steroid hormone | 882 | 4 hours | 2014[100] |
| Progesteron | Sex steroid hormone | 1,195 | 8 hours | 2014[101] |
| Erythropoietin | Antiapoptotic, anti-inflammatory, erytropoietic | 895 | 6 hours | 2014[102] |

## PHARMACOLOGIC NEUROPROTECTION IN SUBARACHNOID HEMORRHAGE

SAH carries a significant risk of morbidity and mortality due to the initial bleeding. In survivors, however, there is risk of cerebral ischemia that develops within days to weeks of the initial event and confers additional injury burden. Delayed ischemia has traditionally been attributed to vasospasm, a vessel narrowing that can be visualized by angiography. Prevention or reduction of vasospasm, therefore, is a crucial target for intervention, with the expected benefit of improving cerebral perfusion and reducing the ischemic burden.

### Clinical Trials Targeting Vasospasm and Delayed Ischemia

Several agents have been tested for vasospasm prevention following SAH. Among them, nimodipine was tested with the hypothesis that it would impede vasospasm by reducing intracellular calcium entry into vascular smooth muscle within the intracerebral arterial circulation. Two RCTs demonstrated some outcome benefit with nimodipine, and although ischemic lesions were less frequent, the incidence of angiographic vasospasm was not.[13–14] Protection was therefore attributed to prevention of excessive intracellular calcium instead of a direct vascular effect. In these initial trials, nimodipine was interpreted to be potentially protective without major side effects. In trials conducted in patients with continuous arterial pressure monitoring in the ICU, however, it was observed that arterial hypotension occurred frequently and that the hypotensive episodes could be severe and associated with decreased tissue oxygenation.[15]

Nicardipine, another calcium entry blocker, was tested in two large studies (906 and 356 patients, respectively).[16–17] The data showed a reduction in angiographic vasospasm but no difference in outcome. Endothelin antagonists (clazosentan and TAK-044) were tested to inhibit vasoconstriction in SAH in small case series and RCTs. These agents have been found to be associated with a measurable reduction in angiographic vasospasm, but no outcome benefits.[18–20]

## Clinical Trials Targeting Multiple Mechanisms of Injury

A broader approach targeting multiple mechanisms of secondary injury in SAH has been investigated in several trials. Magnesium, which blocks N-methyl-D-aspartate (NMDA) and glutamate receptors and voltage-dependent calcium channels, appeared to reduce vasospasm and improve outcomes in a phase II study, but the findings were not confirmed in larger phase III trials.[21–23] Statins have pleiotropic effects on vascular and endothelial function. Their mechanism of action in neuroprotection is not completely understood. They most likely act as anti-inflammatory agents, changing the lipid composition of cells and reducing adhesiveness of monocytes to the endothelium, but other targets include oxidative stress damage and platelet activation. Statin consumption is associated with decreased risk of cognitive impairment and dementia, a feature that could be related to increased neurogenesis and decreased neuronal death.[24]

The 21-aminosteroid tirilazad reduces lipid peroxidation and may protect cerebral tissue from focal ischemia.[25] Despite promising preclinical data, when tested in randomized trials, tirilazad failed to improve outcomes.[26]

More recently, volatile anesthetics, such as isoflurane, have been proposed as neuroprotectants for SAH because they reduce metabolic expenditure, decrease ischemic release of neurotransmitters, and may increase and/or redistribute cerebral blood flow. At this time, however, conclusive data are lacking.[27]

## PHARMACOLOGIC NEUROPROTECTION IN ISCHEMIC STROKE

Stroke is a leading cause of death and disability in Western countries, with approximately 80% of strokes due to ischemia. Following arterial occlusion, a core zone of hypoperfused brain tissue is irreversibly injured and will necrose. In the surrounding area, known as the *ischemic penumbra*, cell survival depends on residual blood flow and the duration of ischemia. Treatment of ischemic stroke, therefore, is based on the possibility of rescuing tissue within the penumbra. A search for pharmacologic interventions targeting molecular mechanisms of secondary injury in ischemic stroke has been in progress over the past two decades.

Pharmacologic interventions for ischemic stroke include restoring blood flow or interrupting molecular cascades that amplify damage. Restoration of flow does not strictly qualify as pharmacologic neuroprotection, but it represents the only therapy with proven tissue-sparing capabilities. Indeed, intravenous recombinant tissue plasminogen activator (Alteplase, rTPA) is the only approved pharmacologic agent to treat ischemic stroke. Several studies have shown improved outcomes in patients receiving rTPA compared to placebo, and a meta-analysis has confirmed its benefit when administered within 270 minutes of symptom onset.[28] Due to stringent eligibility criteria and the relatively short therapeutic time window, however, less than 5% of ischemic stroke patients receive rTPA.[29] Current clinical and experimental research efforts are thus focused on expanding the therapeutic time window, with intra-arterial administration of the drug and increasing use of devices for mechanical clot removal.[28] Current guidelines incorporate thrombectomy as part of ischemic stroke therapy, provided accurate patient selection by rapid computed tomography (CT)-guided diagnosis and a well-organized system of care.[30]

## Oxidative Stress

Overproduction of reactive oxygen species (ROS) causes damage to brain tissue and vasculature after ischemic insults.[31] Pharmacologic agents that act as free radical scavengers have therefore been tested for neuroprotection for ischemic stroke.

Citicoline, a precursor of phosphatidylcholine (a phospholipid component of cellular membranes), stabilizes lipid membranes in response to ischemia and acts as an ROS scavenger. A few clinical trials performed in the 1990s showed conflicting results, but a meta-analysis of the individual patient data that standardized the outcome measures indicated that treated patients had a more favorable 90-day outcome.[32] Subsequently, a large multicenter trial performed in Europe in 2,298 patients with moderate to severe middle cerebral artery stroke failed to confirm benefit.[33]

Tirilazad inhibits iron-dependent lipid peroxidation and preserves cell viability. A meta-analysis of six RCTs showed no benefit compared to placebo.[34] Ebselen is a selenium compound with antioxidant activity. A small placebo-controlled trial was successful in improving outcome; a larger study is ongoing.[35] Edaravone is a ROS scavenger and a blocker of lipid peroxidation that has shown promising results in small clinical trials; a larger trial is ongoing.[36] NXY-059, a nitrone free radical scavenger, has shown promising histological and functional effects in laboratory studies; however, it did not show efficacy in two clinical trials.[37-38]

Overall, free radical scavengers have not emerged as neuroprotective in the clinical setting in the cohorts of patients studied.

## Calcium Channel Blockade

The excessive influx of calcium into cells causes apoptosis through multiple pathways.[39] Calcium channel blockade has been shown to result in improved neurological outcome in animal models of cerebral ischemia. Neither nimodipine nor flunarizine (an organic calcium channel blocker), however, has been associated with improved outcome when compared to placebo in clinical trials.[40-41]

## Inflammation

The role of the inflammatory cascade following cerebral ischemia has been well investigated.[42] Several drugs have been found to be efficacious in modulating the inflammatory response in experimental studies. Enlimomab is a murine monoclonal antibody against ICAM-1, an adhesion molecule that acts to reduce neutrophil adhesion to endothelium and migration into the parenchyma. In a clinical trial, 625 patients were randomized to receive enlimomab or placebo within 6 hours after ischemic stroke onset. Patients treated with enlimomab experienced worse functional outcome and mortality.[43] UK 279,276, another antibody with a similar proposed mechanism that inhibits the CD11b/CD18 receptor, was tested in a clinical trial, but that trial was stopped for futility.[44]

While an aggressive inflammatory response may be detrimental, inflammation also promotes reparative processes and wound healing. Basic fibroblastic growth factor is a protein involved in neuronal differentiation as well as maintenance and proliferation of vascular and glial cells, making it a promising reparative mediator. Despite strong preclinical data, two subsequent phase II–III studies were interrupted due to worse mortality and outcome in the treatment groups.[45]

## Excitotoxicity

The metabolic crisis of an ischemic neuron results in the release of high amounts of glutamate (and other excitatory neurotransmitters) into the extracellular space. Glutamate, through activation of its receptors, increases intracellular calcium to a toxic level and eventually promotes apoptosis. In several preclinical stroke models, glutamate blockade was found to be a successful neuroprotective strategy. In clinical trials, however, neither inhibition of excitatory neurotransmitters nor facilitation of inhibitory neurotransmitters has resulted in outcome benefit. Such trials have investigated the noncompetitive NMDA receptor antagonist aptiganel and the competitive NMDA antagonist Selfotel.[46–48] Other trials have investigated gavestinel, an antagonist that acts at the glycine site on the NMDA receptor complex; the γ-aminobutyric acid (GABA) receptor agonists clomethiazole and diazepam; and lubeluzole, an antagonist of glutamate-activated nitric oxide synthase.[49–52]

## Agents Targeting Multiple Mechanisms

Magnesium is an optimal neuroprotective candidate because it has multiple effects, including calcium antagonism and NMDA receptor blockade. As a smooth muscle relaxant, it ameliorates vasospasm. Additionally, it is safe and inexpensive. It has been extensively studied in stroke; however, a large study (N = 857) showed no benefit in magnesium-treated patients compared to placebo, even when administered in the pre-hospital setting an average of 45 minutes after the initial onset of symptoms.[53]

Table 2.3 lists drugs with multiple mechanisms of action that have been investigated in clinical trials of neuroprotection for ischemic stroke, none of which showed outcome benefit.[54]

Table 2.3 Neuroprotective trials of compounds with multiple mechanisms of action in stroke

| Compound Study Name | Multiple Mechanisms of Action | Patients Enrolled | Therapeutic Window | Publication Year |
| --- | --- | --- | --- | --- |
| BMS-204352 | Potassium channel activator | 1,978 | 6 hours | Unpublished |
| Fosphenytoin | Sodium channel blocker, anticonvulsivant | 462 | 4 hours | Unpublished |
| Repinotan | 5-HT1A receptor agonist | 240 | 6 hours | Unpublished |
| Piracetam | Membrane fluidity modifier | 927 | 12 hours | 1997[103] |
| Cervene | Opioid antagonist | 368 | 6 hours | 2000[104] |

# PHARMACOLOGIC NEUROPROTECTION FOR HYPOXIC-ISCHEMIC ENCEPHALOPATHY IN ADULTS

Hypoxic-ischemic encephalopathy after cardiac arrest is a frequent medical emergency. In Europe it is estimated to affect more than 300,000 patients per year and have a survival rate less than 10%.[55] Even in cases of successful cardiopulmonary resuscitation (CPR), most survivors suffer a poor neurological outcome. Neuroprotection in this patient population has therefore been sought since the beginning of CPR in the 1970s.[56]

## Barbiturates

In the past, barbiturates were used extensively following cardiac arrest, based on the findings of experimental studies performed in the 1970s showing neuroprotective effects. This practice, however, was abandoned 30 years ago after the multicenter Brain Resuscitation Clinical Trial I, in which 262 comatose survivors of cardiac arrest were randomized to receive either thiopental in bolus or placebo.[57] Thiopental therapy showed no neurological outcome benefit.

## Glucocorticoids

In the past, glucocorticoids were commonly administered to patients with global brain ischemia. A retrospective analysis of the patient data from the Brain Resuscitation Clinical Trial I, in which glucocorticoid therapy was left to the discretion of the hospital investigators, compared patients who, within the first 8 hours after arrest, received either no glucocorticoid, low-dose glucocorticoids, medium-dose glucocorticoids, or high-dose glucocorticoids.[58] None of the glucocorticoid regimens was associated with improved survival rate or neurological recovery rate.

## Hemodynamic Optimization During Cardiopulmonary Resuscitation

A randomized, double-blind, placebo-controlled, parallel-group trial comparing vasopressin plus epinephrine (1 mg/CPR cycle) versus saline placebo plus epinephrine (1 mg/CPR cycle) administered during CPR in patients suffering in-hospital cardiac arrest (N = 268) found improved outcomes in the vasopressin treatment group, as reflected by higher probabilities of return of spontaneous circulation for 20 minutes or longer and survival to hospital discharge with a Cerebral Performance Category (CPC) score of 1 or 2.[59] It remains unclear, however, whether the improvement in early survival was due to cerebral neuroprotection per se as opposed to better preservation of cerebral flow during resuscitative efforts.

## Drugs with Varied Mechanisms of Action

Magnesium has been shown to act synergistically with hypothermia in preclinical outcome studies.[60] Clinical studies of magnesium administered to patients suffering in-hospital or out-of-hospital cardiac arrest have found, however, that it was ineffective in improving neurological outcome and reducing mortality.[61–62]

Two calcium-channel blockers, lidoflazine and nimodipine, did not show any neuroprotective effect in patients suffering from hypoxic-ischemic encephalopathy.[63–64]

Erythropoietin is a promising drug based on experimental studies and a case-control trial. It is a hormone with multiple mechanisms of action that include erythropoiesis, anti-inflammatory, anti-apoptotic, and anti-oxidant properties. A randomized clinical trial of this agent, however, was unsuccessful (unpublished, quoted in Taccone).[65]

The noble gas xenon, which has calcium-stabilizing and anti-NMDA receptor properties, was found to confer neuroprotection in a pig model of cardiac arrest.[66] A clinical feasibility study was positive.[67] No randomized clinical trial assessing the efficacy of this treatment has been published.

Current preclinical research is investigating many potential neuroprotective agents for hypoxic-ischemic encephalopathy.[68] These include growth-stimulating hormones, proteins (e.g., estrogen, brain-derived growth factor, granulocyte colony stimulating factor), and gases (e.g., oxygen in hyperbaric environments, molecular hydrogen) that have anti-apoptotic and anti-oxidant properties. To date, however, the only intervention with demonstrated neuroprotective efficacy in this patient population is targeted temperature management.

## SUMMARY

Pharmacologic neuroprotection has been demonstrated consistently for a variety of agents in animal models of TBI, SAH, ischemic stroke, and hypoxic-ischemic encephalopathy. Translation of these findings to clinical practice, however, has not been successful. No large randomized trial has demonstrated pharmacologic neuroprotection in these patient populations. With the exception of early revascularization after stroke by thrombolytic agents, currently there are no compounds for clinical use for neuroprotection.

The discrepancy between the preclinical and clinical study findings has been surprising and requires explanation.[54,69-70] These failures have prompted a critical revision of the translational process, and recommendations for means of better translating preclinical research into clinical trials have been proposed.[71-73] Issues that may underlie discrepancies between preclinical and clinical study findings include pharmacodynamic and pharmacokinetic limitations, the therapeutic time window, differences between animal models and human brain injury, weaknesses in the design of experimental studies and clinical trials, and faulty assumptions underlying the translation of experimental evidence into clinical studies.

With regard to pharmacokinetics, interpretation of the findings of many clinical trials of neuroprotection is limited by the fact that penetration of the investigated compound into the CNS at proper concentrations was not verified. With regard to pharmacodynamics, the targeted mechanism(s) of neuronal damage and its temporal evolution often has not been fully clarified. For instance, a surge of excitatory amino acid release immediately after traumatic neuronal injury is known to be detrimental to neuronal survival. It has therefore been assumed that NMDA receptor antagonists administered for several days following neuronal injury would be protective. On the contrary, it has been demonstrated that glutamate at normal concentrations promotes neuronal survival.[74] Thus, prolonged complete NMDA receptor blockade may be harmful rather than helpful.

It is important to consider the applicability of animal models of neuronal injury to clinical neuroprotection. Experimental models are designed to induce a degree of neuronal injury where neuronal recovery is possible but not inevitable. (Consider the steep part of the curve of a sigmoidal dose-response relationship between insult and injury.) The clinical scenario, however, is a much more heterogeneous situation, with a wide spectrum ranging from trivial neuronal injuries that are destined to recover without intervention through injuries that are so severe that recovery is impossible. It is therefore likely that the proportion of patients in clinical trials who are likely to benefit from pharmacologic and other clinical interventions may only be a small subset of the patients studied. The effectiveness of the intervention, therefore, may only be applicable to a subset of patients in clinical settings, which limits the capacity of the study to detect meaningful clinical changes.

Secondary brain injury often occurs by multiple pathways. The repeated failure of studies testing single agents may be analogous to the findings in cancer trials, where mono-drug therapies are often less efficacious than multidrug regimens. It is possible that combination therapies with complementary targets and effects may be beneficial.[75]

The timing of pharmacologic intervention is a critical factor. Late administration of putative neuroprotective agents, after the majority of primary and secondary injury has occurred, may also explain some discrepancies between laboratory and clinical studies. In laboratory studies, the pharmacologic agents under investigation typically have been administered very soon after injury (i.e., within minutes). In clinical studies, however, the pharmacologic agents typically are administered several hours after onset of the acute brain insult. Indeed, the duration of the "therapeutic window" for many of the experimental pharmacologic interventions has never been defined, and studies have varied greatly in terms of the treatment window employed.

Weaknesses in experimental design include lack of rigorous blinded outcome assessments in the laboratory leading to investigator bias. The need for better design of clinical trials has also been advocated, including the need for adaptive designs that explore and identify optimal dosing prior to proceeding with phase III trials appropriately powered for clinical outcome. Improvements in inclusion criteria, outcome assessments, and statistical methods that account for important confounding variables are also needed.[76]

## CONCLUSION

Effective pharmacologic protection of the brain after traumatic, vascular, or hypoxic-ischemic brain injury has proven elusive. The large number of studies conducted in search of pharmacologic neuroprotection for acute cerebral injury indicates the extent of the investment made in this field. The quest is ongoing.

Many factors may explain why the translation from bench to clinical practice has been unsuccessful. Despite all the lessons learned, however, no new efficacious treatments are on the horizon, and pharmacologic neuroprotection is not yet available. In current practice, neuroprotection at the bedside of patients with traumatic, vascular, or hypoxic-ischemic brain injury should be based on prevention of secondary neuronal injury related to hypoxia, hypotension, hypoglycemia, and intracranial hypertension; early revascularization by thrombolytic agents after ischemic stroke; and targeted temperature management in patients with hypoxic-ischemic encephalopathy after cardiac arrest.[77]

## REFERENCES

1. Kunz A, Dirnagl U, Mergenthaler P. Acute pathophysiological processes after ischaemic and traumatic brain injury. *Best Pract Res Clin Anaesthesiol.* 2010;24(4):495–509.

2. Corps KN, Roth TL, McGavern DB. Inflammation and neuroprotection in traumatic brain injury. *JAMA Neurol.* 2015;72(3):355–62.

3. Roozenbeek B, Maas AI, Menon DK. Changing patterns in the epidemiology of traumatic brain injury. *Nat Rev Neurol.* 2013;9(4):231–6.

4. McConeghy KW, Hatton J, Hughes L, Cook AM. A review of neuroprotection pharmacology and therapies in patients with acute traumatic brain injury. *CNS Drugs.* 2012;26(7):613–36.

5. Bullock MR, Lyeth BG, Muizelaar JP. Current status of neuroprotection trials for traumatic brain injury: lessons from animal models and clinical studies. *Neurosurgery.* 1999;45(2):207–17.

6. Loane DJ, Faden AI. Neuroprotection for traumatic brain injury: translational challenges and emerging therapeutic strategies. *Trends Pharmacol Sci.* 2010;31(12):596–604.

7. Kochanek PM, Bramlett HM, Dixon CE, et al. Approach to modeling, therapy evaluation, drug selection, and biomarker assessments for a multicenter pre-clinical drug screening consortium for acute therapies in severe traumatic brain injury: Operation Brain Trauma Therapy. *J Neurotrauma.* 2016;33(6):513–22.

8. Kabadi SV, Faden AI. Neuroprotective strategies for traumatic brain injury: improving clinical translation. *Int J Mol Sci.* 2014;15(1):1216–36.

9. Faden AI. Neuroprotection and traumatic brain injury: the search continues. *Arch Neurol.* 2001;58(10):1553–5.

10. Ward JD, Becker DP, Miller JD, et al. Failure of prophylactic barbiturate coma in the treatment of severe head injury. *J Neurosurg.* 1985;62(3):383–8.

11. Roberts I, Sydenham E. Barbiturates for acute traumatic brain injury. *Cochrane Database Syst Rev.* 2012;12:CD000033.

12. Knoller N, Levi L, Shoshan I, et al. Dexanabinol (HU-211) in the treatment of severe closed head injury: a randomized, placebo-controlled, phase II clinical trial. *Crit Care Med.* 2002;30(3):548–54.

13. Petruk KC, West M, Mohr G, et al. Nimodipine management in poor-grade aneurysm patients. Results of a multicenter double-blind placebo-control trial. *J Neurosurg.* 1988;68(4):505–17.

14. Pickard JD, Murray GD, Illingworth R, et al. Effect of oral nimodipine on cerebral infarction and outcome after subarachnoid haemorrhage: British aneurysm nimodipine trial. *BMJ.* 1989;298(6674):636–42.

15. Stiefel MF, Heuer GG, Abrahams JM, et al. The effect of nimodipine on cerebral oxygenation in patients with poor grade subarachnoid hemorrhage. *J Neurosurg.* 2004;101(4):594–9.

16. Haley EC Jr, Kassell NF, Torner JC. A randomized controlled trial of high-dose intravenous nicardipine in aneurysmal subarachnoid hemorrhage: a report of the cooperative aneurysm study. *J Neurosurg.* 1993;78(4):537–47.

17. Haley EC Jr, Kassell NF, Torner JC, Truskowski LL, Germanson TP. A randomized trial of two doses of nicardipine in aneurysmal subarachnoid hemorrhage. A report of the Cooperative Aneurysm Study. *J Neurosurg.* 1994;80(5):788–96.

18. Macdonald RL, Kassell NF, Mayer S, et al.; CONSCIOUS-1 Investigators. Clazosentan to overcome neurological ischemia and infarction occurring after subarachnoid hemorrhage (CONSCIOUS-1): randomized, double-blind, placebo-controlled phase 2 dose-finding trial. *Stroke.* 2008;39(11):3015–21.

19. Macdonald RL, Higashida RT, Keller E, et al. Clazosentan, an endothelin receptor antagonist, in patients with aneurysmal subarachnoid haemorrhage undergoing surgical

clipping: a randomised, double-blind, placebo-controlled phase 3 trial (CONSCIOUS-2). *Lancet Neurol.* 2011;10(7):618–25.

20. Laskowitz DT, Kolls BJ. Neuroprotection in subarachnoid hemorrhage. *Stroke.* 2010;41(10 Suppl):S79–84.

21. van den Bergh WM, Algra A, van Kooten F, et al.; MASH Study Group. Magnesium sulfate in aneurysmal subarachnoid hemorrhage: a randomized controlled trial. *Stroke.* 2005;36(5):1011–5.

22. Wong GK, Poon WS, Chan MT, et al.; IMASH Investigators. Intravenous magnesium sulphate for aneurysmal subarachnoid hemorrhage (IMASH). A randomized, double-blinded, placebo-controlled, multicenter phase III trial. *Stroke.* 2010;41(5):921–6.

23. Westermaier T, Stetter C, Vince GH, et al. Prophylactic intravenous magnesium sulfate for treatment of aneurysmal subarachnoid hemorrhage: a randomized, placebo-controlled, clinical study. *Crit Care Med.* 2010;38(5):1284–90.

24. Wong GKC, Poon WS. The biochemical basis of hydroxymethylglutaryl-CoA reductase inhibitors as neuroprotective agents in aneurysmal subarachnoid hemorrhage. *Pharmaceuticals.* 2010;3(10):3186–99.

25. Wong GK, Chan DY, Siu DY, et al.; HDS-SAH Investigators. High-dose simvastatin for aneurysmal subarachnoid hemorrhage multicenter randomized controlled double-blinded clinical trial. *Stroke.* 2015;46(2):382–8.

26. Jang YG, Ilodigwe D, Macdonald RL. Metaanalysis of tirilazad mesylate in patients with aneurysmal subarachnoid hemorrhage. *Neurocrit Care.* 2009;10(1):141–7.

27. Villa F, Iacca C, Molinari AF, et al. Inhalation versus endovenous sedation in subarachnoid hemorrhage patients: effects on regional cerebral blood flow. *Crit Care Med.* 2012;40(10):2797–804.

28. Prabhakaran S, Ruff I, Bernstein RA. Acute stroke intervention: a systematic review. *JAMA.* 2015;313(14):1451–62.

29. Adeoye O, Hornung R, Khatri P, Kleindorfer D. Recombinant tissue-type plasminogen activator use for ischemic stroke in the United States: a doubling of treatment rates over the course of 5 years. *Stroke.* 2011;42(7):1952–5.

30. Powers WJ, Derdeyn CP, Biller J, et al.; American Heart Association Stroke Council. 2015 American Heart Association/American Stroke Association Focused Update of the 2013 Guidelines for the Early Management of Patients with Acute Ischemic Stroke Regarding Endovascular Treatment: a guideline for healthcare professionals from the American Heart Association/American Stroke Association. *Stroke.* 2015;46(10):3020–35.

31. Shirley R, Ord ENJ, Work LM. Oxidative stress and the use of antioxidants in stroke. *Antioxidants.* 2014;3(3):472–501.

32. Davalos A, Castillo J, Alvarez-Sabín J, et al. Oral citicoline in acute ischemic stroke: an individual patient data pooling analysis of clinical trials. *Stroke.* 2002;33(12):2850–7.

33. Davalos A, Alvarez-Sabín J, Castillo J, et al.; International Citicoline Trial on acUte Stroke (ICTUS) trial investigators. Citicoline in the treatment of acute ischaemic stroke: an international, randomised, multicentre, placebo-controlled study (ICTUS trial). *Lancet.* 2012;380(9839):349–57.

34. Desk R, Williams L, Health K. Tirilazad mesylate in acute ischemic stroke: a systematic review. Tirilazad International Steering Committee. *Stroke.* 2000;31(9):2257–65.

35. Ogawa A, Yoshimoto T, Kikuchi H, et al. Ebselen in acute middle cerebral artery occlusion: a placebo-controlled, double-blind clinical trial. *Cerebreovasc Dis.* 1999;9(2):112–8.

36. Kikuchi K, Tancharoen S, Takeshige N, et al. The efficacy of edaravone (radicut), a free radical scavenger, for cardiovascular disease. *Int J Mol Sci.* 2013;14(7):13909–30.

37. Lees KR, Zivin JA, Ashwood T, et al.; Stroke-Acute Ischemic NXY Treatment (SAINT I) Trial Investigators. NXY-059 for acute ischemic stroke. *N Engl J Med.* 2006;354(6):588–600.

38. Shuaib A, Lees KR, Lyden P, et al.; SAINT II Trial Investigators. NXY-059 for the treatment of acute ischemic stroke. *N Engl J Med.* 2007;357(6):562–71.

39. Orrenius S, Zhivotovsky B, Nicotera P. Regulation of cell death: the calcium-apoptosis link. *Nat Rev Mol Cell Biol.* 2003;4(7):552–65.

40. Horn J, de Haan RJ, Vermeulen M, Limburg M. Very Early Nimodipine Use in Stroke (VENUS): a randomized, double-blind, placebo-controlled trial. *Stroke.* 2001;32(2):461–5.

41. Franke CL, Palm R, Dalby M, et al. Flunarizine in stroke treatment (FIST): a double-blind, placebo-controlled trial in Scandinavia and the Netherlands. *Acta Neurol Scand.* 1996;93(1):56–60.

42. Nilupul Perera M, Ma HK, Arakawa S, et al. Inflammation following stroke. *J Clin Neurosci.* 2006;13(1):1–8.

43. Enlimomab Acute Stroke Trial Investigators. Use of anti-ICAM-1 therapy in ischemic stroke: results of the Enlimomab Acute Stroke Trial. *Neurology.* 2001;57(8):1428–34.

44. Krams M, Lees KR, Hacke W, et al.; ASTIN Study Investigators. Acute Stroke Therapy by Inhibition of Neutrophils (ASTIN): an adaptive dose-response study of UK-279,276 in acute ischemic stroke. *Stroke.* 2003;34(11):2543–8.

45. Bogousslavsky J, Victor SJ, Salinas EO, et al.; European-Australian Fiblast (Trafermin) in Acute Stroke Group. Fiblast (Trafermin) in acute stroke: results of the European Australian phase II/III safety and efficacy trial. *Cerebrovasc Dis.* 2002;14(3-4):239–51.

46. Albers GW, Goldstein LB, Hall D, Lesko LM; Aptiganel Acute Stroke Investigators. Aptiganel hydrochloride in acute ischemic stroke: a randomized controlled trial. *JAMA.* 2001;286(21):2673–82.

47. Davis SM, Albers GW, Diener HC, Lees KR, Norris J. Termination of Acute Stroke Studies Involving Selfotel Treatment. ASSIST steering committee. *Lancet.* 1997;349(9044):32.

48. Davis SM, Lees KR, Albers GW, et al. Selfotel in acute ischemic stroke: possible neurotoxic effects of an NMDA antagonist. *Stroke.* 2000;31(2):347–54.

49. Sacco RL, DeRosa JT, Haley EC Jr, et al.; Glycine Antagonist in Neuroprotection Americas Investigators. Glycine antagonist in neuroprotection for patients with acute stroke: GAIN Americas: a randomized controlled trial. *JAMA.* 2001;285(13):1719–28.

50. Lyden P, Shuaib A, Ng K, et al.; CLASS-I/H/T Investigators. Clomethiazole Acute Stroke Study in ischemic stroke (CLASS-I): final results. *Stroke.* 2002;33(1):122–8.

51. Lodder J. Diazepam to improve acute stroke outcome: results of the early GABA-Ergic activation study in stroke trial. A randomized double-blind placebo-controlled trial. *Cerebrovasc Dis.* 2006;21(1-2):120–7.

52. Gandolfo C, Sandercock P, Conti M. Lubeluzole for acute ischaemic stroke. *Cochrane Database Syst Rev* 2002;(1):CD001924.

53. Saver JL, Starkman S, Eckstein M, et al.; FAST-MAG Investigators and Coordinators. Prehospital use of magnesium sulfate as neuroprotection in acute stroke. *N Engl J Med.* 2015;372(6):528–36.

54. Ginsberg MD. Neuroprotection for ischemic stroke: past, present and future. *Neuropharmacology.* 2008;55(3):363–89.

55. Kudenchuk PJ, Sandroni C, Drinhaus HR, et al. Breakthrough in cardiac arrest: reports from the 4th Paris International Conference. *Ann Intensive Care.* 2015;5:22.

56. Safar P, Bleyaert A, Nemoto EM, Moossy J, Snyder JV. Resuscitation after global brain ischemia-anoxia. *Crit Care Med.* 1978;6(4):215–27.

57. Brain Resuscitation Clinical Trial I Study Group. Randomized clinical study of thiopental loading in comatose survivors of cardiac arrest. *N Eng J Med.* 1986;314(7):397–403.

58. Jastremski M, Sutton-Tyrrell K, Vaagenes P. Glucocorticoid treatment does not improve neurological recovery following cardiac arrest. Brain Resuscitation Clinical Trial I Study Group. *JAMA.* 1989;262(24):3427–30.

59. Mentzelopoulos SD, Malachias S, Chamos C, et al. Vasopressin, steroids, and epinephrine and neurologically favorable survival after in-hospital cardiac arrest: a randomized clinical trial. *JAMA.* 2013;310(3):270–9.

60. Meloni BP, Campbell K, Zhu H, Knuckey NW. In search of clinical neuroprotection after brain ischemia: the case for mild hypothermia (35 degrees C) and magnesium. *Stroke.* 2009;40(6):2236–40.

61. Thel MC, Armstrong AL, McNulty SE, Califf RM, O'Connor CM. Randomised trial of magnesium in in-hospital cardiac arrest. Duke Internal Medicine Housestaff. *Lancet.* 1997;350(9087):1272–6.

62. Longstreth WT Jr, Fahrenbruch CE, Olsufka M, Walsh TR, Copass MK, Cobb LA. Randomized clinical trial of magnesium, diazepam, or both after out-of-hospital cardiac arrest. *Neurology.* 2002;59(4):506–14.

63. Abramson N. A randomized clinical-study of a calcium-entry blocker (lidoflazine) in the treatment of comatose survivors of cardiac-arrest. *N Engl J Med.* 1991;324(18):1225–31.

64. Roine R, Kaste M, Kinnunen A, Nikki P, Sarna S, Kajaste S. Nimodipine after resuscitation from out-of-hospital ventricular-fibrillation – a placebo-controlled, double-blind randomized trial. *JAMA.* 1990;264(24):3171–7.

65. Taccone FS, Crippa IA, Dell'Anna AM, Scolletta S. Neuroprotective strategies and neuroprognostication after cardiac arrest. *Best Pract Res Clin Anaesthesiol.* 2015;29(4):451–64.

66. Fries M, Brücken A, Çizen A, et al. Combining xenon and mild therapeutic hypothermia preserves neurological function after prolonged cardiac arrest in pigs. *Crit Care Med.* 2012;40(4):1297–303.

67. Arola OJ, Laitio RM, Roine RO, et al. Feasibility and cardiac safety of inhaled xenon in combination with therapeutic hypothermia following out-of-hospital cardiac arrest. *Crit Care Med.* 2013;41(9):2116–24.

68. Huang L, Applegate PM, Gatling JW, Mangus DB, Zhang J, Applegate RL 2nd. A systematic review of neuroprotective strategies after cardiac arrest: from bench to bedside (part II-comprehensive protection). *Med Gas Res.* 2014;4:10.

69. Narayan RK, Michel ME, Ansell B, et al. Clinical trials in head injury. *J Neurotrauma.* 2002;19(5):503–57.

70. Maas AI, Steyerberg EW, Murray GD, et al. Why have recent trials of neuroprotective agents in head injury failed to show convincing efficacy? A pragmatic analysis and theoretical considerations. *Neurosurgery.* 1999;44(6):1286–98.

71. Xu SY, Pan SY. The failure of animal models of neuroprotection in acute ischemic stroke to translate to clinical efficacy. *Med Sci Monit Basic Res.* 2013;19:37–45.

72. Grupke S, Hall J, Dobbs M, Bix GJ, Fraser JF. Understanding history, and not repeating it. Neuroprotection for acute ischemic stroke: from review to preview. *Clin Neurol Neurosurg.* 2015;129:1–9.

73. Stroke Therapy Academic Industry Roundtable (STAIR). Recommendations for standards regarding preclinical neuroprotective and restorative drug development. *Stroke.* 1999;30(12):2752–8.

74. Ikonomidou C, Turski L. Why did NMDA receptor antagonists fail clinical trials for stroke and traumatic brain injury? *Lancet Neurol.* 2002;1(6):383–6.

75. Margulies S, Hicks R; The Combination Therapies for Traumatic Brain Injury Workshop Leaders. Combination therapies for traumatic brain injury: prospective considerations. *J Neurotrauma.* 2009;26(6):925–39.

76. Stocchetti N, Taccone FS, Citerio G, et al. Neuroprotection in acute brain injury: an up-to-date review. *Critical Care.* 2015;19:186.

77. Nolan JP, Soar J, Cariou A, et al. European Resuscitation Council and European Society of Intensive Care Medicine 2015 guidelines for post-resuscitation care. *Intensive Care Med.* 2015;41(12):2039–56.

78. Teasdale G, Bailey I, Bell A, et al. A randomized trial of nimodipine in severe head injury: HIT I. British/Finnish Co-operative Head Injury Trial Group. *J Neurotrauma.* 1992;9 Suppl 2:S545–50.

79. Young B, Runge JW, Waxman KS, et al. Effects of pegorgotein on neurologic outcome of patients with severe head injury. A multicenter, randomized controlled trial. *JAMA.* 1996;276(7):538–43.

80. Marshall LF, Maas AI, Marshall SB, et al. A multicenter trial on the efficacy of using tirilazad mesylate in cases of head injury. *J Neurosurg.* 1998;89(4):519–25.

81. Marmorou A, Nichols J, Burgess J, et al. Effects of the bradykinin antagonist Bradycor (deltibant, CP-1027) in severe traumatic brain injury: results of a multi-center, randomized, placebo-controlled trial. American Brain Injury Consortium Study Group. *J Neurotrauma.* 1999;16(6):431–44.

82. Morris GF, Bullock R, Marshall SB, Marmarou A, Maas A, Marshall LF. Failure of the competitive N-methyl-D-aspartate antagonist Selfotel (CGS 19755) in the treatment of severe head injury: results of two phase III clinical trials. The Selfotel Investigators. *J Neurosurg.* 1999;91(5):737–43.

83. Ohman J, Braakman R, Legout V; Traumatic Brain Injury Study Group. Repinotan (BAY x 3702): a 5HT1A agonist in traumatically brain injured patients. *J Neurotrauma.* 2001;18(12):1313–21.

84. Lepeintre JF, D'Arbigny P, Mathé JF, et al. Neuroprotective effect of gacyclidine. A multicenter double-blind pilot trial in patients with acute traumatic brain injury. *Neurochirurgie.* 2004;50(2-3 Pt 1):83–95.

85. Yurkewicz L, Weaver J, Bullock MR, Marshall LF. The effect of the selective NMDA receptor antagonist traxoprodil in the treatment of traumatic brain injury. *J Neurotrauma.* 2005;22(12):1428–43.

86. Marmarou A, Guy M, Murphey L, et al.; American Brain Injury Consortium. A single dose, three-arm, placebo-controlled, phase I study of the bradykinin B2 receptor antagonist Anatibant (LF16-0687Ms) in patients with severe traumatic brain injury. *J Neurotrauma.* 2005;22(12):1444–55.

87. Cotton BA, Snodgrass KB, Fleming SB, et al. Beta-blocker exposure is associated with improved survival after severe traumatic brain injury. *J Trauma.* 2007;62(1):26–35.

88. Hatton J, Rosbolt B, Empey P, Kryscio R, Young B. Dosing and safety of cyclosporine in patients with severe brain injury. *J Neurosurg.* 2008;109(4):699–707.

89. Narayan RK, Maas AI, Marshall LF, Servadei F, Skolnick BE, Tillinger MN; rFVIIa Traumatic ICH Study Group. Recombinant factor VIIA in traumatic intracerebral hemorrhage: results of a dose-escalation clinical trial. *Neurosurgery.* 2008;62(4):786–8.

90. Mazzeo AT, Brophy GM, Gilman CB, et al. Safety and tolerability of cyclosporin A in severe traumatic brain injury patients: results from a prospective randomized trial. *J Neurotrauma.* 2009;26(12):2195–206.

91. Shroeppel TJ, Fischer PE, Zarzaur BL, et al. Beta-adrenergic blockade and traumatic brain injury: protective? *J Trauma.* 2010;69(4):776–82.

92. Giacino JT, Whyte J, Bagiella E, et al. Placebo-controlled trial of amantadine for severe traumatic brain injury. *N Engl J Med.* 2012;366(9):819–26.

93. Zafonte RD, Bagiella E, Ansel BM, et al. Effect of citicoline on functional and cognitive status among patients with traumatic brain injury: Citicoline Brain Injury Treatment Trial (COBRIT). *JAMA.* 2012;308(19):1993–2000.

94. Grumme T, Baethmann A, Kolodziejczyk D, et al. Treatment of patients with severe head injury by triamcinolone: a prospective, controlled multicenter clinical trial of 396 cases. *Res Exp Med (Berl).* 1995;195(4):217–29.

95. Roberts I, Yates D, Sandercock P, et al.; CRASH trial collaborators. Effect of intravenous corticosteroids on death within 14 days in 10008 adults with clinically significant head injury (MRC CRASH trial): randomised placebo-controlled trial. *Lancet.* 2004;364(9442):1321–8.

96. Maas AI, Murray G, Henney H 3rd, et al.; Pharmos TBI investigators. Efficacy and safety of dexanabinol in severe traumatic brain injury: results of a phase III randomised, placebo-controlled, clinical trial. *Lancet Neurol.* 2006;5(1):38–45.

97. Temkin NR, Anderson GD, Winn HR, et al. Magnesium sulfate for neuroprotection after traumatic brain injury: a randomised controlled trial. *Lancet Neurol.* 2007;6(1):29–38.

98. Firsching R, Piek J, Skalej M, Rohde V, Schmidt U, Striggow F; KN38-7271 Study Group. Early survival of comatose patients after severe traumatic brain injury with the dual cannabinoid CB1/CB2 receptor agonist KN38-7271: a randomized, double-blind, placebo-controlled phase II trial. *J Neurol Surg A Cent Eur Neurosurg.* 2012;73(4):204–16.

99. Xiao G, Wei J, Yan W, Wang W, Lu Z. Improved outcomes from the administration of progesterone for patients with acute severe traumatic brain injury: a randomized controlled trial. *Crit Care.* 2008;12(2):R61.

100. Wright DW, Yeatts SD, Silbergleit R, et al.; NETT Investigators. Very early administration of progesterone for acute traumatic brain injury. *N Engl J Med.* 2014;371(26):2457–66.

101. Skolnick BE, Maas AI, Narayan RK, et al.; SYNAPSE Trial Investigators. A clinical trial of progesterone for severe traumatic brain injury. *N Engl J Med.* 2014;371(26):2467–76.

102. Robertson CS, Hannay HJ, Yamal JM, et al.; Epo Severe TBI Trial Investigators. Effect of erythropoietin and transfusion threshold on neurological recovery after traumatic brain injury: a randomized clinical trial. *JAMA.* 2014;312(1):36–47.

103. De Deyn PP, Reuck JD, Deberdt W, Vlietinck R, Orgogozo JM. Treatment of acute ischemic stroke with piracetam. Members of the Piracetam in Acute Stroke Study (PASS) Group. *Stroke.* 1997;28(12):2347–52.

104. Clark WM, Raps EC, Tong DC, Kelly RE. Cervene (Nalmefene) in acute ischemic stroke: final results of a phase III efficacy study. The Cervene Stroke Study Investigators. *Stroke.* 2000;31(6):1234–9.

# PART II
# CLINIMETRICS OF NEUROPROTECTION

# 3 Imaging Assessment of Brain Injury

Matthew A. Warner,

Carlos Marquez de la Plata,

David S. Liebeskind, and

Ramon Diaz-Arrastia

## INTRODUCTION

Brain injury due to trauma, ischemic stroke, and hemorrhagic stroke is very common in both the developed and developing world. Numerous animal models of brain injuries have led to identification of several promising experimental therapeutic neuroprotective options. Success in these studies, however, has yet to translate to effective clinical therapies and likely reflects the inherent heterogeneity of each of these conditions. In recent years, major advances in neuroimaging have resulted in improved detection and classification of acquired brain injuries based on recognizable patterns of acute structural damage and secondary deterioration. It is likely that the success of any future clinical trials of neuroprotective therapies will be dependent on reliable and validated neuroimaging biomarkers of injury and recovery. This chapter describes neuroimaging modalities that are currently being utilized in clinical and experimental settings.

With regard to traumatic brain injury (TBI), this discussion focuses on a subtype of injury called diffuse traumatic axonal injury (TAI). This mechanism of injury is very common and is poorly imaged by computed tomography (CT) and conventional structural magnetic resonance imaging (MRI). Recently developed imaging modalities, both clinical and experimental, have allowed for vast improvements in the initial detection and subsequent observation of this type of injury.

The increasing use of neuroimaging in general, and the more recent dissemination of multimodal CT or MRI, noninvasive angiography, and perfusion maps, has transformed our understanding of stroke. Consequently, the potential for neuroprotection has markedly advanced in recent years.[1] The introduction of minimally invasive hematoma evacuation and the establishment of endovascular therapy for ischemic stroke have prompted standardized approaches to emergency brain imaging in acute stroke.

## COMPUTED TOMOGRAPHY
### Traumatic Brain Injury

CT is the most common imaging modality used in the acute phase of head injury to detect skull fractures, hemorrhage, and parenchymal injury. Conventionally, CT has been used for the acute identification of focal injuries that are potentially life-threatening and may require emergent neurosurgical interventions, such as extra-axial or parenchymal hemorrhage with the potential for midline shift and/or incipient herniation. CT is also used for identification of conditions that may require intensive care monitoring, such as small hematomas that may subsequently expand or traumatic subarachnoid or intraventricular hemorrhages that may result in posttraumatic hydrocephalus.[2-4] CT scans also reflect the extent of vasogenic edema and depict the demarcation of boundaries between normal and damaged brain tissue, information that may be useful prognostically during rehabilitation and community reintegration.[5-6]

Assessment of injury severity with CT is critical for initial neurosurgical and ICU-based management of care, but these initial imaging results are only modestly associated with long-term functional outcomes. CT is most informative in patients with severe TBI as abnormalities identified by this modality have a predictive value of 75% for identifying patients likely to have a favorable outcome.[4,7] In mild to moderate brain injury, CT is useful in identifying focal lesions that may affect clinical disposition, but it is not an optimal tool for prediction of long-term outcome. In this population, the number of abnormalities identified by acute CT is not associated with Glasgow Outcome Score or Glasgow Outcome Score-Extended.[4,8] This may be due, in part, to the inadequate sensitivity of CT to detect the diffuse microstructural white matter damage that is characteristic of TAI.

### Stroke

In acute stroke, hemorrhage is easily detected on CT, whereas the stigmata of ischemia are much more subtle. Various forms of intracranial hemorrhage may be identified, prompting quite divergent treatment strategies. For instance, the presence of subarachnoid hemorrhage may trigger an evaluation for a ruptured aneurysm, whereas spontaneous intracerebral hematoma diagnosis may focus attention on prevention of early expansion and treatment of concomitant cerebral edema. In acute ischemic stroke, hemorrhagic transformation of an ischemic lesion is relatively uncommon; however, hemorrhage patterns in the subacute phase are important in guiding management in the ICU.

CT findings of early ischemia center on relative changes in local water concentrations caused by cytotoxic edema, followed by vasogenic edema and blood–brain barrier derangements. Early ischemic injury in the first few hours after stroke onset has been recognized for decades, including loss of the insular ribbon sign and subtle changes that may be best assessed with use of the Alberta Stroke Program Early CT Score (ASPECTS) rating system. Loss of the insular ribbon refers to a lack of gray–white matter differentiation in the lateral margin of the insular cortex; it is an early CT sign of middle cerebral artery (MCA) infarction as a result of this region's lack of collateral supply and susceptibility to ischemia. The ASPECTS rating system provides a framework to score regional changes associated with the extent of hypodensity in the MCA territory.[9] Although most patients have relatively preserved ASPECTS in the first few hours (scaled as 10 = no early infarction, 0 = complete hemispheric brain infarction), lower ASPECTS or more extensive injury may be used to gauge expectations regarding potential salvage with reperfusion therapies, neuroprotective opportunities, and prognoses.

It has become standard to acquire noncontrast CT or other parenchymal imaging at 24 hours after intravenous and endovascular reperfusion therapies. This standard imaging measure has been used in recent clinical trials as a surrogate endpoint.[10] CT lesion size at 24 hours has been assessed by ASPECTS rating, as well as final infarct volume calculated by planimetry and slice-by-slice region of interest (ROI) analysis.

When hemorrhage is observed at 24 hours, the type of bleeding has been used as a routine measure in clinical trials. The Heidelberg bleeding classification system, an adaptation of the earlier European Cooperative Acute Stroke Study (ECASS) classification, divides the types of bleeding into petechiae or parenchymal hematomas based on the degree of mass effect, as well as subarachnoid or remote hemorrhages.[11] For both ischemic and hemorrhagic parenchymal lesions, the change from baseline to 24 hours has become an important quantitative parameter to differentiate the course of stroke patients within a population or study.

## CONVENTIONAL MAGNETIC RESONANCE IMAGING

MRI is an imaging modality that provides higher spatial and contrast resolution than CT, allowing for better delineation of soft tissues and improved detection of less obvious traumatic lesions, such as microhemorrhages, small contusions, and TAI.[2,12–15] This modality may be used in the subacute phase of injury or when the neurologic status of the patient indicates a more serious injury than suggested by CT findings. Conventional MRI sequences include T1-weighted, T2-weighted, fluid attenuated inversion recovery (FLAIR), diffusion weighted imaging (DWI), and susceptibility weighted imaging (SWI).

### T1-Weighted and T2-Weighted MRI

T1-weighted sequences are susceptible to the presence of blood or fat in brain tissue, which are depicted by high signal intensities. This imaging modality, however, offers minimal diagnostic specificity as abnormalities seen on T1 sequences generally indicate multiple types of pathology, such as hematomas, parenchymal lesions, or vascular tumors.[6,16] T2-weighted and gradient recalled echo (GRE) MR imaging detects brain hemorrhage more effectively than T1 images, but high signal intensities from the cerebrospinal fluid (CSF) in these images complicates the identification of TAI lesions.

### FLAIR-Weighted MRI

FLAIR imaging has some clear advantages over CT and other conventional MRI sequences. FLAIR MRI imaging detects cerebral edema and allows for easier identification of injured tissue as it nullifies the CSF signal and greatly increases the contrast between normal and abnormal brain matter.[12,17–18] FLAIR-weighted MRI also can be used to quantify the degree of white matter damage after trauma.[19–21] In addition to improved sensitivity for areas of white matter microstructural damage acutely after injury, FLAIR MRI can also be used to quantify changes in lesion volume over time and detect the appearance of new lesions.[20,22–23]

Several studies have investigated the prognostic value of quantifying white matter hyperintensities by FLAIR MRI after TBI, concluding that identified lesions are significantly associated with long-term outcome.[20] Scheid et al. examined a sample of 18 patients with severe TBI and showed that the number of hyperintensities seen on FLAIR correlated with functional outcome.[21] Marquez de la Plata et al. utilized a method to quantify the volume of white matter FLAIR hyperintensities among patients with moderate to severe TAI and found poorer outcomes among patients with greater lesion volumes.[19] FLAIR imaging results are also associated with chronic alterations in brain structure. The hyperintensities identified acutely after injury are strongly predictive of posttraumatic tissue atrophy 6 months after injury.[23] Figure 3.1 illustrates the different patterns of FLAIR and diffusion abnormalities found on MRIs done within the first several days of injury in patients with severe TBI. In each case the CT scan failed to reveal the extent of trauma-related pathology.

In patients with mild to moderate brain injury, however, MRI is a modest predictor of long-term recovery and return-to-work status.[15,24–25] Recent MRI advances,

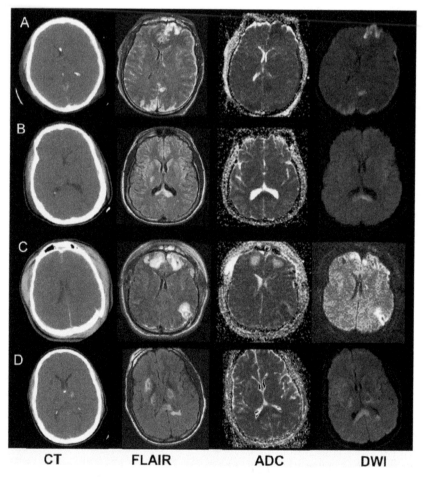

CT      FLAIR      ADC      DWI

FIGURE 3.1 Patterns of traumatic edema lesions. A. Cytotoxic edema in cortical structures. B. Cytotoxic edema in deep white matter structures (corpus callosum; CC). C. Mixed cytotoxic and vasogenic edema in cortical and subcortical structures. D. Mixed cytotoxic and vasogenic edema in deep white matter structures.

as discussed later, have resulted in enhanced sensitivity for microstructural axonal damage and improved the prognostic value.

## Diffusion Weighted Imaging

DWI is another widely used MRI modality that allows for spatial identification and quantification of cytotoxic and vasogenic edema that accompanies brain injuries. In particular, DWI is extremely effective for detecting early tissue ischemia in acute ischemic stroke. Within the first few hours of vessel occlusion, downstream tissue progresses from showing the earliest signs of restricted water diffusion (which appears black on apparent diffusion coefficient [ADC] images), to early cellular swelling with cytotoxic edema (which appears bright on DWI images), to tissue infarction (which appears bright on FLAIR images). Rather than relying on conventional MRI contrast mechanisms such as T1 and T2 relaxation, DWI relies on differences in the random thermal or self-diffusion of protons in water throughout the brain and quantifies these differences using the ADC. Areas with restricted proton diffusion appear hyperintense on DWI images and have low ADC values, whereas the reverse is true in regions with increased diffusion. Vasogenic edema, a consequence of fluid leakage from the local vasculature into the extracellular space, results in areas of increased water diffusion and higher ADC values, whereas cytotoxic edema is characterized by a shift of water from extracellular to intracellular compartments and results in restricted diffusion, hyperintense DWI-weighted MRI signal, and lower (darker) ADC values.[2,26] Both cytotoxic and vasogenic edema contribute to long-term functional outcome. Distinguishing these two types of edema can be useful for guiding neuroprotection strategies as they are likely to respond to different therapies.

DWI can also detect diffusion abnormalities within days or even hours after TAI in patients with mild and severe head injury.[3,26–28] DWI has higher sensitivity for edematous lesions than FLAIR and T2-weighted MRI, although it is less sensitive for detecting hemorrhagic TAI than T2 sequences.[26] With regard to prognosis, the volume of lesions identified acutely by DWI is more strongly correlated with clinical outcome than the aforementioned MRI sequences, supporting the use of acute DWI as a radiologic biomarker for outcome after TAI.[29–30]

## Susceptibility Weighted Imaging

SWI is a recently developed MRI technique, based on conventional GRE MRI, which provides increased sensitivity for the detection of hemorrhagic lesions associated with TAI. SWI utilizes the differing magnetic susceptibility properties of brain tissue and blood (or products of hemolysis, such as hemosiderin) in order to identify microscopic areas of extravasated blood early after trauma.[31] It is now apparent that SWI substantially increases the sensitivity for detection and quantification of hemorrhagic lesions over T2-weighted MRI.[31–34] Moreover, while conventional MRI sequences and even CT may be useful in identifying large hemorrhagic lesions after closed head injury, many small hemorrhages associated with the shearing forces of TAI may only be detected by SWI.[31–32] Chastain et al. compared SWI with CT and FLAIR in 38 patients with acute TBI.[35] They concluded that although SWI is more sensitive than FLAIR for identifying small lesions, it is not as good in discriminating the likelihood of recovery. The discriminate ability of SWI was comparable to CT.

In pediatric TBI, the number and volume of lesions identified by SWI are associated with poor neuropsychological outcomes and decreased intelligence quotient (IQ) scores several years after injury.[34] Moreover, children with moderate or severe disability between 6 and 12 months after TBI have a greater number and volume of SWI-identified lesions than do those with mild disability or normal outcome.[33]

## MRI in Stroke

The use of MRI to characterize brain injuries was prominently forged by the use of the described techniques in the setting of acute stroke. Although MRI is far less practical as a routine modality for widespread use in acute stroke, the degree of information and detection of subtle lesions is superior to CT. The combination of DWI, GRE or SWI, and FLAIR sequences is standardly applied to patients with suspected brain injuries, including stroke. DWI may assess the extent of ischemia, typically quantified as the volume of tissue with apparent diffusion coefficient values of less than 620. GRE or SWI may reveal the presence of hemorrhage, but the use of these sequences has been far more useful in detecting early vessel signs of arterial occlusion and flow changes associated with varying degrees of collateral circulation, including deoxygenation in downstream vessels.[36] FLAIR may only detect parenchymal injury several hours after stroke onset, but relatively subtle findings of vessel occlusion and slow flow in leptomeningeal collateral vessels may be seen. DWI-FLAIR mismatch in different brain regions has been used to estimate the duration and severity of ischemic injury, including the potential to evaluate the therapeutic potential for neuroprotection or reperfusion.

## ADVANCED IMAGING MODALITIES
### Diffusion Tensor Imaging

Diffusion tensor imaging (DTI) has received increasing attention over the past 15 years as a biomarker for white matter injury in several neurologic conditions, including TBI. DTI utilizes the magnetic properties of water to measure thermally induced molecular diffusion occurring within the tissue compartments of the brain (i.e., the intra- and extracellular spaces). The amounts and spatial distribution of diffusion can be measured in one given direction at a time. By successive manipulation of the MRI system, the average amount of water diffusion occurring across all directions measured can be obtained and is termed *mean diffusivity* (MD). The relative directionality of water diffusion can be computed as the normalized standard deviation of these measurements and is referred to as its *fractional anisotropy* (FA).

FA is calculated by measuring the amount of diffusion in multiple directions and computing the composite 3D tensor value for each voxel in the brain. From a diagonalization of this tensor, three eigenvalues are obtained and used to compute MD, FA, and other scalar mappings. Diffusion is said to be *isotropic* if water diffuses in a nonrestricted and random manner (in this case, all three eigenvalues are equal). Diffusion is said to be *anisotropic* if water molecules diffuse in a relatively directional or restricted manner, as is the case when water diffuses along the length of a bundle of axons but not in a perpendicular fashion (in this case, one eigenvalue is much larger than the other two).

DTI has demonstrated clear differences in MD and FA within several clinical populations, including TBI.[37–42] Several investigations have examined the distribution of DTI-derived metrics for voxels throughout the brain to identify gross structural integrity differences between TBI patients and normal control subjects.[43-45] Benson and colleagues examined white matter integrity of patients with chronic TBI and found that the shape of the FA histograms were more peaked (kurtotic) and skewed in TBI patients compared to normal subjects.[44] Bazarian et al. also showed that patients with TBI had FA distributions that were significantly shifted toward lower values compared to normal control subjects, indicating more isotropic diffusion.[43] Furthermore, they noted that these measures of microstructural integrity correlated with postconcussive symptoms 1 month after injury.

DTI has also demonstrated microstructural compromise in centroaxial white matter regions commonly impacted in TAI using a whole-brain analysis technique called *voxel-based analysis* (VBA).[44,46-48] Xu et al. studied a sample of 9 patients scanned 4 years after TBI and 11 control subjects using VBA.[47] They found that TBI patients had lower FA within major white matter structures than did control subjects. Specifically, they found compromise to the integrity of the corpus callosum (CC), internal capsule, superior and inferior longitudinal fasiculi, and the fornix. Bendlin et al. and Nakayama et al. found similar results in patients whose brains were imaged approximately 1 year post-TBI.[46,48] DTI data from moderately to severely injured patients with TAI scanned approximately 8 months after injury revealed compromise to various white matter regions as compared to control subjects. Furthermore, the degree of white matter compromise correlated well with functional and neurocognitive outcomes.[49]

Using a basic ROI approach, Sidaros et al. showed longitudinal changes in white matter integrity after moderate to severe TBI.[50] Specifically, FA was reduced 5 to 11 weeks post-injury due to decreased parallel diffusivity and increased perpendicular diffusivity. Additionally, FA in certain structures improved over time due to an interval increase of parallel diffusivity to normal levels, and this increase primarily occurred in patients with favorable outcomes. Bendlin et al. also examined a cohort of patients with TBI longitudinally, once at approximately 2 months post-injury and again within 1 year of injury.[48] Using VBA analysis on DTI-derived data in this longitudinal fashion, they observed significant white matter volume loss within the CC, cingulum, longitudinal fasciculi, uncinate fasciculi, and brainstem fiber tracts over time. Furthermore, they found gray matter loss over time, suggestive of Wallerian degeneration. Figure 3.2 illustrates data from one of our injured study participants. It shows the evolution of white matter compromise, as measured by FA over a 6-month period, and demonstrates relatively greater sensitivity for white matter lesions using DTI compared to FLAIR.

Nakayama and colleagues studied a group of carefully selected patients who had experienced a nonmissile TBI and demonstrated significant injury-related cognitive impairment without detectible lesions on conventional neuroimaging.[46] Using VBA on DTI scans acquired an average of 14 months post-injury, they observed significant decreases in FA of the CC. Given the stringent inclusion criteria in their study, the results strongly suggest that a voxel-based approach to analyzing white matter integrity can detect areas of damage that may be associated with clinical outcome after TAI. Additionally, Nakayama et al. reconstructed the CC and fornix using diffusion tensor tractography and observed qualitative differences in the length and volume of these structures between patients and control subjects.[46]

Diffusion tensor tractography is a technique used to three-dimensionally reconstruct white matter structures based on the directionality of water diffusion within each voxel. White matter tracts are reconstructed using either deterministic or

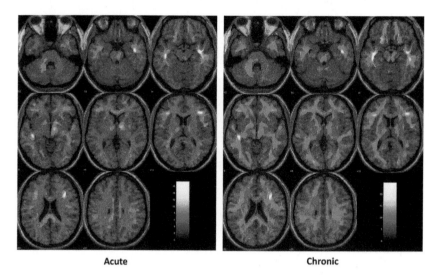

Acute        Chronic

FIGURE 3.2 Statistical parametric mapping (SPM) maps from a representative patient with severe traumatic brain injury, imaged 2 days (acute) and 6 months (chronic) after injury, demonstrating the characteristic increase in white matter regions with low fractional anisotropy values during this period.

probabilistic methods.[51–52] Because water diffuses more anisotropically along axons than perpendicular to them, adjacent voxels within subcortical regions with similar FA values and similar directions of maximal or preferred diffusion can be tracked and are said to be structurally connected. Diffusion tensor tractography has shown sensitivity to compromised white matter in TAI.[46–47,53–55] Wilde et al. examined 16 children at an average of 3 years following severe TBI and found that the reconstructed CC in this group had lower average FA values than did age-matched uninjured counterparts.[53] Additionally, they found that higher FA in the CC is associated with better functional outcomes among patients. Nakayama et al. and Xu et al. used tractography and voxel-based approaches to examine the integrity of the CC and fornix post-TBI.[46–47] Their studies allowed for comparison between approaches, concluding that compromise to the CC can be observed using either approach. Interestingly, Nakayama and colleagues found that tractography was sensitive to compromise within the fornix, whereas FA within this structure measured using VBA was not different from control subjects.[46] Their results suggest that TAI-related white matter compromise in certain structures may be best detected by different DTI techniques, such as trading in-plane resolution with slice thickness to maintain signal but increase structural resolution.

Wang et al. reconstructed several white matter tracts among moderately to severely injured patients with TAI, in acute and chronic phases, and age- and gender-matched control subjects.[55] They demonstrated significantly lower FA within the CC (genu, posterior body, splenium), fornix, and peduncular projections to occipital and parietal cortices of patients. Additionally, they found that the integrity of the splenium of the CC was strongly associated with Glasgow Outcome Score-Extended. Data from our group was used to examine the integrity of several white matter structures, finding that FA within the CC, fornix, right inferior longitudinal fasciculus, and bilateral inferior fronto-occipital fasiculi was strongly correlated with neurocognitive performance approximately 8 months post-injury (see Figure 3.3).[56]

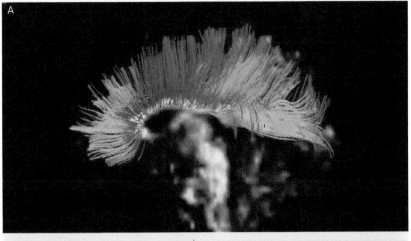

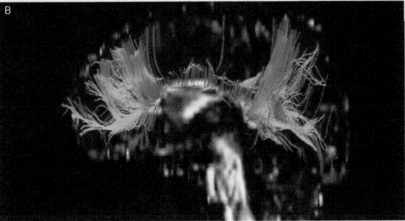

FIGURE 3.3 Reconstructed corpus callosum (CC) using diffusion tensor tractography. A. Reconstructed CC in a healthy, non–brain injured participant. B. CC of age- and gender-matched participant 6 months after a severe traumatic brain injury.

## CT and MR Angiography

In the setting of stroke, multimodal CT and MRI offer the potential of noninvasive angiography and perfusion imaging to identify the location and extent of arterial occlusion and corresponding collateral flow patterns. CT angiography (CTA) and MR angiography (MRA) now have a diverse spectrum of techniques that may be readily applied in routine clinical practice. CTA is most commonly employed, and a variety of approaches have developed to assess vascular changes, depending on the extent of coverage and relative focus on different phases of arterial inflow.[57] Conventional or single-phase CTA is still most commonly used, whereas multiphase CTA has been increasingly used to delineate the extent of collaterals at later venous phases.

MRA may be used akin to CTA to detect proximal arterial occlusions, although the distal leptomeningeal collateral circulation is harder to image with MRA. The overwhelming focus of CTA and MRA has been on detecting complete occlusions during triage of stroke patients, yet the degree of luminal obstruction on the

**Table 3.1** The Original Thrombolysis in Cerebral Infarction Perfusion Scale

| Category | Title | Description |
|---|---|---|
| Grade 0 | No Perfusion | No antegrade flow beyond the point of occlusion. |
| Grade 1 | Penetration with Minimal Perfusion | The contrast material passes beyond the area of obstruction but fails to opacify the entire cerebral bed distal to the obstruction. |
| Grade 2 | Partial Perfusion | The contrast material passes beyond the obstruction and opacifies the arterial bed distal to the obstruction. However, the rate of entry of contrast into the vessel distal to the obstruction and/or its rate of clearance from comparable areas not perfused by the previously occluded vessel. |
| Grade 2a | | Only partial filling (less than two-thirds) of the entire vascular territory is visualized.) |
| Grade 2b | | Complete filling of all of the expected vascular territory is visualized but the filling is slower than normal. |
| Grade 3 | Complete Perfusion | Antegrade flow into the bed distal to the obstruction occurs as promptly as into the obstruction and clearance of contrast material from the involved bed is as rapid as from an uninvolved other bed of the same vessel or the opposite cerebral artery |

modified arterial occlusive lesion scoring system and relative change from baseline to 24 hours has been used in clinical trials. The Thrombolysis in Cerebral Infarction (TICI) scale (Table 3.1), modeled after a similar scale for judging the degree of angiographic reperfusion after treatment for myocardial infarction, is the current standard for reporting the extent of revascularization after acute ischemic stroke.[58]

## CT and MR Perfusion Imaging

Perfusion imaging may be performed with either exogenous or endogenous contrast-based methods on CT or MRI. The acquisition of contrast-based perfusion imaging on CT and MRI is similar, leveraging similar mathematical calculations to generate parameter maps including mean transit time (MTT), $T_{max}$, cerebral blood volume (CBV), and cerebral blood flow (CBF). Endogenous contrast may be used on arterial spin-labeled MRI to map perfusion in various brain regions. Perfusion imaging is not as commonly used as noninvasive angiography during evaluation of the acute stroke patient, yet these techniques have been used for assessment of potential penumbral salvage in clinical trials of neuroprotection and reperfusion. The threshold of $T_{max}$ of greater than 6 seconds on either CT or MRI has been used to measure lesions at risk of ischemic injury. More severe measures of $T_{max}$, such as the relative ratios of $T_{max}$ threshold volumes, have been used as the hypoperfusion intensity ratios to estimate likely benefit with therapeutic interventions. Similar to the use of serial changes in ASPECTS or the modified Arterial Occlusive Lesion score from baseline to 24 hours, changes in repeated perfusion imaging with CT or MRI have been used to estimate the degree of reperfusion.

## Chronic Brain Injury

Cerebral atrophy, progressing for months and possibly years, is a common consequence of TBI and stroke and is associated with poor patient outcomes.[23,50,59–60] While the predominant view is that loss of structural volume results from direct insult to neuron bodies, it is possible that atrophy, in the absence of focal trauma, may originate primarily from axonal damage with subsequent Wallerian degeneration and neuronal cell death.[23] With regard to TAI, recent evidence indicates that posttraumatic atrophy is not globally diffuse, but rather some brain regions are highly susceptible to volume loss while others show marked resilience.[60] Moreover, atrophy in particular brain regions may hold prognostic value for disability or functional recovery. Thus, accurate measurement of in vivo structural changes utilizing 3D structural MRI may potentially serve as a biomarker for outcome after TBI.

Numerous neuroimaging techniques have been proposed for measurement of atrophy. Cross-sectional methods compare the volume of brain tissue (typically gray and white matter, excluding CSF) against a common normalization volume, such as total intracranial volume (ICV) for patient versus control group comparisons. Longitudinal studies utilize repeated MRI scans for between-scan comparisons and tend to incur lower absolute measurement error than cross-sectional studies.[61] There are relatively few longitudinal studies of atrophy after TBI.[48,50,60,62–64] Of these, the majority assessed volume loss occurring between the subacute and chronic time periods, finding volume loss between 1% and 4%.[48,50,62–63] A study of TBI patients with an injury mechanism consistent with TAI (i.e., involving high-speed acceleration-deceleration or rotational forces) assessed atrophy occurring between the acute time period (within 1 week) and a median of 7.9 months (range 6–14) post-injury. Patients exhibited substantial global atrophy, with mean brain parenchymal volume loss of 4.5%.[60] Clearance of acute brain edema did not account for the observed volume decreases. Another study that followed patients for up to 2.5 years after injury found that atrophy of the thalamus and white matter continues beyond 12 months in a subset of patients and that DTI metrics correlated with functional outcomes.[65] It is probable that the rate of posttraumatic volume loss is also related to functional outcome. In order to determine the best time for intervention in future clinical trials of therapies targeted at preserving brain parenchyma, it will be essential to determine the progression of whole-brain volume loss occurring at shorter time intervals and over a longer study period.

Quantifying regional variations in atrophy rates represents a formidable challenge. This is due in large part to regional morphometric distortions caused by focal lesions, leading to complications with image registration, intensity normalization, and tissue segmentation. Nevertheless, several quantitative techniques utilizing 3D structural T1-weighted MRI images for quantifying regional atrophy have been applied to TBI. One of the earliest approaches is ROI analysis, a morphometric procedure that relies heavily on manual tracing of readily identifiable cerebral structures. While ROI studies provide evidence for atrophy in a variety of brain regions, methodological limitations greatly undermine their ability to identify brain regions that are highly susceptible to atrophy after TBI and stroke.[66] Because ROI analyses rely on manual identification and delineation of cerebral structures, they are limited in their ability to quantify brain regions lacking clear structural boundaries. Moreover, ROI analyses typically focus on only a small set of structures and are unable to provide a complete assessment of changes in brain morphometry.

Recognizing these limitations, several quantitative and automated MRI approaches have been developed for the calculation of tissue volume per brain voxel, thereby achieving a more comprehensive picture of structural changes after acquired brain injury. Voxel-based morphometry (VBM) registers structural MRI images to a common 3D reference space; segments tissue based on signal intensities to delineate gray matter, white matter, and CSF; and smooths neighboring voxels for the creation of composite brain tissue maps. Tensor-based morphometry (TBM) allows for improved nonlinear image registration and may be less sensitive to inaccuracies in tissue segmentation than VBM.[50,67] The FreeSurfer image analysis suite (http://surfer.nmr.mgh.harvard.edu) permits high-resolution quantification of thickness, surface area, curvature, and volume of numerous atlas-derived brain regions, increasing the sensitivity to cortical morphometric changes over other voxel-wise approaches.

Employing these techniques, posttraumatic atrophy has been noted in a variety of brain regions, including the amygdala, brainstem, corpus callosum, hippocampus, thalamus, putamen, precuneus cortex, and several regions of the parietal and frontal cortices.[48,50,60,67] Interestingly, many of the regions that are highly susceptible to atrophy after trauma are heavily involved in the default mode network, a network of interacting brain regions that is active when the brain is at wakeful rest. These same regions also undergo particularly high rates of volume loss in Alzheimer's disease. This similarity in regional vulnerability to atrophy hints toward a neurodegenerative mechanism that is shared by both diseases.[68] Future studies are needed to advance our understanding of the implications of regional variations in atrophy rates after TBI and opportunities for intervention (see Figure 3.4).

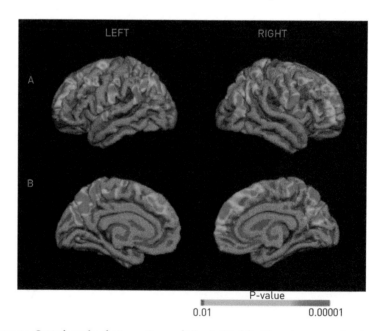

FIGURE 3.4 Cortical atrophy after traumatic axonal injury in 25 adults. Magnetic resonance imaging scans were obtained within 1 week of injury and repeated 8 months later. Highlighted regions represent areas of significant brain volume loss between the two time periods as measured by FreeSurfer morphometry. A. Lateral view, inflated to show extent of cortical surface. B. Lateral view, displayed at the pial layer.

Resting state functional connectivity MRI (fcMRI) is an imaging modality used to determine the functional relatedness of selected brain regions while the brain is at rest. It is based on the temporal correlation of blood oxygenation level-dependent (BOLD) signals among various regions.[68–70] In healthy individuals, functional connectivity patterns demonstrate a functional link between various regions that are known to communicate during various tasks and at rest. In clinical populations with compromise to white matter, connectivity patterns deviate considerably from those observed in healthy brains.

The relationship between CC integrity and functional connectivity was demonstrated by Quigley and colleagues who found that patients with agenesis of the CC had significantly reduced interhemispheric connectivity compared to healthy control subjects, as determined by fcMRI.[71] Likewise, Johnston et al. demonstrated significantly reduced interhemispheric functional connectivity after a complete callosotomy, whereas intrahemispheric connectivity was relatively preserved. These observations indicate that the CC plays a significant role in the degree of interhemispheric functional connectivity patterns determined by fcMRI.[72]

Given that the CC is the most commonly injured white matter structure after TAI, and compromise to the integrity of the CC results in compromised interhemispheric functional connectivity in clinical populations, fcMRI may be useful for detecting functional compromise among patients with TAI as well.[73–76]

McDonald and colleagues examined a 21-year-old woman with a remote history of severe TBI (initial Glasgow Coma Score [GCS] score of 4) with craniotomy and subdural hematoma evacuation 6 years prior, who presented to the outpatient TBI clinic with memory and concentration difficulties affecting her school performance and everyday life.[77] Examinations revealed that she had a moderately severe verbal memory deficit with otherwise intact cognition, as well as decreased functional connectivity in the left hippocampal network on fcMRI. On a group level, patients with moderate to severe TAI have been found to have significantly lower interhemispheric functional connectivity of both the hippocampi and the anterior cingulate cortex compared to control subjects.[78] Furthermore, interhemispheric functional connectivity of the hippocampi was significantly correlated with memory test performance. These findings support the hypothesis that white matter damage due to TAI negatively impacts functional network connectivity that has consequences for neurological function.

Patients with ischemic stroke also exhibit reductions in network functional connectivity. A study that examined spontaneous resting state activity in distributed attention and somatomotor networks found that ischemic stroke patients have reduced interhemispheric coherence in both of these networks that was related to cognitive and behavioral deficits.[79] Disruption of interhemispheric functional connectivity in the attention network correlated with abnormal performance on a test of visual attention, while disruption of interhemispheric functional connectivity in the somatomotor network correlated with upper extremity impairment.

Future studies using resting state fcMRI will examine the degree to which compromise in functional network connectivity results in neurological impairment.

## CONCLUSION

Conventional structural brain imaging is becoming increasingly useful in identifying gross focal injuries at the acute stage. Many of these CT and MRI techniques were pioneered in the triage of acute stroke patients, but they are now routinely used clinically to assess serial changes in ischemic and hemorrhagic lesions, recanalization, and reperfusion. Systematic and quantitative evaluation of such information is useful in characterizing the course of individual stroke patients over time.

Advanced imaging modalities have increased our understanding of the structural and functional changes that occur following TBI, particularly in axonal injuries. DTI shows significant promise as an imaging biomarker of outcome following TBI because it has the ability to identify structural lesions that are not identified via conventional imaging modalities. The emerging knowledge that inefficient functional connectivity is associated with adverse clinical outcome merits further study.

At the current stage of clinical brain imaging, morphologic changes have shown limited prognostic value beyond the detection of moderate to severe injuries. The promise of the more advanced techniques described in this chapter is that sensitive and specific imaging biomarkers of injury will be developed. Ultimately, objective and region-specific assessments of brain injury and recovery will guide the application of clinical neuroprotection techniques. As it has in other areas of medicine, brain imaging holds tremendous potential for revolutionizing clinical care of patients to improve outcomes following acquired brain injury.

## REFERENCES

1. Lin MP, Liebeskind DS. Imaging of ischemic stroke. *Continuum (Minneap Minn)*. 2016;22:1399–1423.
2. Suskauer SJ, Huisman TA. Neuroimaging in pediatric traumatic brain injury: current and future predictors of functional outcome. *Dev Disabil Res Rev.* 2009;15(2):117–23.
3. Kurca E, Sivak S, Kucera P. Impaired cognitive functions in mild traumatic brain injury patients with normal and pathologic magnetic resonance imaging. *Neuroradiology.* 2006;48(9):661–9.
4. Corral L, Herrero JI, Monfort JL, et al. First CT findings and improvement in GOS and GOSE scores 6 and 12 months after severe traumatic brain injury. *Brain Inj.* 2009;23(5):403–10.
5. Schwartz RB. Neuroradiology of brain tumors. *Neurol Clin.* 1995;13(4):723–56.
6. Cenic AC, Nabavi DG, Craen RA, et al. A CT method to measure hemodynamics in brain tumors: validation and application of cerebral blood flow maps. *AJNR Am J Neuroradiol* 2000;21(3):462–70.
7. van der Naalt J, van Zomeren AH, Sluiter WJ, Minderhoud JM. One year outcome in mild to moderate head injury: the predictive value of acute injury characteristics related to complaints and return to work. *J Neurol Neurosurg Psychiatry.* 1999;66(2):207–13.
8. Metting Z, Rodiger LA, De Keyser J, van der Naalt J. Structural and functional neuroimaging in mild-to-moderate head injury. *Lancet Neurol.* 2007;6(8):699–710.
9. Menon BK, Puetz V, Kochar P, Demchuk AM. ASPECTS and other neuroimaging scores in the triage and prediction of outcome in acute stroke patients. *Neuroimaging Clin N Am.* 2011;21:407–23, xii.
10. Liebeskind DS, Jahan R, Nogueira RG, et al. Serial Alberta Stroke Program early CT score from baseline to 24 hours in Solitaire Flow Restoration with the Intention for Thrombectomy study: a novel surrogate end point for revascularization in acute stroke. *Stroke.* 2014;45:723–7.
11. von Kummer R, Broderick JP, Campbell BC, et al. The Heidelberg bleeding classification: classification of bleeding events after ischemic stroke and reperfusion therapy. *Stroke.* 2015;46:2981–6.

12. Lagares A, Ramos A, Pérez-Nuñez A, et al. The role of MR imaging in assessing prognosis after severe and moderate injury. *Acta Neurochir (Wien)*. 2009;151(4):341–56.

13. Gentry LR, Godersky JC, Thompson B, Dunn VD. Prospective comparative-study of intermediate-field MR and CT in the evaluation of closed head trauma. *AJR Am J Roentgenol*. 1988;150(3):673–82.

14. Orrison WW, Gentry LR, Stimac GK, et al. Blinded comparison of cranial CT and MR in closed head injury evaluation. *AJNR Am J Neuroradiology*. 1994;15(2):351–6.

15. Provenzale JM. Imaging of traumatic brain injury: a review of the recent medical literature. *AJR Am J Roentgenol*. 2010;194(1):16–9.

16. Sundaram M, McGuire MH, Schajowicz F. Soft-tissue masses: histological basis for decreased signal (short T2) on T2-weighted MR images. *AJR Am J Roentgenol*. 1987;148(6):1247–50.

17. Chan JHM, Tsui EYK, Peh WCG, et al. Diffuse axonal injury: detection of changes in anisotropy of water diffusion by diffusion-weighted imaging. *Neuroradiology*. 2003;45(1):34–8.

18. Ashikaga R, Araki Y, Ishida O. MRI of head injury using FLAIR. *Neuroradiology*. 1997;39(4):239–42.

19. Marquez de la Plata C, Ardelean A, Koovakkattu D, et al. Magnetic resonance imaging of diffuse axonal injury: quantitative assessment of white matter lesion volume. *J Neurotrauma*. 2007;24(4):591–8.

20. Pierallini A, Pantano P, Fantozzi LM. Correlation between MRI findings and long-term outcome in patients with severe brain trauma. *Neuroradiology*. 2000;42(12):860–7.

21. Scheid R, Walher K, Guthke T, et al. Cognitive sequelae of diffuse axonal injury. *Arch Neurol*. 2006;63(3):418–24.

22. Hofman PAM, Stapert SZ, van Kroonenburgh MJPG, et al. MR imaging, single-photon emission CT, and neurocognitive performance after mild traumatic brain injury. *AJNR Am J Neuroradiol*. 2001;22(3):441–9.

23. Ding K, Marquez de la Plata C, Wang JY, et al. Cerebral atrophy after traumatic white matter injury: correlation with acute neuroimaging and outcome. *J Neurotrauma*. 2008;25(12):1433–40.

24. Hughes D, Jackson A, Mason D, et al. Abnormalities on magnetic resonance imaging seen acutely following mild traumatic brain injury: correlation with neuropsychological tests and delayed recovery. *Neuroradiology*. 2004;46(7):550–8.

25. Lee H, Wintermark M, Gean AD, et al. Focal lesions in acute mild traumatic brain injury and neurocognitive outcome: CT versus 3T MRI. *J Neurotrauma*. 2008;25(9):1049–56.

26. Huisman TA, Sorensen AG, Hergan K, Gonzalez RG, Schaefer PW. Diffusion-weighted imaging for the evaluation of diffuse axonal injury in closed head injury. *J Comput Assist Tomogr*. 2003;27(1):5–11.

27. Goetz P, Blamire A, Rajagopalan B, Cadoux-Hudson T, Young D, Styles P. Increase in apparent diffusion coefficient in normal appearing white matter following human traumatic brain injury correlates with injury severity. *J Neurotrauma*. 2004;21(6):645–54.

28. Liu AY, Maldjian JA, Bagley LJ, Sinson GP, Grossman RI. Traumatic brain injury: diffusion-weighted MR imaging findings. *AJNR Am J Neuroradiol*. 1999;20(9):1636–41.

29. Schaefer PW, Huisman TA, Sorensen AG, Gonzalez RG, Schwamm LH. Diffusion-weighted MR imaging in closed head injury: high correlation with initial Glasgow coma scale score and score on modified Rankin scale at discharge. *Radiology*. 2004;233(1):58–66.

30. Hudak, AM, Peng, L, Marquez de la Plata, C, et al. Cytotoxic and vasogenic cerebral oedema in traumatic brain injury: assessment with FLAIR and DWI imaging. *Brain Inj*. 2014;28(12):1602–9.

31. Mittal S, Wu Z, Neelavalli J, Haacke EM. Susceptibility-weighted imaging: technical aspects and clinical applications, part 2. *AJNR Am J Neuroradiol.* 2009;30(2):232–52.

32. Tong KA, Ashwal S, Holshouser BA, et al. Hemorrhagic shearing lesions in children and adolescents with posttraumatic diffuse axonal injury: improved detection and initial results. *Radiology.* 2003;227(2):332–9.

33. Tong KA, Ashwal S, Holshouser BA, et al. Diffuse axonal injury in children: clinical correlation with hemorrhagic lesions. *Ann Neurol.* 2004;56(1):36–50.

34. Babikian T, Freier MC, Tong KA, et al. Susceptibility weighted imaging: neuropsychologic outcome and pediatric head injury. *Pediatr Neurol.* 2005;33(3):184–94.

35. Chastain CA, Oyoyo UE, Zipperman M, et al. Predicting outcomes of traumatic brain injury by imaging modality and injury distribution. *J Neurotrauma.* 2009;26(8):1183–96.

36. Sheth SA, Liebeskind DS. Imaging evaluation of collaterals in the brain: physiology and clinical translation. *Curr Radiol Rep.* 2014;2:29.

37. Saindane AM, Law M, Ge Y, et al. Correlation of diffusion tensor and dynamic perfusion MR imaging metrics in normal appearing corpus callosum: support for primary hypoperfusion in multiple sclerosis. *AJNR Am J Neuroradiol.* 2007;28(4):467–72.

38. Schmierer K, Wheeler-Kinshott CA, Boulby PA, et al. Diffusion tensor imaging of post mortem multiple sclerosis brain. *NeuroImage.* 2007;35(2):467–77.

39. Budde MD, Kim JH, Liang HF, et al. Toward accurate diagnosis of white matter pathology using diffusion tensor imaging. *Magn Reson Med.* 2007;57(4):688–95.

40. Pfefferbaum A, Rosenbloom MJ, Adalsteinsson E, Sullivan EV. Diffusion tensor imaging with quantitative fibre tracking in HIV infection and alcoholism comorbidity: synergistic white matter damage. *Brain.* 2007;130(1):48–64.

41. Thurnher MM, Castillo M, Stadler A, et al. Diffusion-tensor MR imaging of the brain in human immunodeficiency virus-positive patients. *AJNR Am J Neuroradiol.* 2005;26(9):2275–81.

42. Wang, JY, Bakhadirov, K, Devous, MD, et al. Diffusion tensor tractography of traumatic diffuse axonal injury. *Arch Neurol* 2008;65(5):619–26.

43. Bazarian JJ, Zhong J, Blyth B, et al. Diffusion tensor imaging detects clinically important axonal damage after mild traumatic brain injury: a pilot study. *J Neurotrauma.* 2007;24(9):1447–59.

44. Benson RR, Meda SA, Vasudevan S, et al. Global white matter analysis of diffusion tensor images is predictive of injury severity in traumatic brain injury. *J Neurotrauma.* 2007;24(3):446–59.

45. Lipton ML, Gellella E, Lo C, et al. Multifocal white matter ultrastructural abnormalities in mild traumatic brain injury with cognitive disability: a voxel-wise analysis of diffusion tensor imaging. *J Neurotrauma.* 2008;25:1335–42.

46. Nakayama N, Okamura A, Shinoda J, et al. Evidence for white matter disruption in traumatic brain injury without macroscopic lesions. *J Neurol Neurosurg Psychiatry.* 2006;77(7):850–5.

47. Xu J, Rasmussen I-A, Lagopoulos J, Haberg A. Diffuse axonal injury in severe traumatic brain injury visualized using high-resolution diffusion tensor imaging. *J Neurotrauma.* 2007;24(5):753–65.

48. Bendlin BB, Ries ML, Lazar M, et al. Longitudinal changes in patients with traumatic brain injury assessed with diffusion-tensor and volumetric imaging. *NeuroImage.* 2008;42(2):503–14.

49. Marquez de la Plata CD, Yang FG, Wang JY, et al. Diffusion tensor imaging biomarkers for traumatic axonal injury: analysis of three analytic methods. *J Int Neuropsychol Soc.* 2011;17(1):24–35.

50. Sidaros A, Skimminge A, Liptrot MG, et al. Long-term global and regional brain volume changes following severe traumatic brain injury: a longitudinal study with clinical correlates. *Neuroimage.* 2009;44(1):1–8.

51. Mori S, Crain BJ, Chacko VP, van Zijl PC. Three dimensional tracking of axonal projections in the brain by magnetic resonance imaging. *Ann Neurol.* 1999;45(2):265–69.

52. Behrens TE, Woolrich MW, Jenkinson M, et al. Characterization and propagation of uncertainty in diffusion-weighted MR imaging. *Magn Reson Med.* 2003;50(5):1077–88.

53. Wilde EA, Chu Z, Bigler ED, et al. Diffusion tensor imaging in the corpus callosum in children after moderate to severe traumatic brain injury. *J Neurotrauma.* 2006;23:1412–26.

54. Rutgers DR, Toulgoat F, Cazejust J, et al. White matter abnormalities in mild traumatic brain injury: a diffusion tensor imaging study. *AJNR Am J Neuroradiol.* 2008;29(3):514–9.

55. Wang JY, Bakhadirov K, Abdi, H, et al. Longitudinal changes of structural connectivity in traumatic axonal injury. *Neurology.* 2011;77(9):818–26.

56. Perez,AM, Adler, J, Kulkarni, N, et al. Longitudinal white matter changes after traumatic axonal injury. *J Neurotrauma.* 2014;31(17):1478–85.

57. Jia B, Scalzo F, Agbayani E, et al. Multimodal CT techniques for cerebrovascular and hemodynamic evaluation of ischemic stroke: occlusion, collaterals, and perfusion. *Expert Rev Neurother.* 2016;16:515–25.

58. Higashida RT, Furlan AJ, Roberts H, et al.; Technology Assessment Committee of the American Society of Interventional and Therapeutic Neuroradiology; Technology Assessment Committee of the Society of Interventional Radiology. Trial design and reporting standards for intra-arterial cerebral thrombolysis for acute ischemic stroke. *Stroke.* 2003;34(8):e109–37. Erratum in: *Stroke.* 2003;34(11):2774.

59. Gale SD, Baxter L, Roundy N, Johnson SC. Traumatic brain injury and grey matter concentration: a preliminary voxel based morphometry study. *J Neurol Neurosurg Psychiatry.* 2005;76(7):984–8.

60. Warner M, Youn T, Davis T, et al. Regionally selective atrophy after traumatic axonal injury. *Arch Neurol.* 2010;67(11):1336–44.

61. Smith SM, Zhang Y, Jenkinson M, et al. Accurate, robust, and automated longitudinal and cross-sectional brain change analysis. *Neuroimage.* 2002;17(1):479–89.

62. MacKenzie JD, Siddiqi F, Babb JS, et al. Brain atrophy in mild or moderate traumatic brain injury: a longitudinal quantitative analysis. *AJNR Am J Neuroradiol.* 2002;23(9):1509–15.

63. Trivedi MA, Ward MA, Hess TM, et al. Longitudinal changes in global brain volume between 79 and 409 days after traumatic brain injury: relationship with duration of coma. *J Neurotrauma.* 2007;24(5):766–71.

64. Xu Y, McArthur DL, Alger JR, et al. Early nonischemic oxidative metabolic dysfunction leads to chronic brain atrophy in traumatic brain injury. *J Cereb Blood Flow Metab.* 2010;30(4):883–94.

65. Newcombe, VFJ, Correia, MM, Ledig, C, et al. Dynamic changes in white matter abnormalities correlate with late improvement and deterioration following TBI: a diffusion tensor imaging study. *Neurorehabil Neural Repair* 2016;30(1):49–62.

66. Fox NC, Freeborough PA, Rossor MN. Visualisation and quantification of rates of atrophy in Alzheimer's disease. *Lancet.* 1996;348(9020):94–7.

67. Bigler ED. Quantitative magnetic resonance imaging in traumatic brain injury. *J Head Trauma Rehabil.* 2001;16(2):117–34.

68. Buckner RL, Sepulcre J, Talukdar T, et al. Cortical hubs revealed by intrinsic functional connectivity: mapping, assessment of stability, and relation to Alzheimer's disease. *J Neurosci.* 2009;29(6):1860–73.

69. Biswal B, Yetkin FZ, Haughton VM, et al. Functional connectivity in the motor cortex of resting human brain using echo-planar MRI. *Magn Reson Med.* 1995;34(4):537–41.

70. Peltier SJ, Noll DC. T2 dependence of low frequency functional connectivity. *Neuroimage.* 2002;16(4):985–92.

71. Quigley M, Cordes D, Turski P, et al. Role of the corpus callosum in functional connectivity. *AJNR Am J Neuroradiol.* 2003;24(2):208–12.

72. Johnston JM, Vaishnavi SN, Smyth MD, et al. Loss of resting interhemispheric functional connectivity after complete section of the corpus callosum. *J Neurosci.* 2008;28(25):6453–8.

73. Meythaler JM, Peduzzi JD, Eleftheriou E, Novack TA. Current concepts: diffuse axonal injury-associated traumatic brain injury. *Arch Phys Med Rehabil.* 2001;82(10):1461–71.

74. Adams JH, Graham DI, Murray LS, Scott G. Diffuse axonal injury due to nonmissile head injury in humans: an analysis of 45 cases. *Ann Neurol.* 1982;12(6):557–63.

75. Ng HK, Mahaliyana RD, Poon WS. The pathological spectrum of diffuse axonal injury in blunt head trauma: assessment with axon and myelin strains. *Clin Neurol Neurosurg.* 1994;96(1):24–31.

76. Amaral DG, Insausti R, Cowan WM. The commissural connections of the monkey hippocampal formation. *J Comp Neurol.* 1984;224(3):307–36.

77. MacDonald CL, Schwarze N, Vaishnavi SN, et al. Verbal memory deficit following traumatic brain injury: assessment using advanced MRI methods. *Neurology.* 2008;71(15):1199–201.

78. Marquez de la Plata CD, Garces J, Shokri KE, et al. Deficits in functional connectivity of hippocampal and frontal lobe circuits after traumatic axonal injury. *Archives of Neurology.* 2011;68(1):74–84.

79. Carter AR, Astafiev SV, Lang CE, et al. Resting interhemispheric functional magnetic resonance imaging connectivity predicts performance after stroke. *Ann Neurol.* 2010;67(3):365–75.

# 4 Tissue Biomarkers and Neuroprotection

Axel Petzold

## INTRODUCTION

This chapter will review the use of tissue biomarkers to objectively assess the effects of neuroprotective treatment strategies on tissue preservation. The clinical problem is that an insult coupled with a failure of neuroprotection results in central nervous system (CNS) tissue damage, which may lead to temporary or permanent disability. Tissue biomarkers can be viewed as objective and quantitative measures of CNS injury that complement clinical and imaging assessments in the settings of critical care and perioperative medicine.

Tissue biomarkers permit the detection of neural tissue injury because degeneration of neuronal and glial cells results in release of intracellular compounds that provide indirect evidence for CNS tissue damage. These biomarker compounds diffuse from disintegrating cells into the adjacent body fluid compartment and can readily be quantified from body fluids such as the extracellular fluid (ECF), cerebrospinal fluid (CSF), and blood (plasma and serum). Body fluid tissue biomarkers are particularly useful in the acute phase of tissue injury.

Tissue damage that causes degeneration will eventually result in atrophy. Structural imaging biomarkers can confirm the presence of atrophy once it has been established, but this takes time. Therefore, as time passes, the usefulness of structural imaging biomarkers increases and gains over body fluid biomarkers. Taken together, the combined and longitudinal assessments of body fluid biomarkers and structural imaging biomarkers provide powerful tools to monitor the efficacy and success of neuroprotective treatment strategies.

This chapter will review body fluid biomarkers of CNS tissue damage. The previous decades of investigation have yielded significant advances in biomarker discovery, but the process of development from laboratory validation to clinical correlation studies takes many years.

**Table 4.1** Biomarker terminology

| Terminology | Definition |
| --- | --- |
| Biomarker | "A characteristic that is objectively measured and valuated as an indicator of normal biologic processes, pathogenic processes, or pharmacological responses to therapeutic intervention"[43] |
| Cell type–specific | Distinguish neuroaxonal from glial and other CNS tissue damage |
| Prognostic | Predict clinical outcome |
| Predictive | Narrow choices of treatment options: Process |
| | Monitor dynamics of pathology: Safety |
| | Control treatment: Safety |

## TERMINOLOGY

The terminology used to refer to body fluid biomarkers of tissue damage is summarized in Table 4.1. It is important to be clear about the cell type specificity of various biomarkers used to monitor neurodegeneration and neuroprotection. Assessment of a biomarker that is only or predominantly expressed by one cell type will give very specific information about damage to these cells. In the case of neuroprotection, this implies a particular focus on biomarkers specific to the neuroaxonal compartment.

There is, however, an advantage to the use of nonspecific tissue biomarkers as well. Because they are expressed more broadly throughout the body, any type of damage will cause an increase in these biomarkers. A classic example is the S100B protein.[1–3] The advantages of S100B are its stability and sensitivity. The S100B protein is so stable that routine sampling techniques can be used for ECF, CSF, and blood. The S100B protein is also so prevalent in tissues that concentrations will increase with even small amounts of nonspecific tissue damage, such as following the running of a marathon.[4] Therefore, S100B can be used as a sensitive screening test for tissue injury (e.g., following cardiac arrest or poisoning), but requires follow-up with cell type–specific biomarker tests to confirm whether or not CNS damage has occurred.[5–6]

Likewise, S100B has been used as a prognostic biomarker because of its potential to predict clinical outcomes, but its prognostic value is limited by its lack of tissue specificity.[5,7–9] Finally, S100B has been used successfully as a process biomarker to monitor the dynamics of pathology, although it has some limitations.[10–13] These limitations can be overcome by use of cell type–specific biomarkers.

## CELL TYPE–SPECIFIC BIOMARKERS AND NONSPECIFIC BIOMARKERS

There is no single biomarker that is ideal for all purposes. Some biomarkers have high sensitivity but less specificity, while others have high specificity but less sensitivity. An overview of CNS biomarkers and their cell type specificity is provided in Table 4.2. It is beyond the scope of this chapter to discuss all biomarkers. This chapter will review representative cell type–specific biomarkers for neurons, astrocytes, and microglia.

**Table 4.2** Tissue biomarkers for central nervous system damage and neuroprotection

| Biomarker | Neuron | Astrocyte | Microglia | Oligodendrocyte |
|---|---|---|---|---|
| 14-3-3γ | ++ | + | + | + |
| ABP | + | | | |
| AD7c-NTP | + | | | |
| Albumin | | | | |
| α spectrin | + | + | + | + |
| α(1) BG | | + | | |
| α–internexin | + | | | |
| ApoE | | | + | |
| β–tubulin | + | | | |
| β-2-Microglobulin | | | + | |
| β-trace | | | | (+) |
| CHI3L1 | | + | + | |
| Clusterin | + | + | | + |
| Cystatin C | + | | | |
| EDG-8 | | | | + |
| FABPs | + | + | + | + |
| FFA | + | + | + | + |
| Ferritin | | | + | |
| GFAP | | + | | |
| Glucose | + | + | + | + |
| Glutamate | + | + | + | + |
| HK6 | | | | |
| HNE | + | + | + | + |
| Hypocretin–1 | + | | | |
| Isoprostanes | + | + | + | + |
| Lactate | + | + | + | + |
| MAG | | | | + |
| MBP | | | | + |
| MDA | + | + | + | + |
| MOBP | | | | + |
| MOG | | | | + |
| NAA | ++ | + | + | + |
| NCAM | + | | | + |
| NOx | + | + | + | |
| NSE | + | | | |
| Neurotrophins | + | + | + | + |
| Nf | ++ | | | |
| OMgp | | | | + |
| PLP | | | | + |
| Pyruvate | + | + | + | + |
| S100B | | ++ | | |

*(continued)*

Table 4.2 Continued

| Biomarker | Neuron | Astrocyte | Microglia | Oligodendrocyte |
|---|---|---|---|---|
| SFas (sCD95) | + | | | |
| Tau | + | + | + | + |
| Ubiquitin | + | + | + | + |
| UCHL-1 | ++ | | | |
| Vimentin | + | + | + | |

ABP, amyloid β-peptide; AD7c-NTP, neuronal thread protein AD7c; EDG8/S1P5, sphingolipid G-protein–coupled receptor 8; FABPs, fatty acid binding proteins; FFA, Free fatty acids; GFAP, glial fibrillary acidic protein; HK6, human kallikrein 6; HNE, 4-hydroxynonenal; MAG, myelin-associated glycoprotein; MBP, myelin basic protein; MDA, malondialdehyde; MOBP, myelin–associated oligodendrocytic protein; MOG, myelin/oligodendrocyte glycoprotein; NAA, N–acetyl aspartate; Nf, neurofilament; NfH, neurofilament heavy chain; NfL, neurofilament light chain; NfM, neurofilament medium chain; NCAM, neural cell adhesion molecule; NSE, neuron-specific enolase; OMgp, oligodendrocyte/myelin glycoprotein; PLP, proteolipid protein; UCH-L1, ubiquitin carboxyl-terminal hydrolase L1.

Modified from Petzold A. CSF biomarkers for improved prognostic accuracy in acute CNS disease. Neurol Res. 2007;29(7):691–708.

## Neuronal Biomarkers

Neurofilament (Nf) proteins are one of the most extensively studied brain tissue biomarkers (Table 4.2). Other well-characterized examples of neuron-specific protein biomarkers include neuron-specific enolase (NSE), a glycolytic enzyme that is also applicable as a biomarker for lung cancer, and ubiquitin carboxyl-terminal hydrolase L1 (UCH-L1), a Parkinson disease susceptibility gene.[14–18]

The advantage of measuring Nf proteins is the high cell type–specificity for the neuroaxonal compartment.[19–21] There are five Nf proteins: (1) Nf heavy chain (NfH), (2) Nf medium chain (NfM), (3) Nf light chain (NfL), (4) a-internexin, and (5) peripherin, a biomarker for peripheral nervous system injury (see Figure 4.1). Neurofilaments are obligate heteropolymers, requiring NfL, NfM, and NfH subunits, each of which serves a specific function. NfL is believed to function as the backbone of the heteropolymer and is the only Nf isoform that can self-assemble. The NfM isoform is key to radial growth. The NfH isoform is responsible for charge repulsion and interaction with other axonal organelles, such as mitochondria. All of these Nf proteins are released into the ECF following axonal injury. Activation of proteases, such as the axonal membrane-bound enterokinase, causes cleavage of Nf peptides, which then diffuse into the CSF or blood.[22] These Nf peptides can readily be quantified with validated and commercially available enzyme-linked immunosorbent assay (ELISA) kits.[23–25]

## Astrocytic Biomarkers

The major clinically relevant cell type–specific protein biomarker for astrocytes is glial fibrillary acidic protein (GFAP). Like the Nf proteins, GFAP is classified by fiber diameter (8–12 nm) as intermediate in size between microfilaments and microtubules.[26] In contrast to most Nf isoforms, GFAP can readily self–assemble, as summarized in Figure 4.2.[27] This can be a problem for quantification because the presence of GFAP aggregates may cause a GFAP hook effect and inaccurate biomarker level readings.

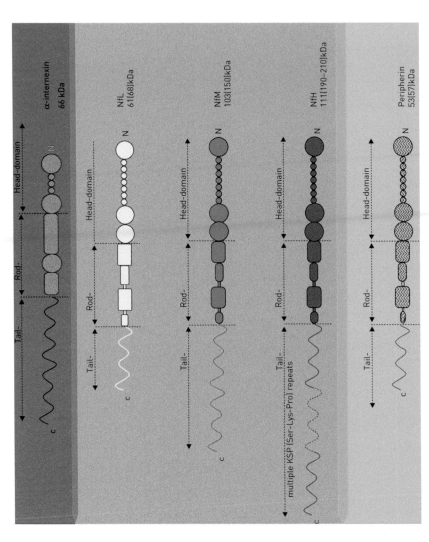

FIGURE 4.1 Neurofilament subunits. In axons, neurofilament light chain (NfL), medium chain (NfM), and heavy chain (NfH) are predominantly expressed. In the central nervous system there is also α-internexin, and in the peripheral nervous system there is also peripherin. The figure shows that the Nf subunits are essentially different in their tail domain. A long tail contributes to a heavier weight, which is calculated from the DNA (in kDa). Because of post-translational modifications such as phosphorylation, the in vivo weight is higher (shown in brackets). There is less difference in the protein head domain, except for α-internexin, which is shorter.

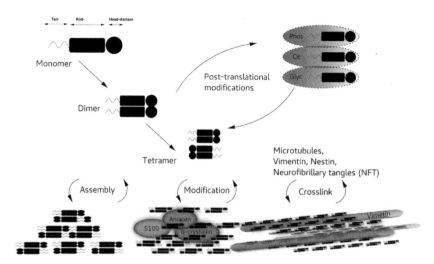

FIGURE 4.2 Intracellular organization of glial fibrillary acidic protein (GFAP). The dynamic and reversible steps between the GFAP monomer and the assembled, functional and cross–linked cytoskeletal network are shown in this simplified sketch. *Phos*, phosphorylation; *Cit*, citrullination; *Glyc*, glycosylation.

Reproduced with permission from Petzold A. Glial fibrillary acidic protein is a body fluid biomarker for glial pathology in human disease. *Brain Res.* 2015;1600:17–31.

Figure 4.2 also highlights important posttranslational modifications, such as phosphorylation, glycosylation, and citrullination, which may be relevant in neurodegeneration and apoptosis but that have not yet been sufficiently investigated. It is thought that the same processes that damage axons also damage axonal proteins. Therefore, analyses of posttranslational modifications of protein biomarkers might give as valuable information as simple quantification of these protein biomarkers.

Figure 4.2 illustrates important interactions among different biomarkers listed in Table 4.2, such as how S100 and vimentin interact with the GFAP polymer. Similar structural interactions also apply to the more complex family of Nf proteins.

## Microglial Biomarkers

Microglia are the resident macrophages of the CNS.[28] Almost any disturbance of CNS homoeostasis can lead to microglial activation. Molecules associated with microglial activation include CR3, MHC, CD68, FcR, interleukin-1β (IL-1β), tumor necrosis factor (TNF), nitric oxide, and ferritin. S100B is expressed in microglia and released when there is structural injury.[28–29] None of these biomarkers, however, is tissue-specific for CNS microglia, and many can also be found in circulating macrophages. A highly specific biomarker for CNS microglial activation that is stable and readily quantifiable would be of great clinical value.

## COMPREHENSIVE VIEW OF TISSUE BIOMARKERS

Whether one is assessing acute tissue damage, neurodegeneration, or the effect of a specific neuroprotection strategy, the choice of biomarker is not a trivial one. In this review, the long list of biomarkers reported in the literature has been condensed to include only those that have the advantage of cell type specificity.

Figure 4.3 is a unified model that shows the relative quantities of biomarkers over time, illustrating the importance of timing of tissue biomarker assessment. Prior to injury or disease onset, patients are assumed to have a healthy CNS. The blue shaded area shows the volume of the CNS, as assessed by structural imaging over time. The green curve reflects clinical injuries, such as stroke, traumatic brain injury (TBI), or cardiac arrest with CNS tissue damage. Sampling of blood or CSF during the acute period, shown in Figure 4.3 as yellow area (a), will permit accurate quantification of cell type–specific biomarkers and estimate how much neuronal or glial damage is likely to have occurred (red curve). Of note, during the acute phase, edema formation can mask any potential loss of CNS tissue (as demonstrated by an elevation of the blue curve). Thus, it will take time before a more definite assessment of the final extent of CNS atrophy can be determined with an imaging biomarker (declining size of blue line). As the acute phase of injury progresses, body fluid biomarker levels decrease (red curve). Single-point sampling in the acute phase is sufficient for most cross-sectional studies.

The yellow area (b) gives an example of "poor" timing for sampling of a body fluid biomarker, but good timing for sampling an imaging biomarker. Imaging demonstrates CNS atrophy compared to baseline (blue shaded area decreased). A more robust assessment occurs with combined sampling of body fluid and imaging biomarkers at both time points. A successful neuroprotective treatment strategy should result in less CNS tissue atrophy (blue shaded area) in comparison to a patient with a comparable primary injury (red shaded area).

In circumstances where injury or disease progression continues, CNS complications occur (hydrocephalus, vasospasm, infection), or new adverse clinical events have occurred, biomarker assessments will demonstrate more tissue damage. In these cases, frequent longitudinal sampling will strengthen the assessment but is much more demanding of resources. A pragmatic strategy to limit resource utilization is to use one final outcome assessment, as illustrated by the yellow area (c) of Figure 4.3. In the common critical care setting that involves a long progression of serial injuries to the brain, body fluid biomarkers will ultimately return to normal levels. At this point in time, it is necessary to use imaging technologies to assess the extent of CNS atrophy and determine the efficacy of a course of therapy designed to provide neuroprotection.

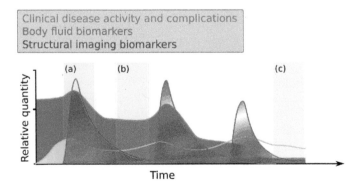

FIGURE 4.3  Biomarkers and clinical events in critical care.

## CLINICAL APPLICATIONS

A unique advantage of applying tissue biomarkers to critical care and perioperative medicine is that patients are seen in the acute phase of CNS tissue injury, which is optimally timed to the window during which biomarkers have their strongest prognostic and predictive value (Table 4.1). Likewise, these biomarkers can be applied to monitoring the process of CNS injury and enable early recognition of complications in intubated and ventilated patients who cannot readily be assessed by a detailed neurological examination.

### Stroke

The prognostic value of body fluid biomarkers has been demonstrated in studies of ischemic stroke. Larger ischemic strokes are associated with greater biomarker release and worse clinical outcomes than smaller ischemic strokes.[30-37] A longitudinal study of patients with cervical artery dissection presenting with stroke found that serum NfL levels measured in the first week after the insult correlated with clinical severity.[38] Blood Nf levels have also been found to detect perioperative brain injury after carotid endarterectomy.[39] Serum NfH and NfL levels have been observed to be transiently elevated in the first week after ischemic stroke in two longitudinal studies, highlighting the importance of timing of biomarker sampling.[37-38]

There also is strong evidence for the prognostic value of biomarkers in intracerebral hemorrhage (ICH).[40] ICH has been consistently associated with an increase of GFAP in CSF and blood samples taken within 1–6 hours after onset of ICH.[30-33,37,40-41]

Subarachnoid hemorrhage (SAH) can be devastating, particularly if complicated by systemic complications such as hydrocephalus, cerebral salt wasting syndrome, shunt infection, or vasospasm resulting in delayed cerebral ischemia (DCI). There is moderate evidence supporting the use of neuroprotective treatment options for SAH, such as nimodipine prophylaxis and hypertensive/hypervolemic rescue therapy for reducing DCI.[42-46] It is likely that longitudinal studies will provide evidence that body fluid biomarkers are useful for prognosis, monitoring, and early detection of complications, as well as for safety and outcome assessments.[47-48] Elevated CSF levels of NfL and NfH after SAH have consistently been reported.[17,24,49-53] State-of-the-art proteomics studies have been confirmatory.[54] The European Federation of Neurological Societies (EFNS) guidelines rated the prognostic value of CSF Nf levels in SAH as class I evidence.[55]

New candidate biomarkers for stroke continue to be discovered, but their clinical relevance remains to be determined.[33,56-57]

### Traumatic Brain Injury

The association of TBI with axonal injury has been firmly established. In recent years, the field has been advanced by research support from the US military to develop biomarkers to detect blast wave–induced TBI. Further interest has been spurred by the public debate about sports-related concussion and chronic traumatic encephalopathy (CTE).[58-59] The potential utility of quantitative biomarkers to detect subclinical and mild brain injury is clear.

The complex pathophysiology of TBI ranges from massive impact-related hemorrhage and contusion, to diffuse axonal injury (DAI), to more subtle dysfunction of brain homoeostasis and metabolism. Whereas hemorrhage is readily detected with brain imaging, DAI is only detectable using magnetic resonance imaging (MRI) diffusion tensor imaging (DTI), although the characteristic "shearing lesions" found in the dorsolateral midbrain, posterior corpus callosum, and centrum semiovale represent a "tip of the iceberg" phenomenon. Measurement of more subtle biochemical and metabolic disturbances associated with CNS injury requires sophisticated functional imaging techniques such as functional MRI (fMRI) and positron emission tomography (PET), as well as assessment of body fluid biomarkers.

Disruption of the blood–brain barrier (BBB) is readily detected using the CSF-to-serum albumin ratio.[2] Associated neuroinflammation can be monitored in the CSF with IL-6, IL-8, and IL-10, but a potential confound for interpretation of the data is that these interleukins can leak from the blood into the CSF.

Axonal biomarkers provide important prognostic information. There is an extensive literature on CSF total τ protein, myelin basic protein (MBP), NfL, NfH, NSE, spectrin breakdown products, and ubiquitin carboxyl-terminal hydrolase L1 (UCH-L1).[2,60] Of these biomarkers, blood, CSF, and ECF Nf levels most consistently provide prognostic information in TBI.[22,61–62] ECF τ protein is also informative and correlates with later structural imaging data.[63–64] It should be remembered that τ is not solely expressed by neurons, but also by glial cells (Table 4.2).

The glial biomarker GFAP was also found to be of value in TBI prognosis.[65–69] In fact, GFAP was superior to S100B in a number of studies.[70–72] There are data indicating that continued increases in body fluid GFAP concentration precede a sustained increase of intracranial pressure (ICP) and subsequent secondary brain damage.[71,73] Serum GFAP is the main body fluid biomarker under investigation in the TRACK-TBI trial (NCT01565551).[74]

## Guillain-Barré Syndrome

The first description of Guillain-Barré Syndrome (GBS) in 1916 was occasioned by the discovery of a biomarker. Three French neurologists observed CSF hyperalbuminosis in the absence of a cytologic reaction in two soldiers within a 1-day period. Both soldiers had presented clinically with ascending generalized weakness, and both made a full recovery. Since that time, much research had been done on CSF proteins in GBS.[75] A review of the literature shows that many of the CSF biomarkers found in GBS are nonspecific markers of inflammation.[75] Only CSF Nf proteins have been consistently found to have prognostic relevance.[23,76–79] Additionally, CSF Nf levels are predictors of axonal injury at clinical presentation. In one longitudinal case series, CSF Nf levels also gave information regarding the process of ongoing axonal injury in complicated GBS.[76] Taken together, these data suggest a relationship of Nf proteins with GBS pathology, as summarized in Figure 4.4.

In patients with GBS who have a good prognosis and a monophasic disease course, the pathology is thought to be predominantly demyelination (see Figure 4.4A). Some distal axonotmesis may coexist, but full recovery is typical due to the potential for peripheral nerves to regenerate. A poor prognosis may, however, follow in the presence of proximal axonotmesis or retrograde axonal degeneration after severe distal axonotmesis (see Figure 4.4B). Loss of the motor neuron likely continues by means of trans-synaptic retrograde degeneration from the spinal cord to the cortex; however, this remains to be demonstrated by studies combining body fluid biomarkers and structural imaging (Figure 4.3).

(A) Good prognosis    (B) Poor prognosis

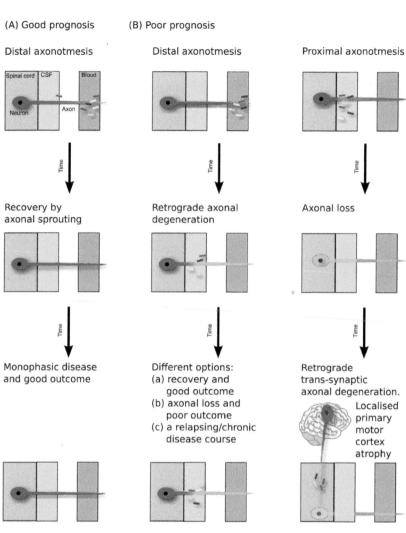

FIGURE 4.4 Conceptual relationships of body fluid neurofilament (Nf) levels to prognosis and disease course in Guillain-Barré syndrome. A. A good prognosis for a patient with a monophasic disease course who suffers from demyelination alone and/or distal axonotmesis and makes a full recovery. B. A poor prognosis may follow extensive distale axonotmesis leading to retrograde axonal degeneration and loss or be caused by proximal axonotmesis. In those cases where the motor neuron is lost, trans-synaptic retrograde axonal degeneration might follow and should be demonstrable by longitudinal structural imaging evidence for localized atrophy in the pyramidal tracts and corresponding area of the primary motor cortex.

Figure reproduced with permission of the Peripheral Nerve Society.

Figure 4.4 illustrates how the combined use of all five Nf subunits can be informative. Acutely, proximal axonotmesis causes high CSF NfL, NfM, and NfH levels. Next, presence of trans-synaptic retrograde axonal degeneration will cause an increase of CSF *a*-internexin levels, which should precede potentially preventable CNS atrophy. The added value of measuring blood peripherin levels is in distinguishing distal from proximal axonotmesis in the acute phase of GBS.

## Cardiac Arrest and Cardiac Surgery

An important complication of cardiac arrest and cardiac surgery is CNS damage. This poses an important prognostic challenge in critical care.[80] Body fluid and structural imaging biomarkers have an important role to play, alongside oxygenation and electrophysiological monitoring.[81-83]

Cardiac arrest causes an increase of CSF NfL levels, which are predictive of outcome 1 year later.[84] However, CSF is not readily available in the setting of acute cardiac arrest. Therefore, it was important to learn that blood NfH and NfL levels also have prognostic value following cardiac arrest.[85-86]

NSE levels above a cutoff of 33 µg/L have been recommended as a poor prognostic sign by a systematic literature review.[87] However, a prospective cohort study of 391 adult patients with persisting coma after cardiopulmonary resuscitation treated with therapeutic hypothermia (32–34°C) found that NSE levels (sampled on ICU admission, 12 hours after reaching the target temperature, and 36 and 48 hours after collapse) did not reliably predict poor outcomes.[88] Of note, NSE is not entirely cell type–specific, an important preanalytical limitation for this biomarker.

An interesting neuroprotective treatment approach to the predictable problem of surgically induced arrest of the circulation is remote ischemic preconditioning (RIPC). There are good experimental data showing that body fluid biomarkers for axonal damage (i.e., Nf proteins) are decreased following RIPC.[89-90] A prospective multicenter trial, however, did not reveal any clinical meaningful treatment effect of upper-limb RIPC prior to open heart surgery.[91] The accompanying editorial cautions that there may also be deleterious side effects of RIPC, as suggested by the observed elevations of biomarkers C-reactive protein and cardiac troponin.[92] The use of Nf proteins and GFAP as a safety biomarker (as suggested in Table 4.1) will be important for testing future neuroprotective treatment strategies.

## Critical Illness Brain Syndrome and Delirium

One of the most important and frequent management problems in the ICU is delirium.[93-94] The incidence of delirium or critical illness brain syndrome (CIBS) has likely been greatly underestimated.[95-96] The difficulty of assessing CNS function acutely is reflected by the research focus on outcomes.[94] It remains unclear what etiologic factors cause CNS dysfunction or injury during critical illness.

It has been proposed that multimodal monitoring, including use of biomarkers, will eventually contribute to an unravelling of the complex, multicausal pathogenesis of CIBS.[95-98] One hypothesis is that loss of neurons, axons, and dendritic branches impairs CNS network function.[96] Activation of primed microglia by systemic inflammation is a likely explanation for the clinical observation that delirium/CIBS occurs in some patients with apparently minor infections.[28] A typical example might be delirium/CIBS in an elderly patient with a previous stroke who develops a minor urinary tract infection. Patients treated in critical care units with no known chronic or acute CNS pathology frequently suffer from cognitive deficits after discharge.[99]

Among survivors of critical illness with poor cognitive outcome, it frequently remains uncertain whether this is the consequence of diffuse hypoxic brain injury, unrecognized status epilepticus, or metabolic, nutritional, toxic or infectious complications. Severe clinical complications, such as single- or multiorgan failure, may also take their toll on the CNS. Compared to the other clinical entities discussed in this chapter, delirium/CIBS remains the least well understood. Studies of CNS tissue biomarkers in this vulnerable patient population may lead to a better understanding of the pathophysiology underlying CIBS and methods for monitoring development of CIBS. The ultimate aim is successful neuroprotection using treatments targeted to biomarker findings.

## CONCLUSION

There is an important role for tissue biomarkers in the detection and monitoring of acute brain injury and in assessing the efficacy of various neuroprotection strategies. An informed selection of well-validated, cell type–specific biomarkers from a large list of candidates will lead to more effective use of laboratory resources and enhanced precision in future research studies. In isolation and based on cross-sectional data only, tissue biomarker studies are of more limited value. The most robust approach to diagnosis and monitoring of brain injury will undoubtedly combine longitudinal observations of body fluid biomarkers and structural imaging biomarkers that are targeted to specific clinical scenarios.

## REFERENCES

1. Donato R. S100: a multigenic family of calcium-modulated proteins of the EF-hand type with intracellular and extracellular functional roles. *Int J Biochem Cell Biol.* 2001;33(7):637–68.

2. Petzold A. CSF biomarkers for improved prognostic accuracy in acute CNS disease. *Neurological Research.* 2007;29(7):691–708.

3. Sen J, Belli A. S100B in neuropathologic states: the CRP of the brain? *J. Neurosci. Res.* 2007;85(7):1373–80.

4. Hasselblatt M, Mooren FC, von Ahsen N, et al. Serum S100beta increases in marathon runners reflect extracranial release rather than glial damage. *Neurology.* 2004;62(9):1634–6.

5. Mayer SA, Linares G. Can a simple blood test quantify brain injury? *Crit Care.* 2009;13(4):166.

6. Züngün C, Yilmaz FM, Tutkun E, Yilmaz H, Uysal S. Assessment of serum S100B and neuron specific enolase levels to evaluate the neurotoxic effects of organic solvent exposure. *Clin Toxicol.* 2013;51(8):748–51.

7. Berger RP, Bazaco MC, Wagner AK, Kochanek PM, Fabio A. Trajectory analysis of serum biomarker concentrations facilitates outcome prediction after pediatric traumatic and hypoxemic brain injury. *Dev Neurosci.* 2010;32(5-6):396–405.

8. Anderson R, Hansson L, Nilsson O, Dijlai-Merzoug R, Settergren G. High serum S100B levels for trauma patients without head injuries. *Neurosurgery.* 2001;48(6):1255-8; discussion 1258–60.

9. Bouzat P, Francony G, Declety P, et al. [Can serum protein S100beta predict neurological deterioration after moderate or minor traumatic brain injury?]. *Ann Fr Anesth Reanim.* 2009;28(3):135–9.

10. Kleindienst A, Meissner S, Eyupoglu IY, Parsch H, Schmidt C, Buchfelder M. Dynamics of S100B release into serum and cerebrospinal fluid following acute brain injury. *Acta Neurochir Suppl.* 2010;106:247–50.

11. Murillo-Cabezas F, Muñoz-Sánchez MA, Rincón-Ferrari MD, et al. The prognostic value of the temporal course of S100beta protein in post-acute severe brain injury: a prospective and observational study. *Brain Inj.* 2010;24(4):609–19.

12. Sen J, Belli A, Petzold A, et al. Extracellular fluid S100B in the injured brain: a future surrogate marker of acute brain injury? *Acta Neurochir (Wien).* 2005;147(8):897–900.

13. Kleindienst A, Ross Bullock M. A critical analysis of the role of the neurotrophic protein S100B in acute brain injury. *J Neurotrauma.* 2006;23(8):1185–200.

14. Mokuno K, Kato K, Kawai K, Matsuoka Y, Yanagi T, Sobue I. Neuron-specific enolase and S-100 protein levels in cerebrospinal fluid of patients with various neurological diseases. *J Neurol Sci.* 1983;60(3):443–51.

15. Schmechel D, Marangos P, Zis A, Brightman M, Goodwin FK. Brain endolases as specific markers of neuronal and glial cells. *Science.* 1978;199(4326):313–5.

16. Yokobori S, Hosein K, Burks S, Sharma I, Gajavelli S, Bullock R. Biomarkers for the clinical differential diagnosis in traumatic brain injury-a systematic review. *CNS Neurosci Ther.* 2013;19(8):556–65.

17. Lewis SB, Wolper R, Chi YY, et al. Identification and preliminary characterization of ubiquitin C terminal hydrolase 1 (UCHL1) as a biomarker of neuronal loss in aneurysmal subarachnoid hemorrhage. *J Neurosci Res.* 2010;88(7):1475–84.

18. Neher MD, Keene CN, Rich MC, Moore HB, Stahel PF. Serum biomarkers for traumatic brain injury. *South Med J.* 2014;107(4):248–55.

19. Comabella M, Montalban X. Body fluid biomarkers in multiple sclerosis. *Lancet Neurol.* 2014;13(1):113–26.

20. Friese MA, Schattling B, Fugger L. Mechanisms of neurodegeneration and axonal dysfunction in multiple sclerosis. *Nat Rev Neurol.* 2014;10(4):225–38.

21. Petzold A. Neurofilament phosphoforms: surrogate markers for axonal injury, degeneration and loss. *J Neurol Sci.* 2005;233(1-2):183–98.

22. Petzold A, Tisdall MM, Girbes AR, et al. In vivo monitoring of neuronal loss in traumatic brain injury: a microdialysis study. *Brain.* 2011;134(Pt 2):464–83.

23. Gaiottino J, Norgren N, Dobson R, et al. Increased neurofilament light chain blood levels in neurodegenerative neurological diseases. *PLoS One.* 2013;8(9):e75091.

24. Petzold A, Keir G, Green AJ, Giovannoni G, Thompson EJ. A specific ELISA for measuring neurofilament heavy chain phosphoforms. *J Immunol Methods.* 2003;278(1-2):179–90.

25. Petzold A, Altintas A, Andreoni L, et al. Neurofilament ELISA validation. *J Immunol Methods.* 2010;352(1-2):23–31.

26. Fuchs E, Cleveland D. A structural scaffolding of intermediate filaments in health and disease. *Science.* 1998;279(5350):514–9.

27. Petzold A. Glial fibrillary acidic protein is a body fluid biomarker for glial pathology in human disease. *Brain Res.* 2015;1600:17–31.

28. Perry VH, Holmes C. Microglial priming in neurodegenerative disease. *Nat Rev Neurol.* 2014;10(4):217–24.

29. Adami C, Sorci G, Blasi E, Agneletti AL, Bistoni F, Donato R. S100B expression in and effects on microglia. *Glia.* 2001;33(2):131–42.

30. Dvorak F, Haberer I, Sitzer M, Foerch C. Characterisation of the diagnostic window of serum glial fibrillary acidic protein for the differentiation of intracerebral haemorrhage and ischaemic stroke. *Cerebrovasc Dis.* 2009;27(1):37–41.

31. Foerch C, Curdt I, Yan B, et al. Serum glial fibrillary acidic protein as a biomarker for intracerebral haemorrhage in patients with acute stroke. *J Neurol Neurosurg Psychiatry.* 2006;77(2):181–4.

32. Foerch C, Niessner M, Back T, et al.; BE FAST Study Group. Diagnostic accuracy of plasma glial fibrillary acidic protein for differentiating intracerebral hemorrhage and cerebral ischemia in patients with symptoms of acute stroke. *Clin Chem.* 2012;58(1):237–45.

33. Martínez-Morillo E, García Hernández P, Begcevic I, et al. Identification of novel biomarkers of brain damage in patients with hemorrhagic stroke by integrating bioinformatics and mass spectrometry-based proteomics. *J Proteome Res.* 2014;13(2):969–81.

34. Norgren N, Rosengren L, Stigbrand T. Elevated neurofilament levels in neurological diseases. *Brain Res.* 2003;987(1):25–31.

35. Petzold A, Michel P, Stock M, Schluep M. Glial and axonal body fluid biomarkers are related to infarct volume, severity, and outcome. *J Stroke Cerebrovasc Dis.* 2008;17(4):196–203.

36. Reynolds M, Kirchick H, Dahlen J, et al. Early biomarkers of stroke. *Clin Chem.* 2003;49(10):1733–9.

37. Sellner J, Patel A, Dassan P, Brown MM, Petzold A. Hyperacute detection of neurofilament heavy chain in serum following stroke: a transient sign. *Neurochem Res.* 2011;36(12):2287–91.

38. Traenka C, Disanto G, Seiffge DJ, et al. Serum neurofilament light chain levels are associated with clinical characteristics and outcome in patients with cervical artery dissection. *Cerebrovasc Dis.* 2015;40(5-6):222–7.

39. Sellner J, Petzold A, Sadikovic S, et al. The value of the serum neurofilament protein heavy chain as a biomarker for peri-operative brain injury after carotid endarterectomy. *Neurochem Res.* 2009;34(11):1969–74.

40. Zhang J, Zhang CH, Lin XL, Zhang Q, Wang J, Shi SL. Serum glial fibrillary acidic protein as a biomarker for differentiating intracerebral hemorrhage and ischemic stroke in patients with symptoms of acute stroke: a systematic review and meta-analysis. *Neurol Sci.* 2013;34(11):1887–92.

41. Sun Y, Qin Q, Shang YJ, et al. The accuracy of glial fibrillary acidic protein in acute stroke differential diagnosis: a meta-analysis. *Scand J Clin Lab Invest.* 2013;73(8):601–6.

42. Lantigua H, Ortega-Gutierrez S, Schmidt JM, et al. Subarachnoid hemorrhage: who dies, and why? *Crit Care.* 2015;19:309.

43. Mayer S, Fink M, Homma S, et al. Cardiac injury associated with neurogenic pulmonary edema following subarachnoid hemorrhage. *Neurology.* 1994;44(5):815–20.

44. Mayer S, Kreiter K, Copeland D, et al. Global and domain-specific cognitive impairment and outcome after subarachnoid hemorrhage. *Neurology.* 2002;59(11):1750–8.

45. Petzold A. Disorders of plasma sodium. *N Engl J Med.* 2015;372(13):1267.

46. Sen J, Belli A, Albon H, Morgan L, Petzold A, Kitchen N. Triple-H therapy in the management of aneurysmal subarachnoid haemorrhage. *Lancet Neurol.* 2003;2(10):614–21.

47. Hussain S, Barbarite E, Chaudhry NS, et al. Search for biomarkers of intracranial aneurysms: a systematic review. *World Neurosurg.* 2015;84(5):1473–83.

48. Siman R, Giovannone N, Toraskar N, et al. Evidence that a panel of neurodegeneration biomarkers predicts vasospasm, infarction, and outcome in aneurysmal subarachnoid hemorrhage. *PLoS One.* 2011;6(12):e28938.

49. Lewis SB, Wolper RA, Miralia L, Yang C, Shaw G. Detection of phosphorylated NF-H in the cerebrospinal fluid and blood of aneurysmal subarachnoid hemorrhage patients. *J Cereb Blood Flow Metab.* 2008;28(6):1261-71.

50. Nylén K, Csajbok L, Ost M, et al. CSF -neurofilament correlates with outcome after aneurysmal subarachnoid hemorrhage. *Neurosci Lett.* 2006;404(1-2):132–6.

51. Petzold A, Keir G, Kerr M, et al. Early identification of secondary brain damage in subarachnoid hemorrhage: a role for glial fibrillary acidic protein. *J Neurotrauma.* 2006;23(7):1179–84.

52. Petzold A, Rejdak K, Belli A, et al. Axonal pathology in subarachnoid and intracerebral hemorrhage. *J Neurotrauma*. 2005;22(3):407–14.

53. Zanier ER, Refai D, Zipfel JG, et al. Neurofilament light chain levels in ventricular cerebrospinal fluid after acute aneurysmal subarachnoid haemorrhage. *J Neurol Neurosurg Psychiatry*. 2011;82(2):157–9.

54. Lad SP, Hegen H, Gupta G, Deisenhammer F, Steinberg GK. Proteomic biomarker discovery in cerebrospinal fluid for cerebral vasospasm following subarachnoid hemorrhage. *J Stroke Cerebrovasc Dis*. 2012;21(1):30–41.

55. Deisenhammer F, Egg R, Giovanni G, et al.; EFSN. EFNS guidelines on disease specific CSF investigations. *Eur J Neurol*. 2009;16(6):760–70.

56. Baird A. Blood biologic markers of stroke: improved management, reduced cost? *Curr Atheroscler Rep*. 2006;8(4):267–75.

57. Schiff L, Hadker N, Weiser S, Rausch C. A literature review of the feasibility of glial fibrillary acidic protein as a biomarker for stroke and traumatic brain injury. *Mol Diagn Ther*. 2012;16(2):79–92.

58. Gruson D. Football, concussions and biomarkers: ready for more touchdowns? *Clin Biochem*. 2014;47(13-14):1345–6.

59. Shahim P, Linemann T, Inekci D, et al. Serum tau fragments predict return to play in concussed professional ice hockey players. *J Neurotrauma*. 2016;33(22):1995–9.

60. Zetterberg H, Smith DH, Blennow K. Biomarkers of mild traumatic brain injury in cerebrospinal fluid and blood. *Nat Rev Neurol*. 2013;9(4):201–10.

61. Tisdall M, Petzold A. Comment on chronic traumatic encephalopathy in blast-exposed military veterans and a blast neurotrauma mouse model. *Sci Transl Med*. 2012;4(157):157le8; author reply 157lr5.

62. Zetterberg H, Blennow K. Fluid markers of traumatic brain injury. *Mol Cell Neurosci*. 2015;66(Pt B):99–102.

63. Magnoni S, Esparza TJ, Conte V, et al. Tau elevations in the brain extracellular space correlate with reduced amyloid- β levels and predict adverse clinical outcomes after severe traumatic brain injury. *Brain*. 2012;135(Pt 4):1268–80.

64. Magnoni S, Mac Donald CL, Esparza TJ, et al. Quantitative assessments of traumatic axonal injury in human brain: concordance of microdialysis and advanced MRI. *Brain*. 2015;138(Pt 8):2263–77.

65. Czeiter E, Mondello S, Kovacs N, et al. Brain injury biomarkers may improve the predictive power of the IMPACT outcome calculator. *J Neurotrauma*. 2012;29(9):1770–8.

66. Nylen K, Ost M, Csajbok L, et al. Increased serum-GFAP in patients with severe traumatic brain injury is related to outcome. *J Neurol Sci*. 2006;240(1-2):85–91.

67. Papa L, Lewis LM, Falk JL, et al. Elevated levels of serum glial fibrillary acidic protein breakdown products in mild and moderate traumatic brain injury are associated with intracranial lesions and neurosurgical intervention. *Ann Emerg Med*. 2012;59(6):471–83.

68. Papa L, Silvestri S, Brophy GM, et al. GFAP out-performs S100B in detecting traumatic intracranial lesions on CT in trauma patients with mild traumatic brain injury and those with extracranial lesions. *J Neurotrauma*. 2014;31(22):1815–22.

69. Vos PE, Jacobs B, Andriessen TM, et al. GFAP and S100B are biomarkers of traumatic brain injury: an observational cohort study. *Neurology*. 2010;75(20):1786–93.

70. Honda M, Tsuruta R, Kaneko T, et al. Serum glial fibrillary acidic protein is a highly specific biomarker for traumatic brain injury in humans compared with S-100B and neuron-specific enolase. *J Trauma*. 2010;69(1):104–9.

71. Pelinka EL, Kroepfl A, Leixnering M, Buchinger W, Raabe A, Redl H. GFAP versus S100B in serum after traumatic brain injury: relationship to brain damage and outcome. *J Neurotrauma*. 2004;21(11):1553–61.

72. Vos P, Lamers K, Hendriks J, et al. Glial and neuronal proteins in serum predict outcome after severe traumatic brain injury. *Neurology.* 2004;62(8):1303–10.

73. Pelinka LE, Kroepfl A, Schmidhammer R, et al. Glial fibrillary acidic protein in serum after traumatic brain injury and multiple trauma. *J Trauma.* 2004;57(5):1006–12.

74. Yue JK, Vassar MJ, Lingsma HF, et al; TRACK-TBI Investigators. Transforming research and clinical knowledge in traumatic brain injury pilot: multicenter implementation of the common data elements for traumatic brain injury. *J Neurotrauma.* 2013;30(22):1831–44.

75. Brettschneider J, Petzold A, Süssmuth S, Tumani H. Cerebrospinal fluid biomarkers in Guillain-Barré syndrome–where do we stand? *J Neurol.* 2009;256(1):3–12.

76. Dujmovic I, Lunn MP, Reilly MM, Petzold A. Serial cerebrospinal fluid neurofilament heavy chain levels in severe Guillain-Barré syndrome. *Muscle Nerve.* 2013;48(1):132–4.

77. Petzold A, Brettschneider J, Jin K, et al. CSF protein biomarkers for proximal axonal damage improve prognostic accuracy in the acute phase of Guillain-Barré syndrome. *Muscle Nerve.* 2009;40(1):42–9.

78. Petzold A, Hinds N, Murray N, et al. CSF neurofilament levels: a potential prognostic marker in Guillain-Barré syndrome. *Neurology.* 2006;67(6):1071–3.

79. Wang XK, Zhang HL, Meng FH, et al. Elevated levels of S100B, tau and pNFH in cerebrospinal fluid are correlated with subtypes of Guillain-Barré syndrome. *Neurol Sci.* 2013;34(5):655–61.

80. Mayer SA. Outcome prediction after cardiac arrest: new game, new rules. *Neurology.* 2011;77(7):614–5.

81. Bouwes A, Binnekade JM, Zandstra DF, et al. Somatosensory evoked potentials during mild hypothermia after cardiopulmonary resuscitation. *Neurology.* 2009;73(18):1457–61.

82. Hirsch KG, Mlynash M, Eyngorn I, et al. Multi-center study of diffusion-weighted imaging in coma after cardiac arrest. *Neurocrit Care.* 2015;24(1):82–9.

83. Siman R, Roberts VL, McNeil E, et al. Biomarker evidence for mild central nervous system injury after surgically-induced circulation arrest. *Brain Res.* 2008;1213:1–11.

84. Rosén H, Karlsson J, Rosengren L. CSF levels of neurofilament is a valuable predictor of long-term outcome after cardiac arrest. *J Neurol Sci.* 2004;221(1-2):19–24.

85. Rosén C, Rosén H, Andreasson U, et al. Cerebrospinal fluid biomarkers in cardiac arrest survivors. *Resuscitation.* 2014;85(2):227–32.

86. Rundgren M, Friberg H, Cronberg T, Romner B, Petzold A. Serial soluble neurofilament heavy chain in plasma as a marker of brain injury after cardiac arrest. *Crit Care.* 2012;16(2):R45.

87. Wijdicks EF, Hijdra A, Young GB, Bassetti CL, Wiebe S; Quality Standards Subcommittee of the American Academy of Neurology. Practice parameter: prediction of outcome in comatose survivors after cardiopulmonary resuscitation (an evidence-based review): report of the Quality Standards Subcommittee of the American Academy of Neurology. *Neurology.* 2006;67(2):203–10.

88. Bouwes A, Binnekade JM, Kuiper MA, et al. Prognosis of coma after therapeutic hypothermia: a prospective cohort study. *Ann Neurol.* 2012;71(2):206–12.

89. Jensen HA, Loukogeorgakis S, Yannopoulos F, et al. Remote ischemic preconditioning protects the brain against injury after hypothermic circulatory arrest. *Circulation.* 2011;123(7):714–21.

90. Kyrou IE, Papakostas JC, Ioachim E, et al. Early ischaemic preconditioning of spinal cord enhanced the binding profile of heat shock protein 70 with neurofilaments and promoted its nuclear translocation after thoraco-abdominal aortic occlusion in pigs. *Eur J Vasc Endovasc Surg.* 2012;43(4):408–14.

91. Meybohm P, Bein B, Brosteanu O, et al.; RIPHeart Study Collaborators. A multicenter trial of remote ischemic preconditioning for heart surgery. *N Engl J Med.* 2015;373(15):1397–407.

92. Zaugg M, Lucchinetti E. Remote ischemic preconditioning in cardiac surgery–ineffective and risky? *N Engl J Med.* 2015;373(15):1470–2.

93. Gunther ML, Morandi A, Ely EW. Pathophysiology of delirium in the intensive care unit. *Crit Care Clin.* 2008;24(1):45–65, viii.

94. Salluh JIF, Wang H, Schneider EB, et al. Outcome of delirium in critically ill patients: systematic review and meta-analysis. *BMJ.* 2015;350:h2538.

95. Ely EW, Jackson JC, Gordon SM, Hopkins RO. Critical illness brain syndrome: an underestimated entity? *Crit Care Med.* 2005;33(6):1464–5.

96. Petzold A, Downie P, Smith M. Critical illness brain syndrome (CIBS): an underestimated entity? *Crit Care Med.* 2005;33(6):1464; author reply 1464-5.

97. Pustavoitau A, Stevens RD. Mechanisms of neurologic failure in critical illness. *Crit Care Clin.* 2008;24(1):1–24, vii.

98. Stevens RD, Pronovost PJ. The spectrum of encephalopathy in critical illness. *Semin Neurol.* 2006;26(4):440–51.

99. Jackson JC, Hart RP, Gordon SM, et al. Six-month neuropsychological outcome of medical intensive care unit patients. *Crit Care Med.* 2003;31(4):1226–34.

# 5 Neurophysiologic Monitoring and Neuroprotection

Aws Alawi, Michael Reznik,

and Jan Claassen

## INTRODUCTION

Critically ill patients are often at risk of neurological dysfunction, either because of a primary acute brain injury or due to neurological sequelae of their critical illness. One of the most important goals of treating at-risk patients in the intensive care unit (ICU) is the early identification of neurological changes suggesting new or worsening brain injury, so that permanent damage and adverse outcomes may be ameliorated or prevented.

Although the bedside clinical examination remains the gold standard for the evaluation of neurologically ill patients in the ICU, it may not be sufficient in some patients, especially those with impaired consciousness and those who require substantial sedation (e.g., patients with severe intracranial pressure [ICP] elevation, status epilepticus, or acute respiratory distress syndrome [ARDS]). In such patients, significant changes in neurological status might go undetected without other modes of neurological monitoring. Moreover, neuroimaging studies such as computed tomography (CT) scans, magnetic resonance imaging (MRI), and transcranial Doppler (TCD) studies provide clinical data that are often meaningful, but that are restricted to the time of the study.

As a consequence of these limitations, monitoring of various physiologic markers has become essential for the early detection of secondary brain injury and amelioration or prevention of irreversible damage. Current neuromonitoring tools that allow for real-time continuous physiologic assessment of the central nervous system include various invasive and noninvasive techniques. Invasive techniques include ICP and brain tissue oxygen tension ($PbtO_2$). Noninvasive techniques include continuous electroencephalography (cEEG), TCD, and transcranial oximetry.[1] This chapter describes the various neuromonitoring modalities that are employed in the ICU.

ICP is determined by the volume of the intracranial contents (i.e., brain, cerebrospinal fluid CSF, and blood). Normally, ICP ranges from 5 mm Hg to 15 mm Hg. The relationship between ICP and volume of the three components is summarized by the Monro-Kellie doctrine. This fundamental principle states that the total volume of the intracranial contents must remain constant, and that any change in one of the intracranial components must be compensated by a reciprocal change in the volume of one or both of the remaining components in order to keep ICP stable. An increase in the volume of one of the intracranial components, or the emergence of a new space-occupying lesion such as a brain tumor or hematoma, may eventually exhaust the brain's innate compensatory mechanisms, leading to a rise in ICP. Brain injuries, such as traumatic brain injury (TBI), intracranial hemorrhage (ICH), and large ischemic stroke, may cause sustained elevation of ICP that can lead to a significant decrease in cerebral perfusion pressure (CPP) and cerebral blood flow (CBF), and/or cerebral herniation with subsequent secondary brain damage. Refractory ICP elevation is a known predictor of poor outcome and increased mortality.[2–3] Therefore, ICP monitoring is strongly recommended in patients with clinical and/or radiological findings suggestive of increased ICP, such as severe TBI, aneurysmal subarachnoid hemorrhage (SAH), ICH, bacterial meningitis, and fulminant hepatic failure.[1]

## Invasive Intracranial Pressure Monitoring

In contrast to noninvasive methods, invasive monitoring devices provide direct measurements of ICP. There are a variety of such devices, with probes that can be placed in the intraventricular, intraparenchymal, subarachnoid, subdural, or epidural compartments. The most commonly employed invasive ICP monitors are intraparenchymal monitors and external ventricular drains (EVD) which also allow for therapeutic drainage of CSF as needed (Table 5.1).

A unique feature of invasive ICP monitoring is the appearance of a pressure waveform. Normal ICP waveform morphology is characterized by three components: P1 (percussion wave) represents arterial pulsation; P2 (tidal wave) represents the overall state of intracranial compliance; and P3 (dicrotic wave) represents venous pulsation (Figure 5.1). Normally, P1 has the highest amplitude, P2 has intermediate amplitude, and P3 has the lowest amplitude. As intracranial compliance diminishes as a consequence of intracranial hypertension, the P2 amplitude may increase as high as, or even higher than P1.

Lundberg A and B waves refer to pathologic ICP elevation that occurs in patients with reduced intracranial compliance (Figure 5.2). These waves represent a trend of ICP values plotted over time, rather than a single ICP waveform. Lundberg A (plateau) waves represent prolonged periods of profoundly elevated ICP and CPP reduction, and are considered a marker of ongoing brain injury. Lundberg B waves represent elevations in ICP of shorter duration and lower amplitude, and indicate that intracranial compliance reserves are compromised.[4] Abnormal ICP waveforms and pathologic waves carry importance even in the setting of normal ICP values, because they may foreshadow future ICP crises with minor changes in a patient's condition (e.g., changes in head position, agitation, pain, or relative hypotension).

**Table 5.1** Multimodality Devices and Parameters for Monitoring Patients with Acute Brain Injury

| Modality | Measurement | Abnormal Findings | Interpretation |
|---|---|---|---|
| **ICP Monitoring** | | | |
| – ICP monitor (EVD, intraparenchymal) | ICP | Sustained ICP >20 mm Hg | ICP sufficient to cause decreased blood flow and lead to herniation |
| – TCD | Pulsatility Index (PI) | PI >1.4 | Consistent with high resistance blood flow, which may be caused by increased ICP |
| – Optic nerve sheath ultrasound | Optic nerve sheath diameter | Diameter >5 mm | Consistent with increased ICP |
| **CBF Monitoring** | | | |
| – TCD | Mean blood flow velocity | Mean velocity >120 cm/sec in the MCA territory. Diastolic reversal of flow | Consistent with vasospasm or intracranial stenosis (with LR > 3), or hyperemia (LR < 3) May be seen with brain death |
| – Thermal diffusion flowmetry | rCBF in mL/100g/min | rCBF <20 mL/100g/min rCBF >70 mL/100g/min | Indicative of ischemia and decreased cerebral perfusion Indicative of hyperemia and increased cerebral perfusion |
| **Brain Oxygen Monitoring** | | | |
| – Brain tissue Oxygen pressure monitor (Licox $PbtO_2$ probe and Neurovent-P Temp) | Brain tissue partial pressure of oxygen ($PbtO_2$) | $PbtO_2$ <20 mm Hg | Indicative of cerebral ischemia |
| – Jugular Venous Bulb Oximetry | Jugular venous Oxygen saturation ($SjvO_2$) | $SjvO_2$ <55% $SjvO_2$ >75% | Suggestive of either decreased $O_2$ supply due to ischemia or increased $O_2$ extraction (as with seizure and fever) Suggestive of either cerebral hyperemia or decreased $O_2$ consumption (as with hypothermia, sedation, or infarction) |

| | | | |
|---|---|---|---|
| – Near Infrared Spectroscopy | Cerebral oxyhemoglobin ($rSO_2$) | $rSO_2$ <60%, consistent with regional ischemia | Regional ischemia |
| **Cerebral Microdialysis** | Glucose | Trend of decreasing glucose | Most suggestive of hypoxia/ischemia, as well as cerebral hyperglycolysis and decreased glucose delivery. |
| | Lactate | Trend of increasing lactate | Most suggestive of anaerobic metabolism due to hypoxia/ischemia or ICP crisis |
| | Lactate/pyruvate ratio (LPR) | LPR >25–40 | Increasing LPR more suggestive than lactate or pyruvate alone for hypoxia/ischemia, ICP crisis, or increased $O_2$ consumption (e.g., due to inflammation, seizure, or fever) |
| | Glutamate | Trend of increasing glutamate | Suggestive of hypoxia/ischemia and excitotoxicity |
| | Glycerol | Trend of increasing glycerol | Suggestive of destruction of cell membranes (e.g., due to ischemia/hypoxia or seizure) |

*ICP*, intracranial pressure; *EVD*, external ventricular drains; *TCD*, transcranial Doppler; *CBF*, cerebral blood flow; *rCBF*, regional cerebral blood flow; *LR*, Lindegaard ratio; *MCA*, middle cerebral artery; *PbtO₂*, partial pressure of brain tissue oxygen

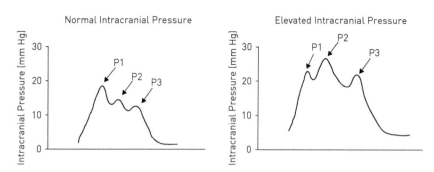

FIGURE 5.1 Intracranial pressure waveform in normal and abnormal intracranial pressure states. *P1*, percussion wave; *P2*, tidal wave; *P3*, dicrotic wave.

One of the main indications for ICP monitoring is in the setting of severe TBI, defined as a Glasgow Coma Scale (GCS) score of less than 8 after initial resuscitation. The Brain Trauma Foundation guidelines recommend ICP monitoring with an EVD in patients with severe TBI and an abnormal head CT scan (Class II evidence).[5] The guidelines also recommend ICP monitoring in patients with a normal head CT scan and two of the following three characteristics: older than 40 years, admission systolic blood pressure of less than 90 mm Hg, or early unilateral or bilateral motor posturing (Class III evidence). The current Brain Trauma Foundation guidelines recommend interventions to reduce ICP in patients with pressures greater than 20–25 mm Hg because elevated ICP is known to be associated with increased mortality in severe TBI.[2] One systematic review showed that mortality increased with the degree of ICP elevation, and that persistently elevated and refractory ICP is a better predictor of mortality than absolute ICP value.[3] A study of 1,426 patients with severe TBI, 388 of whom were treated for elevated ICP, showed that response to

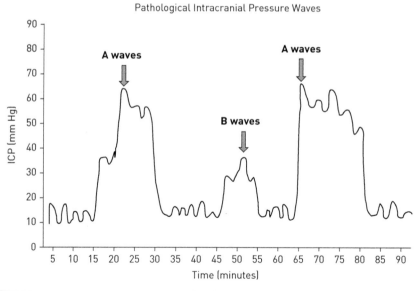

FIGURE 5.2 Pathological intracranial pressure (ICP) waves. Lundberg A and B waves occur in the setting of reduced intracranial compliance. B waves are usually of shorter duration and lower amplitude elevations in ICP than are A waves.

ICP-lowering therapy was independently associated with decreased mortality, with a 64% lower risk of death at 2 weeks as compared to nonresponders.[6] Measuring the ICP enables targeting a CPP range of 50 to 70 mm Hg in severe TBI.[7] CPP values of less than 50 mm Hg should be avoided, since low CPP due to increased ICP and/or arterial hypotension is associated with poor outcome.[8] Similarly, aggressive attempts to maintain CPP above 70 mm Hg with intravenous fluids and vasopressors should be avoided since that strategy can lead to systemic complications and higher risk of developing ARDS.[9]

Whether or not an ICP-guided approach to treatment of severe TBI improves outcomes remains controversial. The Benchmark Evidence from South American Trials: Treatment of Intracranial Pressure (BEST TRIP) was a randomized controlled trial conducted in Bolivia and Ecuador. It showed no difference in mortality or functional outcomes in patients with severe TBI treated using ICP-guided therapy versus treatment strategies based on clinical examination and serial head imaging.[10] The study, however, has been criticized on the grounds that the findings are not generalizable given the significant differences in health care utilization and pre-hospital care of trauma patients between Bolivia/Ecuador and the United States and Europe.

ICP monitoring is also recommended in any patient with nontraumatic brain injury who is suspected to have ICP elevation, such as in SAH, ICH, fulminant bacterial meningitis, and fulminant hepatic failure.[11] In aneurysmal SAH, EVD placement is recommended in patients with a poor-grade aneurysmal SAH and/or acute hydrocephalus to provide ICP monitoring and CSF diversion for ICP control.[12] ICP monitoring is also used at times in patients with spontaneous ICH. Recent guidelines for the management of spontaneous ICH suggest that EVD placement should be considered in patients with a GCS score of less than 9, those with clinical evidence of transtentorial herniation, or those with significant intraventricular hemorrhage or hydrocephalus.[13]

## Noninvasive Intracranial Pressure Monitoring

Noninvasive ICP monitoring techniques may be considered as a surrogate to track increased ICP when invasive measures are contraindicated or unavailable. Examples of noninvasive techniques are transcranial Doppler (TCD), ultrasonographic measurement of optic nerve sheath diameter (ONSD), and pupillometry. Their main advantage is the avoidance of complications associated with invasive monitoring, namely hemorrhage and infection. Their dependence on the operator's skill and poor inter-rater reliability, however, limit the reproducibility of findings from one operator to another.[14]

TCD measures the blood flow velocity of the middle cerebral artery (MCA) and allows for calculation of the pulsatility index (PI), which correlates with ICP (Table 5.1).[15] PI reflects the difference between systolic and diastolic flow velocity, divided by the mean flow velocity. High PI of the MCA has been associated with increased ICP and worse outcome in brain-injured patients, with values greater than 1.4 being predictive of intracranial hypertension with a sensitivity of 88% and specificity of 97%.[16–17] Other studies, however, showed that the PI value is insufficient to provide accurate ICP measurements, thereby limiting its use as a means of guiding management for elevated ICP.[18] In addition to operator dependency, another major limitation of TCD is that 10–15% of patients lack the necessary bone windows to allow insonation of the MCA, rendering TCD impossible.[19]

ONSD is a useful screening tool for detecting increased ICP and can be obtained using bedside transocular ultrasound to measure the width of the optic nerve approximately 3–5 mm behind the globe (Table 5.1).[20] The optic sheath is contiguous with the dura and surrounds the optic nerve; in between the optic nerve and optic sheath is a small subarachnoid space that communicates with the subarachnoid space surrounding the cerebral hemispheres so that increased pressure in the latter leads to sheath expansion. Although not accurate enough to replace invasive ICP monitoring, measurement of ONSD can be useful in distinguishing between normal and increased ICP, with an ONSD of greater than 5 mm having been shown to correlate with an ICP of greater than 20 mm Hg (sensitivity 74–95%, specificity 79–100%).[21]

Another useful screening tool for detecting midbrain or third cranial nerve dysfunction related to intracranial hypertension is the digital pupillometer. Using this handheld device at the bedside yields a measurement called the Neurological Pupil index (NPi), a proprietary algorithm that incorporates several parameters of pupillary reactivity (including size, latency, constriction percentage, and constriction/dilation velocity). The NPi is graded on a scale of 0 to 5, with values less than 3 indicating decreased pupil reactivity, which may be an early indicator of increased ICP.[22] The NPi scale removes subjectivity from the pupillary evaluation and provides a more quantifiable way to assess pupillary reactivity; however, more clinical studies are needed to validate the correlation between the low NPi scores and increases in ICP.

## CEREBRAL BLOOD FLOW MONITORING

CBF is defined as CPP divided by cerebrovascular resistance (CVR). In normal circumstances, cerebrovascular autoregulation keeps CBF relatively constant across a wide range of CPPs through modification of cerebral vascular resistance. Autoregulation will lead to increased CVR via constriction of precapillary arterioles in the setting of high CPP, and decreased CVR via vasodilation in the setting of low CPP. Patients with acute brain injuries may have impaired cerebrovascular autoregulation, which may create conditions in which CBF becomes passively dependent on CPP (i.e., a decrease in CPP leads to a decrease in CBF).

Ischemia due to reduction in CBF is an important cause of neurological deterioration following initial brain injury and therefore is a focus of monitoring techniques. Brain imaging has been the gold standard for quantification of CBF but only provides a snapshot in time, whereas the neurological exam is insufficient to identify impending ischemia and infarction in patients with impaired consciousness. These limitations, as well as the fact that reductions in CBF may precede ischemia, both underscore the need for continuous actionable CBF monitoring.

### Transcranial Doppler Ultrasonography

TCD provides direct measurement of blood flow velocity in the large arteries of the brain. The TCD probe emits high-frequency pulsed-wave ultrasound that penetrates tissue with varying degrees of reflection, and the changes in frequency of the sound waves reflected from intravascular red blood cells are used to determine the direction and velocity of blood flow. Flow velocities are used as a surrogate for vessel diameter, with higher velocities indicating vessel narrowing.

One of the primary practical applications of TCD is the detection of vasospasm following aneurysmal SAH. Studies have shown that up to 70% of patients with aneurysmal SAH may develop vasospasm that may be diagnosed using catheter angiography, CT angiography, or TCD.[12] It is estimated that this vasospasm is symptomatic (defined as focal or global neurological deficits attributable to arterial vasospasm) in only 20-40% of such patients.[23] Delayed cerebral ischemia occurs more frequently with intraventricular hemorrhage and/or with the presence of blood in the basal cistern or any major fissure.[24]

TCD is most reliable for detecting vasospasm of the anterior circulation, especially in the internal carotid artery (ICA) and MCA (as opposed to anterior cerebral artery) distributions. Using a mean velocity threshold of 120 cm/s, the sensitivity of TCD for angiographically documented vasospasm is 73%, while specificity is 80%.[25] Higher mean velocities have even better correlation with catheter angiography in detecting vasospasm, with a positive predictive value of 87% for vasospasm when MCA mean velocity is greater than 200 cm/s, and a negative predictive value of 95% for lack of vasospasm when MCA mean velocity is less than 120 cm/s. Intermediate velocities between 120 and 200 cm/s have lower predictive value in detecting vasospasm.[26]

Increased flow velocity may also occur in hyperemic states, such as fever and increased cardiac output. In such circumstances, measuring the ratio of MCA velocity to extracranial ICA velocity (also known as the Lindegaard ratio [LR]), can help differentiate between vasospasm and hyperemia. LR less than 3 is considered normal, whereas LR between 3 and 6 is consistent with mild to moderate vasospasm, and LR greater than 6 indicates severe vasospasm.[27] As a noncontinuous monitoring device, however, daily TCD may fail to capture changes in CBF that precede ischemia.

## Thermal Diffusion Flowmetry

Thermal diffusion flowmetry (TDF) uses thermal conductive properties of brain tissue to provide quantitative measurements of regional CBF (rCBF) expressed in mL/100 g/min. This can be measured via an intraparenchymal thermal diffusion microprobe, typically inserted through a bolt fixed in the skull with its tip situated 20–25 mm deep to the dura. The microprobe (Hemedex, Inc., Cambridge, MA) carries a distal thermistor that is intermittently heated and a proximal temperature sensor that provides sensitive and continuous absolute values based on dissipation of heat from the distal thermistor (Table 5.1). TDF technology provides real-time, continuous, and dynamic CBF data at the bedside, and TDF-derived rCBF measurements have been shown to correlate well with those obtained simultaneously using stable xenon-enhanced CT scans.[28] Normal rCBF values range between 40 to 70 mL/100 g/min, with rCBF less than 20 mL/100 g/min representing states of ischemia, assuming that metabolic demand is unchanged.[29]

Cerebral blood flow monitoring by TDF, however, has several limitations. The device automatically recalibrates approximately every 30 minutes (this can be adjusted) and results in a loss of data for 2–5 minutes at a time, with the possibility of significant baseline shifts after each recalibration. The system is unable to measure CBF when brain temperature rises above 39°C. Additionally, it relies on proper positioning and only measures CBF in a small region of brain tissue around the probe. Despite these limitations, TDF provides useful information when used in conjunction with other monitoring devices. There is some evidence suggesting that rCBF monitoring using TDF can help detect vasospasm in patients with aneurysmal SAH.[30]

CBF monitoring also allows real-time, bedside measurement of brain water content in acutely brain-injured patients that correlates with brain edema assessments using brain imaging. A practical application of this technology would be to monitor the CBF effects of the reduction in brain water content in response to hyperosmolar therapy for increased ICP.[31] Regional CBF may also predict outcome in TBI; patients with low rCBF on presentation who don't respond well to treatment have poor outcomes.[32] Moreover, rCBF can help target an optimal CPP in brain-injured patients with impaired autoregulation.[33] Using rCBF monitoring in conjunction with other invasive brain monitors may help guide treatment in critically ill patients, but further studies are needed to determine its impact on clinical outcome.

## BRAIN OXYGEN MONITORING

Maintenance of adequate brain oxygenation is a primary objective in the management of patients with acute brain injury, and direct assessment of brain tissue oxygen is feasible via invasive and noninvasive techniques. Brain tissue hypoxia, however, is difficult to interpret because the underlying causes are numerous and include hypoperfusion from arterial occlusion or stenosis, decreased cardiac output, impaired systemic oxygenation or blood oxygen carrying capacity, changes in pH, microvascular changes, or cytotoxicity from cellular energy failure and mitochondrial dysfunction.[34]

### Brain Tissue Oxygen Pressure Measurement

Direct brain tissue partial pressure of oxygen $(PbtO_2)$ monitors provide continuous real-time monitoring of brain oxygenation. The most widely used system utilizes a probe inserted into the subcortical white matter, with $PbtO_2$ measurements that are calculated based on the Clark principle. Oxygen diffuses through the membrane in the probe tip and undergoes electrochemical reduction, with its diffusion proportionally related to oxygen partial pressure.[35] The process is temperature-dependent and requires constant calibration of the system with respect to patient body temperature.

The most widely used invasive probes are the Licox $PbtO_2$ probe (Integra Lifesciences, Plainsboro, NJ) and the Neurovent-P Temp (Raumedic AG, Münchberg, Germany). The Licox system includes a temperature probe that is inserted into the brain tissue with the $PbtO_2$ probe through a triple-lumen bolt, which allows measurement of brain temperature and calibrates automatically (Table 5.1). The Neurovent-P Temp measures $PbtO_2$ and brain temperature using a single catheter. Licox and Neurovent probes have different calibration methods (with Neurovent values that tend to run higher), thus values are not interchangeable between devices.[36] Although the $PbtO_2$ probes sample a small volume of brain tissue $(15 \text{ mm}^3)$ surrounding the tip, local measurements have been shown to correlate well with global brain oxygenation when probe placement is in normal subcortical white matter. When the probe tip is located adjacent to a lesion, however, measurement values are often lower and therefore more reflective of regional rather than global brain oxygenation status.[37]

Most clinical data regarding $PbtO_2$ monitoring are drawn from studies in TBI patients and, to a lesser extent, SAH patients. Values between 25 and 35 mm Hg are considered normal, while those less than 20 mm Hg are suggestive of cerebral ischemia. Studies have shown a correlation between $PbtO_2$ less than 15 mm Hg and poor outcome in patients with TBI and aneurysmal SAH.[38–39] Observational studies have also shown better outcomes with $PbtO_2$-guided ICP/CPP management in patients with severe TBI, especially when interventions are successful in correcting brain hypoxia.[40–41] Similar findings have been observed in aneurysmal SAH patients.[42] As a result, current Brain Trauma Foundation guidelines recommend the use of brain tissue oxygen monitoring in addition to standard ICP monitors in the management of patients with severe TBI (level III evidence).[43]

Interpretation of $PbtO_2$ data requires an understanding of the various factors that may affect cerebral oxygenation, including conditions that alter global oxygen supply and oxygen extraction.[44] In addition to CBF and CPP, many other variables can affect $PbtO_2$, such as $PaCO_2$, $PaO_2$, increased brain oxygen extraction (as in shivering and fever), and decreased local tissue extraction (as in cerebral edema).[45] $PbtO_2$ measurements, therefore, should always be interpreted in the context of other physiologic data. Initial measures to optimize $PbtO_2$ usually consist of raising the mean blood pressure. Other considerations based on the clinical scenario may include packed red blood cell transfusion, sedation, targeted temperature management, and prevention of hypocapnia, among others. Transiently increasing fraction of inspired oxygen ($FiO_2$) can be used to test the validity of $PbtO_2$ measurements, but this should not be used as a method of treatment because it does not address the underlying state of hypoperfusion.[46]

## Jugular Venous Bulb Oximetry

Monitoring of the jugular venous oxygen saturation ($SjvO_2$) provides information about global cerebral hemodynamics and metabolism, with $SjvO_2$ reflecting the balance between brain oxygen supply and consumption. This requires the placement of a catheter in the bulb of the internal jugular vein in order to avoid contamination by venous drainage from extracerebral structures such as the face and neck. Ideally, the catheter should be inserted into the dominant internal jugular vein, as determined by brief manual occlusion of each internal jugular vein while noting the side with a greater increase in ICP after occlusion. Since cerebral metabolic rate of oxygen ($CMRO_2$) can be estimated from CBF and the difference in the arterio-jugular bulb oxygen saturation ($CMRO_2 = CBF \times [SaO_2 - SjvO_2]$), the arteriovenous oxygen saturation difference can be used to assess the CBF. Indeed, when cerebral metabolism is constant, the arteriovenous oxygen saturation difference is inversely related to CBF. In other words, decreased cerebral perfusion results in an increased difference in arteriovenous $O_2$ saturation, and vice-versa.[47]

Measurement of $SjvO_2$ can be accomplished using a fiber-optic probe. Normal $SjvO_2$ ranges between 55% and 75%. Levels less than 55% represent abnormally high oxygen extraction and suggest that cerebral oxygen demand exceeds supply. This can occur in cases of decreased $O_2$ supply or in cases of increased cerebral metabolism and $O_2$ demand, such as seizure or fever. An $SjvO_2$ level greater than 75% may indicate cerebral hyperemia or decreased cerebral $O_2$ consumption, whether due to hypothermia, sedation, or cerebral infarction (Table 5.1).

Studies in patients with TBI have suggested that episodes of low $SjvO_2$ with limited improvement after appropriate treatment may indicate cerebral infarction and predict poor outcome, with both duration and number of jugular venous desaturations found to be associated with outcomes.[48–49] A small study showed that in patients with aneurysmal SAH, jugular venous desaturation may precede symptomatic vasospasm and that treatment of vasospasm resulted in resolution of symptoms and improvement in $SjvO_2$.[50]

In summary, $SjvO_2$ monitoring is more reliable for detecting global cerebral oxygenation abnormalities compared to $PbtO_2$ monitoring, but it is limited in its ability to detect regional cerebral hypoxia.[51]

## Near Infrared Spectroscopy

By measuring the concentration of light-absorbing compounds in brain tissue, near infrared spectroscopy (NIRS) allows for noninvasive continuous bedside monitoring of cerebral oxygenation. High-intensity light in the near infrared wavelength range (680–1,000 nm) is emitted from a probe placed on the scalp. This light penetrates underlying tissues and is subsequently absorbed by oxyhemoglobin, deoxyhemoglobin, and cytochrome oxidase. Reflected light is then detected by the probe, and the degree to which the light is attenuated correlates with the tissue concentration of the above chromophores, thereby providing an estimate of tissue oxygenation.

Cerebral oxyhemoglobin ($rSO_2$) is the chromophore that is most widely used to evaluate changes in regional oxygenation and CBF after brain injury, and $rSO_2$ values less than 60% are considered abnormal (Table 5.1). NIRS has been studied in aneurysmal SAH and TBI patients, with mixed results compared to invasive measures.[52–53] At this time, therefore, NIRS should not be used as the only monitoring parameter in patients with acute brain injury; it is best suited as an adjunct to other neuromonitoring devices.

## MICRODIALYSIS

Cerebral microdialysis (MD) is an increasingly utilized technique that allows for direct biochemical assessment of brain extracellular fluid (ECF). This is accomplished by inserting a fine double-lumen probe with a semipermeable membrane at its tip into the subcortical white matter. Fluid isotonic to the brain ECF, called the *perfusate*, is pumped through the MD catheter, and molecules at high concentration in the ECF equilibrate across the semipermeable membrane at the catheter tip. This fluid, called the *microdialysate*, can be collected at hourly intervals for analysis. Many molecules can be measured, but those of particular interest are energy-related molecules, such as glucose, lactate, and pyruvate; excitatory neurotransmitters such as glutamate (which is believed to be associated with inflammatory cascade responses); and glycerol (a marker of neuronal cellular breakdown that is associated with irreversible cellular death) (Table 5.1).

Glucose is the main source of energy to the brain, and glucose metabolism provides the fuel for physiological brain function through the generation of adenosine triphosphate (ATP). Glycolysis produces pyruvate, which subsequently enters the citric acid cycle for efficient energy production. During ischemic states, pyruvate undergoes anaerobic metabolism and is converted to lactate. Lactate, pyruvate, and the lactate-to-pyruvate ratio (LPR) therefore have been utilized as markers of anaerobic metabolism and energy failure, with LPR considered as the most reliable marker of neuronal energy dysfunction.

As with the other modalities discussed earlier, MD is a tool that can be used for the early detection of secondary events in patients with acute brain injury, and can be useful in any comatose patient with neurological critical illness. Cerebral MD studies reveal significant metabolic changes in TBI and poor-grade aneurysmal SAH patients, including increased levels of lactate, glutamate, glycerol, and LPR, and decreased glucose during periods of sustained, brain tissue hypoxia.[54-55] These abnormalities have also been shown to correlate with poor outcome in these conditions.[39,56-59] Moreover, MD metabolic changes can detect vasospasm in SAH patients and may help prevent delayed cerebral ischemia and neurological deterioration.[60-62]

The MD pattern of cerebral ischemia is typically characterized by a marked increase in LPR combined with a low brain glucose level. This is due to reductions in oxygen and glucose and a subsequent shift to anaerobic metabolism and increased brain lactate. Values of LPR greater than 40 represent a state of cerebral "metabolic distress," whereas the combination of LPR greater than 40 and brain glucose level less than 0.7 mmol/L represents brain "metabolic crisis."[54,63]

It is important to recognize that both metabolic distress and metabolic crisis represent a state of imbalance between cerebral energy supply and consumption that can occur in clinical scenarios other than reduced CBF. In poor-grade SAH patients, abrupt reductions in serum glucose (even to levels within the normal range) can result in brain metabolic crisis, most likely due to dysfunctional active transport of glucose across the blood–brain barrier into the CNS.[64] In patients with severe brain injury, tight glycemic control using intensive insulin therapy reduces extracellular cerebral glucose and may be associated with cerebral metabolic crisis and increased mortality, even when cerebral glucose levels are normal.[65-66] A reduced brain-to-serum glucose ratio itself has been found to be associated with cerebral metabolic distress and increased mortality after severe brain injury.[67]

In summary, MD helps provide early signs of adverse events in comatose patients with brain injury, but it is not yet clear whether therapeutic interventions driven by MD biochemical changes will improve outcome in these patients.

## ELECTROPHYSIOLOGICAL MONITORING

Electroencephalogram (EEG) and evoked potentials (EPs) are the most commonly used electrophysiological techniques in the ICU.

### Electroencephalogram

The main application of the EEG in the ICU is detection and management of seizures and status epilepticus, particularly nonconvulsive seizures (NCSz) and nonconvulsive status epilepticus (NCSE), both of which frequently occur in the ICU setting. These typically manifest as persistent impairment in mental status after cessation of a convulsive seizure or unexplained fluctuation in mental status in critically ill patients with or without subtle clinical findings such as eyelid twitching, nystagmus, or facial twitching. NCSz occur in 48% and NCSE occurs in 14% of persistently unresponsive patients following cessation of convulsive status epilepticus.[68] Approximately 8% of medical ICU patients without a prior history of neurological disorder, 16% of surgical ICU patients, and 34% of neurological ICU patients develop NCSz and/or NCSE.[69–71]

Continuous EEG (cEEG) is usually required to detect electrographic seizures in ICU patients since routine EEG may miss more than half of those electrographic seizures detected by cEEG.[72] Longer duration of recording is usually required in comatose patients because 20% have their first seizure after more than 24 hours of monitoring, as compared to only 5% of noncomatose patients.[73] It is recommended that cEEG monitoring not be delayed in patients with brain injury who have an unexplained or a prolonged decreased level of consciousness.[11,74] Delayed treatment of seizures may result in increased resistance to antiseizure medications and secondary brain damage from ongoing seizures.[75–78]

Continuous EEG is also used to titrate intravenous infusions of anesthetics and sedative/hypnotics (i.e., midazolam, propofol, pentobarbital) in treatment of refractory status epilepticus, in order to use the lowest dose required to achieve seizure suppression or background suppression while minimizing systemic adverse effects.[79] It is also used to achieve the therapeutic goal of a burst-suppression pattern when barbiturate coma is induced for treatment of refractory elevated ICP.[80]

Quantitative EEG (qEEG) utilizes a number of algorithms to transform the raw EEG into data that can be displayed as graphs, and allows for rapid screening of large amounts of EEG data. The most traditional approach applies the fast Fourier transform to the digitally recorded EEG signal, creating power spectra (Figure 5.3). The qEEG is very helpful for seizure quantification and detection of ischemia since it allows for the quick review of several hours of cEEG data and may reveal subtle changes that occur over long periods of time and may not be evident in the raw EEG data.

Certain parameters of qEEG can be used to detect delayed cerebral ischemia and vasospasm after SAH (Figure 5.4).[81–82] Decrease in relative $\alpha$ variability on qEEG may precede the onset of the clinical symptoms of vasospasm in SAH patients and can be resolved with treatment.[83] The post-stimulation $\alpha$-$\delta$ (alpha-delta) power ratio (ADR) can detect delayed cerebral ischemia after poor grade SAH. A prolonged decrease of the ADR by more than 10%, or even a brief reduction by more than 50%, correlates well with development of delayed cerebral ischemia and may detect its development before the onset of clinical deterioration and the appearance of ischemic changes on brain CT scan.[84–85]

Subdural strip electrodes and intracortical depth electrodes are forms of intracranial invasive EEG that can detect abnormal electrophysiological activities that are not visible on scalp EEG, such cortical spreading depression (CSD) and depth seizures. CSD is a slow wave of sustained depolarization in the cortex.[86] These waves are commonly observed after acute brain injury such as severe TBI, SAH, and malignant MCA infarction.[87–88] CSD waves are associated with significant metabolic and hemodynamic changes, such as excitotoxicity, cerebral metabolic crisis, brain tissue hypoxia, and cerebral ischemia, that can cause secondary injury and lead to poor outcome in patients with acute brain injury.[89–93] The full extent to which CSD contributes to brain injury in these and other coma states remains to be elucidated, and no treatments have been tested to date.

Intracortical depth EEG allows for detection of intracortical seizures that are not readily apparent on scalp EEG.[94] Essentially a thin wire with six discrete EEG contacts separated by 4–5 mm, depth EEG is usually utilized in combination with other forms of invasive brain monitoring and has a safety profile similar to other

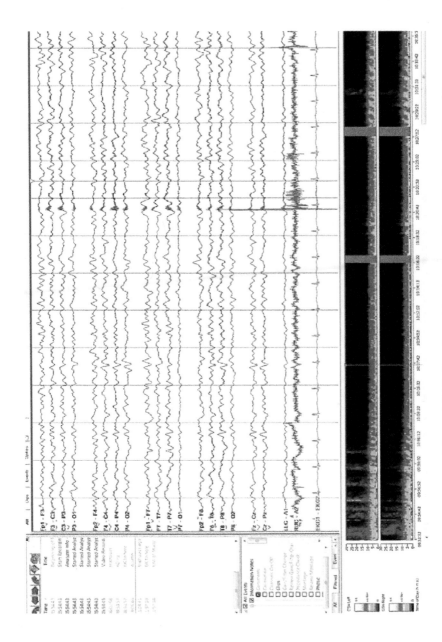

FIGURE 5.3 Quantitative electroencephalogram (qEEG) allows for a quick review of several hours of continuous EEG raw data.

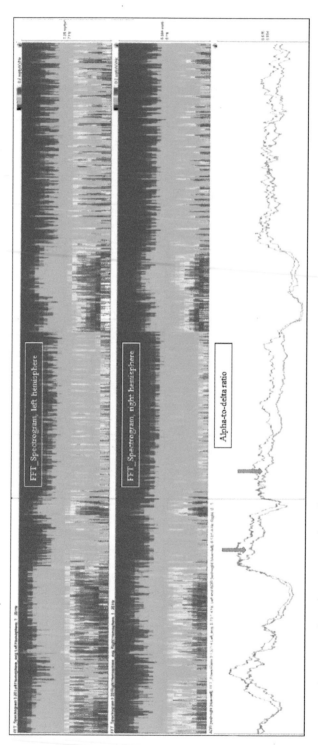

FIGURE 5.4 Quantitative electroencephalogram (qEEG) in patient with aneurysmal subarachnoid hemorrhage. Compressed spectral array (first and second rows from top) and α-to-δ ratio (bottom row) show decreased α-to-δ ratio of the right hemisphere (*arrows*) due to vasospasm.

invasive brain devices.[95–96] The clinical significance of isolated seizures exclusively detected by depth EEG is not yet clear. Studies using multimodality brain monitors, however, have shown that intracortical seizures are associated with metabolic crisis after severe TBI, as well as with sympathetic stimulation (elevated heart rate, blood pressure, and respiratory rate), rising CPP and ICP, and poor outcome after aneurysmal SAH.[76,97]

## Evoked Potentials

Sensory EPs are small electric discharges recorded from cerebral cortex after sensory stimuli (visual, auditory, or somatosensory). The main indication for EPs is to assess the integrity of sensory pathways, from the periphery up to the sensory cortex. The most commonly used EP in the neurological ICU is the median nerve somatosensory evoked potential (SSEP). SSEPs are used to assess the integrity of sensory pathways from the posterior column of the spinal cord, through the medial lemniscus and thalamus, and up to somatosensory cortex. It involves stimulation of a peripheral nerve and recording potentials from the somatosensory cortex. The amplitudes of SSEPs are much smaller than EEGs and therefore require averaging the signals received from multiple stimuli within a limited time period.

The main advantages of using SSEP in neurological ICUs are that it is noninvasive, it can assess the functional status of subcortical structures, and it can be used with mild hypothermia and most sedatives.[98] One of the main indications for SSEP is for prognostication after cardiac arrest and TBI. For instance, absence of the N20s wave bilaterally is an indicator of poor prognosis after cardiac arrest.[99]

## INTERPRETATION OF MULTIPLE MODALITIES

Acute brain injuries are often complex and dynamic. Multimodal monitoring allows for the assessment of a variety of physiological parameters (ICP, cerebral microdialysis, $PbtO_2$, $SjvO_2$, cEEG) to provide a comprehensive assessment that allows for real-time, early detection of secondary cerebral injury, and facilitates interventions to prevent or ameliorate further damage. Ideally, the information obtained from these multiple modalities should be integrated and interpreted collectively, rather than in isolation, so as to guide the management of acute brain injuries. It is a challenge to interpret a drop in $PbtO_2$ in isolation because there are many possible underlying causes. For example, a decrease in $PbtO_2$ in the context of an LPR increase, glucose decrease, rCBF decrease, and a jugular bulb oxygen saturation increase is almost certainly ischemia.

## CONCLUSION

Critically ill patients are often at risk of neurological deterioration due to primary acute brain injury or subsequent secondary brain insults. One of the main goals of monitoring neurologically ill patients in the ICU is detection of secondary brain injury early enough to intervene in order to prevent permanent damage. The bedside neurological examination remains the gold standard for assessment of patients with neurologic disease or injury; however, it may be insufficient or impractical in sedated patients or those with impaired levels of consciousness. Various neuroimaging studies provide valuable clinical information, but the information is restricted to the time of the study.

Monitoring various brain physiologic parameters by invasive and noninvasive means has therefore become an essential tool in the care of critically ill patients. Multimodal physiological monitoring provides a more comprehensive physiological assessment of the injured brain, allows real-time detection of ongoing (secondary) cerebral injury, and may guide interventions to prevent or ameliorate permanent damage. Importantly, these modalities should be interpreted collectively and not in isolation in the management of acute brain injuries, which are often complex and dynamic. Devices should be chosen based on the individual patient's needs and targeted pathophysiology.

## REFERENCES

1. Le Roux P, Menon DK, Citerio G, et al. Consensus summary statement of the International Multidisciplinary Consensus Conference on Multimodality Monitoring in Neurocritical Care: a statement for healthcare professionals from the Neurocritical Care Society and the European Society of Intensive Care Medicine. *Neurocrit Care*. 2014;21 Suppl 2:S1–26.

2. Badri S, Chen J, Barber J, et al. Mortality and long-term functional outcome associated with intracranial pressure after traumatic brain injury. *Intensive Care Med*. 2012;38(11):1800–9.

3. Treggiari MM, Schutz N, Yanez ND, Romand JA. Role of intracranial pressure values and patterns in predicting outcome in traumatic brain injury: a systematic review. *Neurocrit Care*. 2007;6(2):104–12.

4. Lundberg N. Continuous recording and control of ventricular fluid pressure in neurosurgical practice. *Acta Psych Scand*. 1960;36(Suppl 149):1–193.

5. Bratton SL, Chestnut RM, Ghajar J, et al. Guidelines for the management of severe traumatic brain injury. VI. Indications for intracranial pressure monitoring. *J Neurotrauma*. 2007;24 Suppl 1:S37–44.

6. Farahvar A, Gerber LM, Chiu YL, et al. Response to intracranial hypertension treatment as a predictor of death in patients with severe traumatic brain injury. *J Neurosurg*. 2011;114(5):1471–8.

7. Bratton SL, Chestnut RM, Ghajar J, et al. Guidelines for the management of severe traumatic brain injury. IX. Cerebral perfusion thresholds. *J Neurotrauma*. 2007;24 Suppl 1:S59–64.

8. Marmarou A, Saad A, Aygok G, Rigsbee M. Contribution of raised ICP and hypotension to CPP reduction in severe brain injury: correlation to outcome. *Acta Neurochir*. 2005;95(Suppl):277–80.

9. Robertson CS, Valadka AB, Hannay HJ, et al. Prevention of secondary ischemic insults after severe head injury. *Crit Care Med*. 1999;27(10):2086–95.

10. Chesnut RM, Temkin N, Carney N, et al. A trial of intracranial-pressure monitoring in traumatic brain injury. *N Engl J Med*. 2012;367(26):2471–81.

11. Le Roux P, Menon DK, Citerio G, et al. The International Multidisciplinary Consensus Conference on Multimodality Monitoring in Neurocritical Care: a list of recommendations and additional conclusions: a statement for healthcare professionals from the Neurocritical Care Society and the European Society of Intensive Care Medicine. *Neurocrit Care*. 2014;21 Suppl 2:S282–96.

12. Bederson JB, Connolly ES Jr, Batjer HH, et al. Guidelines for the management of aneurysmal subarachnoid hemorrhage: a statement for healthcare professionals from a special writing group of the Stroke Council, American Heart Association. *Stroke*. 2009;40(3):994–1025.

13. Hemphill JC 3rd, Greenberg SM, Anderson CS, et al. Guidelines for the Management of Spontaneous Intracerebral Hemorrhage: A Guideline for Healthcare Professionals from the American Heart Association/American Stroke Association. *Stroke.* 2015;46(7):2032–60.

14. Kristiansson H, Nissborg E, Bartek J Jr, Andresen M, Reinstrup P, Romner B. Measuring elevated intracranial pressure through noninvasive methods: a review of the literature. *J Neurosurg Anesthesiol.* 2013;25(4):372–85.

15. Rasulo FA, De Peri E, Lavinio A. Transcranial Doppler ultrasonography in intensive care. *Eur J Anaesthesiol.* 2008;42(Suppl):167–73.

16. Bellner J, Romner B, Reinstrup P, Kristiansson KA, Ryding E, Brandt L. Transcranial Doppler sonography pulsatility index (PI) reflects intracranial pressure (ICP). *Surg Neurol.* 2004;62(1):45–51; discussion 51.

17. Wang Y, Duan YY, Zhou HY, et al. Middle cerebral arterial flow changes on transcranial color and spectral Doppler sonography in patients with increased intracranial pressure. *J Ultrasound Med.* 2014;33(12):2131–6.

18. Behrens A, Lenfeldt N, Ambarki K, Malm J, Eklund A, Koskinen LO. Transcranial Doppler pulsatility index: not an accurate method to assess intracranial pressure. *Neurosurgery.* 2010;66(6):1050–7.

19. Shen Q, Stuart J, Venkatesh B, Wallace J, Lipman J. Inter observer variability of the transcranial Doppler ultrasound technique: impact of lack of practice on the accuracy of measurement. *J Clin Monitor Comput.* 1999;15(3-4):179–84.

20. Hansen HC, Helmke K. The subarachnoid space surrounding the optic nerves. An ultrasound study of the optic nerve sheath. *Surg Radiol Anat.* 1996;18(4):323–8.

21. Rajajee V, Vanaman M, Fletcher JJ, Jacobs TL. Optic nerve ultrasound for the detection of raised intracranial pressure. *Neurocrit Care.* 2011;15(3):506–15.

22. Chen JW, Gombart ZJ, Rogers S, Gardiner SK, Cecil S, Bullock RM. Pupillary reactivity as an early indicator of increased intracranial pressure: the introduction of the Neurological Pupil index. *Surg Neurol Intern.* 2011;2:82.

23. Frontera JA, Fernandez A, Schmidt JM, et al. Defining vasospasm after subarachnoid hemorrhage: what is the most clinically relevant definition? *Stroke.;* 2009;40(6):1963–8.

24. Claassen J, Bernardini GL, Kreiter K, et al. Effect of cisternal and ventricular blood on risk of delayed cerebral ischemia after subarachnoid hemorrhage: the Fisher scale revisited. *Stroke.* 2001;32(9):2012–20.

25. Suarez JI, Qureshi AI, Yahia AB, et al. Symptomatic vasospasm diagnosis after subarachnoid hemorrhage: evaluation of transcranial Doppler ultrasound and cerebral angiography as related to compromised vascular distribution. *Crit Care Med.* 2002;30(6):1348–55.

26. Vora YY, Suarez-Almazor M, Steinke DE, Martin ML, Findlay JM. Role of transcranial Doppler monitoring in the diagnosis of cerebral vasospasm after subarachnoid hemorrhage. *Neurosurgery.* 1999;44(6):1237–47; discussion 47–8.

27. Lindegaard KF, Nornes H, Bakke SJ, Sorteberg W, Nakstad P. Cerebral vasospasm diagnosis by means of angiography and blood velocity measurements. *Acta Neurochir.* 1989;100(1-2):12–24.

28. Vajkoczy P, Roth H, Horn P, et al. Continuous monitoring of regional cerebral blood flow: experimental and clinical validation of a novel thermal diffusion microprobe. *J Neurosurg.* 2000;93(2):265–74.

29. Phillips SJ, Whisnant JP. Hypertension and the brain. The National High Blood Pressure Education Program. *Arch Intern Med.* 1992;152(5):938–45.

30. Vajkoczy P, Horn P, Thome C, Munch E, Schmiedek P. Regional cerebral blood flow monitoring in the diagnosis of delayed ischemia following aneurysmal subarachnoid hemorrhage. *J Neurosurg.* 2003;98(6):1227–34.

31. Ko SB, Choi HA, Parikh G, et al. Real time estimation of brain water content in comatose patients. *Ann Neurol.* 2012;72(3):344–50.

32. Sioutos PJ, Orozco JA, Carter LP, Weinand ME, Hamilton AJ, Williams FC. Continuous regional cerebral cortical blood flow monitoring in head-injured patients. *Neurosurgery.* 1995;36(5):943–9; discussion 949–50.

33. Miller JI, Chou MW, Capocelli A, Bolognese P, Pan J, Milhorat TH. Continuous intracranial multimodality monitoring comparing local cerebral blood flow, cerebral perfusion pressure, and microvascular resistance. *Acta Neurochir.* 1998;71(Suppl):82–4.

34. Coles JP. Regional ischemia after head injury. *Curr Opin Crit Care.* 2004;10(2):120–5.

35. Siegemund M, van Bommel J, Ince C. Assessment of regional tissue oxygenation. *Intensive Care Med.* 1999;25(10):1044–60.

36. Dengler J, Frenzel C, Vajkoczy P, Wolf S, Horn P. Cerebral tissue oxygenation measured by two different probes: challenges and interpretation. *Intensive Care Med.* 2011;37(11):1809–15.

37. Sarrafzadeh AS, Kiening KL, Bardt TF, Schneider GH, Unterberg AW, Lanksch WR. Cerebral oxygenation in contusioned vs. nonlesioned brain tissue: monitoring of PtiO2 with Licox and Paratrend. *Acta Neurochir.* 1998;71(Suppl):186–9.

38. Maloney-Wilensky E, Gracias V, Itkin A, et al. Brain tissue oxygen and outcome after severe traumatic brain injury: a systematic review. *Crit Care Med.* 2009;37(6):2057–63.

39. Kett-White R, Hutchinson PJ, Al-Rawi PG, Gupta AK, Pickard JD, Kirkpatrick PJ. Adverse cerebral events detected after subarachnoid hemorrhage using brain oxygen and microdialysis probes. *Neurosurgery.* 2002;50(6):1213–21; discussion 1221–2.

40. Spiotta AM, Stiefel MF, Gracias VH, et al. Brain tissue oxygen-directed management and outcome in patients with severe traumatic brain injury. *J Neurosurg.* 2010;113(3):571–80.

41. Narotam PK, Morrison JF, Nathoo N. Brain tissue oxygen monitoring in traumatic brain injury and major trauma: outcome analysis of a brain tissue oxygen-directed therapy. *J Neurosurg.* 2009;111(4):672–82.

42. Bohman LE, Pisapia JM, Sanborn MR, et al. Response of brain oxygen to therapy correlates with long-term outcome after subarachnoid hemorrhage. *Neurocrit Care.* 2013;19(3):320–8.

43. Bratton SL, Chestnut RM, Ghajar J, et al. Guidelines for the management of severe traumatic brain injury. X. Brain oxygen monitoring and thresholds. *J Neurotrauma.* 2007;24 Suppl 1:S65–70.

44. Rosenthal G, Hemphill JC 3rd, Sorani M, et al. Brain tissue oxygen tension is more indicative of oxygen diffusion than oxygen delivery and metabolism in patients with traumatic brain injury. *Crit Care Med.* 2008;36(6):1917–24.

45. Stiefel MF, Udoetuk JD, Spiotta AM, et al. Conventional neurocritical care and cerebral oxygenation after traumatic brain injury. *J Neurosurg.* 2006;105(4):568–75.

46. Hlatky R, Valadka AB, Gopinath SP, Robertson CS. Brain tissue oxygen tension response to induced hyperoxia reduced in hypoperfused brain. *J Neurosurg.* 2008;108(1):53–8.

47. Obrist WD, Langfitt TW, Jaggi JL, Cruz J, Gennarelli TA. Cerebral blood flow and metabolism in comatose patients with acute head injury. Relationship to intracranial hypertension. *J Neurosurg.* 1984;61(2):241–53.

48. Le Roux PD, Newell DW, Lam AM, Grady MS, Winn HR. Cerebral arteriovenous oxygen difference: a predictor of cerebral infarction and outcome in patients with severe head injury. *J Neurosurg.* 1997;87(1):1–8.

49. Robertson CS, Gopinath SP, Goodman JC, Contant CF, Valadka AB, Narayan RK. SjvO2 monitoring in head-injured patients. *J Neurotrauma.* 1995;12(5):891–6.

50. Heran NS, Hentschel SJ, Toyota BD. Jugular bulb oximetry for prediction of vasospasm following subarachnoid hemorrhage. *Can J Neurol Sci.* 2004;31(1):80–6.

51. Gupta AK, Hutchinson PJ, Al-Rawi P, et al. Measuring brain tissue oxygenation compared with jugular venous oxygen saturation for monitoring cerebral oxygenation after traumatic brain injury. *Anesth Analg.* 1999;88(3):549–53.

52. Rosenthal G, Furmanov A, Itshayek E, Shoshan Y, Singh V. Assessment of a noninvasive cerebral oxygenation monitor in patients with severe traumatic brain injury. *J Neurosurg.* 2014;120(4):901–7.

53. Naidech AM, Bendok BR, Ault ML, Bleck TP. Monitoring with the Somanetics INVOS 5100C after aneurysmal subarachnoid hemorrhage. *Neurocrit Care.* 2008;9(3):326–31.

54. Hlatky R, Valadka AB, Goodman JC, Contant CF, Robertson CS. Patterns of energy substrates during ischemia measured in the brain by microdialysis. *J Neurotrauma.* 2004;21(7):894–906.

55. Sarrafzadeh AS, Thomale UW, Haux D, Unterberg AW. Cerebral metabolism and intracranial hypertension in high grade aneurysmal subarachnoid haemorrhage patients. *Acta Neurochir.* 2005;95(Suppl):89–92.

56. Persson L, Valtysson J, Enblad P, et al. Neurochemical monitoring using intracerebral microdialysis in patients with subarachnoid hemorrhage. *J Neurosurg.* 1996;84(4):606–16.

57. Sarrafzadeh A, Haux D, Kuchler I, Lanksch WR, Unterberg AW. Poor-grade aneurysmal subarachnoid hemorrhage: relationship of cerebral metabolism to outcome. *J Neurosurg.* 2004;100(3):400–6.

58. Goodman JC, Valadka AB, Gopinath SP, Uzura M, Robertson CS. Extracellular lactate and glucose alterations in the brain after head injury measured by microdialysis. *Crit Care Med.* 1999;27(9):1965–73.

59. Vespa PM, McArthur D, O'Phelan K, et al. Persistently low extracellular glucose correlates with poor outcome 6 months after human traumatic brain injury despite a lack of increased lactate: a microdialysis study. *J Cerebral Blood Flow Metabol.* 2003;23(7):865–77.

60. Skjøth-Rasmussen J, Schulz M, Kristensen SR, Bjerre P. Delayed neurological deficits detected by an ischemic pattern in the extracellular cerebral metabolites in patients with aneurysmal subarachnoid hemorrhage. *J Neurosurg.* 2004;100(1):8–15.

61. Sarrafzadeh AS, Sakowitz OW, Kiening KL, Benndorf G, Lanksch WR, Unterberg AW. Bedside microdialysis: a tool to monitor cerebral metabolism in subarachnoid hemorrhage patients? *Crit Care Med.* 2002;30(5):1062–70.

62. Helbok R, Madineni RC, Schmidt MJ, et al. Intracerebral monitoring of silent infarcts after subarachnoid hemorrhage. *Neurocrit Care.* 2011;14(2):162–7.

63. Hillered L, Vespa PM, Hovda DA. Translational neurochemical research in acute human brain injury: the current status and potential future for cerebral microdialysis. *J Neurotrauma.* 2005;22(1):3–41.

64. Helbok R, Schmidt JM, Kurtz P, et al. Systemic glucose and brain energy metabolism after subarachnoid hemorrhage. *Neurocrit Care.* 2010;12(3):317–23.

65. Oddo M, Schmidt JM, Carrera E, et al. Impact of tight glycemic control on cerebral glucose metabolism after severe brain injury: a microdialysis study. *Crit Care Med.* 2008;36(12):3233–8.

66. Schlenk F, Graetz D, Nagel A, Schmidt M, Sarrafzadeh AS. Insulin-related decrease in cerebral glucose despite normoglycemia in aneurysmal subarachnoid hemorrhage. *Crit Care.* 2008;12(1):R9.

67. Kurtz P, Claassen J, Schmidt JM, et al. Reduced brain/serum glucose ratios predict cerebral metabolic distress and mortality after severe brain injury. *Neurocrit Care.* 2013;19(3):311–9.

68. DeLorenzo RJ, Waterhouse EJ, Towne AR, et al. Persistent nonconvulsive status epilepticus after the control of convulsive status epilepticus. *Epilepsia.* 1998;39(8):833–40.

69. Oddo M, Carrera E, Claassen J, Mayer SA, Hirsch LJ. Continuous electroencephalography in the medical intensive care unit. *Crit Care Med.* 2009;37(6):2051–6.

70. Kurtz P, Gaspard N, Wahl AS, et al. Continuous electroencephalography in a surgical intensive care unit. *Intensive Care Med.* 2014;40(2):228–34.

71. Jordan KG. Neurophysiologic monitoring in the neuroscience intensive care unit. *Neurol Clin.* 1995;13(3):579–626.

72. Pandian JD, Cascino GD, So EL, Manno E, Fulgham JR. Digital video-electroencephalographic monitoring in the neurological-neurosurgical intensive care unit: clinical features and outcome. *Arch Neurol.* 2004;61(7):1090–4.

73. Claassen J, Mayer SA, Kowalski RG, Emerson RG, Hirsch LJ. Detection of electrographic seizures with continuous EEG monitoring in critically ill patients. *Neurology.* 2004;62(10):1743–8.

74. Brophy GM, Bell R, Claassen J, et al. Guidelines for the evaluation and management of status epilepticus. *Neurocrit Care.* 2012;17(1):3–23.

75. Vespa P, Prins M, Ronne-Engstrom E, et al. Increase in extracellular glutamate caused by reduced cerebral perfusion pressure and seizures after human traumatic brain injury: a microdialysis study. *J Neurosurg.* 1998;89(6):971–82.

76. Claassen J, Perotte A, Albers D, et al. Nonconvulsive seizures after subarachnoid hemorrhage: multimodal detection and outcomes. *Ann Neurol.* 2013;74(1):53–64.

77. Vespa PM, Miller C, McArthur D, et al. Nonconvulsive electrographic seizures after traumatic brain injury result in a delayed, prolonged increase in intracranial pressure and metabolic crisis. *Crit Care Med.* 2007;35(12):2830–6.

78. Vespa PM, O'Phelan K, Shah M, et al. Acute seizures after intracerebral hemorrhage: a factor in progressive midline shift and outcome. *Neurology.* 2003;60(9):1441–6.

79. Claassen J, Hirsch LJ, Emerson RG, Mayer SA. Treatment of refractory status epilepticus with pentobarbital, propofol, or midazolam: a systematic review. *Epilepsia.* 2002;43(2):146–53.

80. Winer JW, Rosenwasser RH, Jimenez F. Electroencephalographic activity and serum and cerebrospinal fluid pentobarbital levels in determining the therapeutic end point during barbiturate coma. *Neurosurgery.* 1991;29(5):739–41; discussion 41-2.

81. Wickering E, Gaspard N, Zafar S, et al. Automation of classical QEEG trending methods for early detection of delayed cerebral ischemia: more work to do. *J Clin Neurophysiol.* 2016;33(3):227–34.

82. Muniz CF, Shenoy AV, O'Connor KL, et al. Clinical development and implementation of an institutional guideline for prospective EEG monitoring and reporting of delayed cerebral ischemia. *J Clin Neurophysiol.* 2016;33(3):217–26.

83. Vespa PM, Nuwer MR, Juhasz C, et al. Early detection of vasospasm after acute subarachnoid hemorrhage using continuous EEG ICU monitoring. *Electroencephalogr Clin Neurophysiol.* 1997;103(6):607–15.

84. Claassen J, Hirsch LJ, Kreiter KT, et al. Quantitative continuous EEG for detecting delayed cerebral ischemia in patients with poor-grade subarachnoid hemorrhage. *Clin Neurophysiol.* 2004;115(12):2699–710.

85. Rots ML, van Putten MJ, Hoedemaekers CW, Horn J. Continuous EEG monitoring for early detection of delayed cerebral ischemia in subarachnoid hemorrhage: a pilot study. *Neurocrit Care.* 2016;24(2):207–16.

86. Dreier JP, Fabricius M, Ayata C, et al. Recording, analysis, and interpretation of spreading depolarizations in neurointensive care: review and recommendations of the COSBID research group. *J Cerebral Blood Flow Metabol.* 2017;37(5):1595-1625.

87. Dohmen C, Sakowitz OW, Fabricius M, et al. Spreading depolarizations occur in human ischemic stroke with high incidence. *Ann Neurol.* 2008;63(6):720–8.

88. Fabricius M, Fuhr S, Willumsen L, et al. Association of seizures with cortical spreading depression and peri-infarct depolarisations in the acutely injured human brain. *Clin Neurophysiol.* 2008;119(9):1973–84.

89. Schiefecker AJ, Beer R, Pfausler B, et al. Clusters of cortical spreading depolarizations in a patient with intracerebral hemorrhage: a multimodal neuromonitoring study. *Neurocrit Care.* 2015;22(2):293–8.

90. Sakowitz OW, Santos E, Nagel A, et al. Clusters of spreading depolarizations are associated with disturbed cerebral metabolism in patients with aneurysmal subarachnoid hemorrhage. *Stroke.* 2013;44(1):220–3.

91. Bosche B, Graf R, Ernestus RI, et al. Recurrent spreading depolarizations after subarachnoid hemorrhage decreases oxygen availability in human cerebral cortex. *Ann Neurol.* 2010;67(5):607–17.

92. Dreier JP, Major S, Manning A, et al. Cortical spreading ischaemia is a novel process involved in ischaemic damage in patients with aneurysmal subarachnoid haemorrhage. *Brain.* 2009;132(Pt 7):1866–81.

93. Hartings JA, Watanabe T, Bullock MR, et al. Spreading depolarizations have prolonged direct current shifts and are associated with poor outcome in brain trauma. *Brain.* 2011;134(Pt 5):1529–40.

94. Waziri A, Claassen J, Stuart RM, et al. Intracortical electroencephalography in acute brain injury. *Ann Neurol.* 2009;66(3):366–77.

95. Mikell CB, Dyster TG, Claassen J. Invasive seizure monitoring in the critically-Ill brain injury patient: current practices and a review of the literature. *Seizure.* 2016;41:201–5.

96. Stuart RM, Schmidt M, Kurtz P, et al. Intracranial multimodal monitoring for acute brain injury: a single institution review of current practices. *Neurocrit Care.* 2010;12(2):188–98.

97. Vespa P, Tubi M, Claassen J, et al. Metabolic crisis occurs with seizures and periodic discharges after brain trauma. *Ann Neurol.* 2016;79(4):579–90.

98. Cruccu G, Aminoff MJ, Curio G, et al. Recommendations for the clinical use of somatosensory-evoked potentials. *Clin Neurophysiol.* 2008;119(8):1705–19.

99. Bouwes A, Binnekade JM, Verbaan BW, et al. Predictive value of neurological examination for early cortical responses to somatosensory evoked potentials in patients with postanoxic coma. *J Neurol.* 2012;259(3):537–41.

# 6 Neurological and Functional Outcomes Assessment

Suzan Uysal and Stephan A. Mayer

## GENERAL CONSIDERATIONS

The evidence base for neuroprotective strategies in critical care and perioperative medicine rests on outcomes research, a critical component of which is the quantitative assessment of the functional effects of neurological injury and disease. Outcome assessment is generally conceptualized hierarchically in terms of *global outcome, impairment, disability, handicap,* and *health-related quality of life (HR-QOL).*[1] *Global outcome* refers to the spectrum from death to complete recovery. *Impairment* refers to specific loss of neurological function. *Disability* refers to the loss of independence in activities of daily living (ADLs) resulting from impairment. Disability can be further broken down into loss of independence in self-care *(ADLs)* such as walking, toileting, and eating, and *instrumental activities of daily living (IADLs)* such as using a phone, shopping, and housekeeping. *Handicap* refers to limitation of social or societal role function because of impairment or disability. HR-QOL is a multidimensional assessment of the patient's perceived physical, social, and emotional health status and well-being. This hierarchy is presented in Box 6.1, with examples of some of the most commonly used measures.

It is important to measure both neurological impairment and global outcome because reduced severity of neurological deficit and improved global outcome are the immediate results of any effective intervention.[2] Reduced severity of neurological impairment, however, is only meaningful to the patient if it results in less disability or handicap or improved QOL. Thus, neuroprotection trials should include outcome measures that are relevant to the patient, such as disability, handicap, and QOL scales.

### Outcome Measure Characteristics

When designing or evaluating clinical neuroprotection outcomes studies, it is important to consider the reliability of the measure, whether the measure is valid

> **Box 6.1** Commonly Used Outcome Measures
>
> **Global Outcome Scales**
> > Glasgow Outcome Scale (GOS)
> > Glasgow Outcome Scale- Extended (GOS-E)
> > Modified Rankin Scale (mRS)
>
> **Impairment Scales**
> > *Neurological Deficit Scales*
> > > Glasgow Coma Scale (GCS)
> > > The Rancho Los Amigos Scale (RLAS)
> > > NIH Stroke Scale (NIHSS)
> >
> > *Neurocognitive Testing*
> > > Montreal Cognitive Assessment (MOCA)
> > > Telephone Interview for Cognitive Status (TICS)
> > > Multidomain neuropsychological testing
>
> **Disability and Handicap Scales**
> > ADL Scales
> > > Barthel Index
> > > Disability Rating Scale (DRS)
> > IADL Scales
> > > Lawton Instrumental Activities of Daily Living Scale
>
> **Quality of Life Scales**
> > EuroQol Five-Dimension Scale (EQ-5D)
> > Sickness Impact Profile 68 (SIP68)
> > Short Form Health Survey 36 (SF-36)
> > Stroke Specific Quality Of Life Scale (SS-QOL)

for the intended purpose, and whether it is responsive to change over time. The reliability of an instrument reflects its *consistency*—the degree to which it is free from measurement error. Test–retest reliability reflects the degree to which a score obtained by a person at one time-point is similar/identical at a second time-point when there has been no change in the underlying construct being measured. Inter-rater reliability reflects the degree to which a score given by one rater is matched by the score given by a second rater. By classical test theory, a person's obtained score on a test is the sum of a true score (error-free score) and an error score. Reliability reflects the proportion of the total observed variance (which is comprised of true score variance plus error variance) that is due to true score variance.

It is also important to use measures of outcome that can be applied to all subjects regardless of their degree of impairment. Combining events to make up a single response variable (i.e., death or severe disability) is an accepted approach for clinical trials that allows the inclusion of all patients in a dichotomized outcome variable.[3]

It is desirable that measures of outcome can be expressed as a single dichotomous, ordinal, or continuous variable for ease of data interpretation.[3] Instruments that generate multiple scores, such as neuropsychological test batteries and multiattribute QOL scales, are problematic in this regard. Categorical analysis of outcome measures is generally preferred to comparing median scores derived from ordinal scales because the results can be expressed in a much more clinically meaningful way (e.g., "the treatment increases the likelihood of survival with minimal or no disability by 30%").

## Statistical Analysis of Ordinal Outcome Scales

Many of the metrics used in outcomes research that assesses efficacy of neuroprotective strategies are ordinal scales. Ordinal scales measure the magnitude of a variable in terms of rank order. The differences between each level of the scale do not reflect quantitative differences, as they do on interval and ratio scales.

There are a variety of methods for comparing the distributions of two groups assessed with an ordinal outcome scale. The simplest and most straightforward approach is to compare the proportion of patients in each group above and below a prespecified cutpoint. For instance, the cutpoint can be used to identify the proportion of survivors who escaped death or severe disability (e.g., modified Rankin Scale [mRS] score of 4–6 versus 0–3), which might be appropriate for a study of devastating illness such as severe traumatic brain injury, or survivors with an extremely good outcome and minimal or no disability (e.g., mRS 3–6 versus 0–2), which might be appropriate for a study of an intervention for mild acute ischemic stroke. The advantage of this approach is its simplicity. The disadvantages are loss of information and the arbitrariness of where the cutpoint is drawn. The latter problem is illustrated by the results of the European Cooperative Acute Stroke Study (ECASS) trial of intravenous thrombolysis using recombinant tissue plasminogen activator (rtPA) for acute ischemic stroke.[4] This was a negative study based on the prespecified cutpoint. However, if the investigators had set the cutpoint just one level higher, the observed trend toward improved outcome with rtPA would have reached statistical significance.

Another approach is to use a "sliding dichotomy." In this prognosis-based approach the cutpoint that identifies patients with "favorable" versus "unfavorable" outcome is different depending on the prognosis that is calculated at the time of randomization. The Surgical Trial in Intracerebral Hemorrhage (STICH) used this approach and found negative results with the cutpoint for patients with a poor prognosis drawn between upper and lower severe disability, and the cutpoint for subjects with a good prognosis drawn between lower moderate and upper severe disability.[5]

The most popular methodology for evaluating global outcome scales in clinical trials today is the "shift analysis" approach. This form analysis compares the proportion of patients across the entire spectrum of outcome except death or severe disability (i.e., mRS levels 5 and 6), which are combined. The reason for this is twofold. First, physicians and families can heavily influence who lives or dies in the ICU based on the different approaches taken regarding "goals of care" that affect decision-making. Second, there is no general agreement whether survival in a neurologically devastated condition (i.e., comatose with a tracheotomy and feeding tube) is "better" or "worse" than death. In shift analysis, a pooled odds ratio that expresses the likelihood of moving from any given outcome level to the next best level is calculated using ordinal logistic regression or a similar statistical test. This methodology is only valid if the direction of change is consistent across all levels of outcome (i.e., it cannot be used if a given intervention results in more patients at the extremes of outcome, such as no disability *and* greater mortality). Finally, the pooled odds ratio can be adjusted by controlling for prespecified covariates that are known to influence outcome at the time of randomization, such as age, Glasgow Coma Scale (GCS) score, National Institutes of Health Stroke Scale (NIHSS) score, or ordinal gradations of lesion volume.

Finally, another approach to assessing outcome in clinical neuroprotection trials is to simultaneously test for a treatment effect using a combination of scales. This was the approach used by the NIH rtPA Stroke Study.[6] This trial, which was the first to demonstrate the benefit of an intervention for ischemic stroke, evaluated outcome using two global outcome scales (the Glasgow Outcome Scale and the mRS), a disability scale that rates dependence in basic ADLs (the Barthel Index), and a neurological impairment scale (the NIHSS). A global test statistic (the Wald test) was generated using generalized estimating equations to simultaneously test for a treatment effect on all four outcome scales, dichotomized at a level of "highly favorable outcome" as the primary outcome measure. The attractiveness of this approach is that it allows a single basic hypothesis to be tested (e.g., Does rtPA improve outcome?) while taking several different measures of outcome into account simultaneously. Because critical illnesses and perioperative insults to the nervous system produce wide-ranging impairments, from devastating neurological deficits to subtle cognitive impairment, neuroprotection research should simultaneously evaluate outcome at different levels along the spectrum, from complete devastation to complete health, rather than using different measures that evaluate the same level of outcome.

## GLOBAL OUTCOME SCALES

Global outcomes scales measure the complete range of functional outcome ranging from death to survival with no disability. Because of their inclusiveness, the global outcome scales described here are the preferred measures of outcome in clinical trials.

### Glasgow Outcome Scale

The Glasgow Outcome Scale (GOS) is a brief descriptive scale used to determine the extent of a brain injury, to assess recovery, and to predict long-term outcome.[7–8] It is comprised of a single-item, five-level ordinal scale with scores ranging from 1 to 5. Higher scores reflect better functional status and are predictive of improved outcomes (Box 6.2).

---

**Box 6.2** Glasgow Outcome Scale (GOS)

1 DEATH
2 PERSISTENT VEGETATIVE STATE: Patient exhibits no obvious cortical function.
3 SEVERE DISABILITY: Conscious but disabled. Patient depends upon others for daily support due to mental or physical disability or both.
4 MODERATE DISABILITY: Disabled but independent. Patient is independent as far as daily life is concerned. The disabilities found include varying degrees of dysphasia, hemiparesis, or ataxia, as well as intellectual and memory deficits and personality changes.
5 GOOD RECOVERY: Resumption of normal activities even though there may be minor neurological or psychological deficits.

_____ GOS SCORE (1–5)

---

## The Glasgow Outcome Scale-Extended

The Extended Glasgow Outcome Scale (GOS-E) expands the GOS scale from 5 to 8 categories by dividing GOS categories 3–5 each into two categories.[9–10] Thus, the GOS-E is a single-item, eight-level ordinal scale, with scores ranging from 1 to 8 and higher scores predicting better outcomes (Box 6.3). The GOS-E was developed for the purpose of overcoming limitations of the GOS attributable to broad categories that are insensitive to change. The GOS-E is more sensitive to change in mild to moderate TBI, compared to the GOS. Use of a structured interview and rating form facilitates rating consistency.[11]

## The Modified Rankin Scale

The mRS is a measure of global disability and dependence in ADLs following stroke and other causes of neurological disability. It is widely used for clinical purposes to assess rehabilitation needs and outpatient course and in clinical trials that include assessment of stroke outcomes. The mRS consists of a single item that is rated on a seven-level ordinal scale (Box 6.4).[12] Scores range from 0 to 6, with lower scores reflecting better outcomes. Objectivity and inter-rater reliability can be enhanced by using structured assessment tools to guide raters in assigning mRS grades, such as the Rankin Focused Assessment (RFA), which provides clear, operationalized criteria to distinguish the seven assignable global disability levels, and the mRS-9Q, which consists of nine questions that each require a simple "yes" or "no" answer.[13–14]

## IMPAIRMENT SCALES

Impairment scales quantify the degree and extent of loss of neurological function. They represent the numerical measure of findings that can only be assessed with bedside examination or neurocognitive testing.

Box 6.4 Modified Rankin Scale (mRS)

0  NO SYMPTOMS AT ALL
1  NO SIGNIFICANT DISABILITY DESPITE SYMPTOMS: Able to carry out all usual duties and activities
2  SLIGHT DISABILITY: Unable to carry out all previous activities, but able to look after own affairs without assistance
3  MODERATE DISABILITY: Requiring some help, but able to walk without assistance
4  MODERATELY SEVERE DISABILITY: Unable to walk without assistance and unable to attend to own bodily needs without assistance
5  SEVERE DISABILITY: Bedridden, incontinent, and requiring constant nursing care and attention
6  DEAD

_____ mRS SCORE (1–6)

## Neurological Deficit Scales

Neurological deficit scales quantify neurological impairment or loss of neurological function. These scales are generated by bedside examination and are best characterized by the GCS, the NIHSS, and a large number of tests that quantify neurocognitive function, such as the Montreal Cognitive Assessment (MoCA) and the Telephone Interview of Cognitive Status (TICS). Such scales provide a structured framework for rating the severity of specific signs or deficits that are characteristic of the condition that the scale is designed to assess. Neurologic deficit scales are used to estimate the severity of acute neurologic injury, to monitor recovery and deterioration, to assess prognosis, and to evaluate the efficacy of therapeutic interventions. Some scales apply to a variety of clinical conditions and therefore can be described as "generic" in nature, while other scales are designed to assess neurologic deficit due to a specific condition (e.g., stroke scales).

## The Glasgow Coma Scale

The GCS is used to assess neurological status by rating the state of consciousness.[15] Three behaviors reflecting responsiveness to the environment are assessed: best eye opening response, best verbal response, and best motor response. Responsivity within each behavioral domain is graded, as indicated in Box 6.5. Eye opening is rated on a 4-point scale, verbal responsivity is graded on a 5-point scale, and motor responsivity is rated on a 6-point scale. Within each domain, the lowest score is 1, reflecting the worst function. The three domain scores are summed to yield the total GCS score. Thus, the lowest possible GCS score is 3, reflecting deep coma or brain death (i.e., no eye opening, no verbal response, no motor response), and the highest possible GCS score is 15, indicating full consciousness. In clinical practice, the total GCS score should be reported with the domain scores, such as GCS-11: E3 V3 M5.

Tracheal intubation makes it impossible to test the verbal response, and severe swelling around or damage to the eye makes it impossible to test eye responses. In these circumstances, a score of 1 is given for the domain with a modifier of "c"

Box 6.5 Glasgow Coma Scale (GCS)

### EYE OPENING

1  NONE: Even to supraorbital pressure
2  T O PAIN: Pain from sternum/limb/supraorbital pressure
3  T O SPEECH: Nonspecific response, not necessarily to command
4  SPONTANEOUS: Eyes open, not necessarily aware

_____  GCS EYE OPENING SUBSCALE SCORE (1–4)

### MOTOR RESPONSE

1  NONE: To any pain; limbs remain flaccid
2  EXTENSION: Shoulder adducted and shoulder and forearm internally rotated
3  FLEXOR RESPONSE: Withdrawal response or assumption of hemiplegic posture
4  WITHDRAWAL: Arm withdraws to pain, shoulder abducts
5  LOCALIZES PAIN: Arm attempts to remove supraorbital/chest pressure
6  OBEYS COMMANDS: Follows simple commands

_____  GCS MOTOR RESPONSE SUBSCALE SCORE (1–6)

### VERBAL RESPONSE

1  NONE: No verbalization of any type
2  INCOMPREHENSIBLE: Moans/groans, no speech
3  INAPPROPRIATE: Intelligible, no sustained sentences
4  CONFUSED: Converses but confused, disoriented
5  ORIENTED: Converses and oriented

_____  GCS VERBAL RESPONSE SUBSCALE SCORE (1–5)

_____  TOTAL GCS SCORE (3–15)

indicating closed eyes and "t" indicating tube. Thus, a composite score "GCS 5tc" would indicate eyes closed because of swelling = 1, intubated = 1, leaving a motor score of 3 for "abnormal flexion." The GCS for intubated patients is scored out of 10, omitting the verbal response grading.

TBI severity is classified based on the initial GCS score. Injuries resulting in initial GCS scores of 8 or lower are classified as severe, 9–12 are classified as moderate, and 13 or higher are classified as mild. Serial assessment of the GCS score is also used to monitor recovery and deterioration.

The GCS was originally developed as an objective, standardized method for rating the severity of TBI and monitoring recovery, but it is applicable in diverse medical contexts.

## The Rancho Los Amigos Scale

The Rancho Los Amigos Scale (RLAS), also known as the Rancho Level of Cognitive Functioning Scale (LCFS), is widely used clinically in the TBI patient

**Box 6.6** Rancho Los Amigos Scale (RLAS)/Rancho Los Amigos

LEVEL OF COGNITIVE FUNCTIONING SCALE (LCFS)

Level I      NO RESPONSE: Patient does not respond to external stimuli and appears asleep.

Level II     GENERALIZED RESPONSE: Patient reacts to external stimuli in nonspecific, inconsistent, and nonpurposeful manner with stereotypic and limited responses.

Level III    LOCALIZED RESPONSE: Patient responds specifically and inconsistently with delays to stimuli, but may follow simple commands for motor action.

Level IV     CONFUSED, AGITATED RESPONSE: Patient exhibits bizarre, nonpurposeful, incoherent, or inappropriate behaviors, has no short-term recall, attention is short, and nonselective.

Level V      CONFUSED, INAPPROPRIATE, NONAGITATED RESPONSE: Patient gives random, fragmented, and nonpurposeful responses to complex or unstructured stimuli. Simple commands are followed consistently, memory and selective attention are impaired, and new information is not retained.

Level VI     CONFUSED, APPROPRIATE RESPONSE: Patient gives context appropriate, goal-directed responses, dependent upon external input for direction. There is carry-over for relearned, but not for new tasks, and recent memory problems persist.

Level VII    AUTOMATIC, APPROPRIATE RESPONSE: Patient behaves appropriately in familiar settings, performs daily routines automatically, and shows carry-over for new learning at lower than normal rates. Patient initiates social interactions, but judgment remains impaired.

Level VIII   PURPOSEFUL, APPROPRIATE RESPONSE: Patient oriented and responds to the environment, but abstract reasoning abilities are decreased relative to premorbid levels.

_____ RLAS LEVEL (I–VIII)

population to describe status and assess recovery.[16] It consists of a single-item 8-point scale (Box 6.6). The eight levels represent the typical sequential progression of recovery from coma to full consciousness. The RLAS is most appropriate for comatose study populations who are entering rehabilitation after the acute treatment period has ended.

## The NIH Stroke Scale

The NIHSS is a structured assessment tool for objectively rating the severity of neurological deficits related to hemispheric infarction.[17] It comprises 11 stroke symptoms, each rated on a 3-, 4-, or 5-point scale, with scores of 0 reflecting normal function (i.e., no symptoms) and higher scores reflecting greater deficit.

The domains and symptoms are: level of consciousness (0–7), extraocular movements (0–2), visual field loss (0–3), facial palsy (0–3), arm strength (0–4 for each arm), leg strength (0–4 for each leg), limb ataxia (0–2), somatosensory loss (0–2), aphasia (0–3), dysarthria (0–2), and hemi-inattention (0–2). Total scores range from 0 (indicating normal function, no stroke) to 42. Severity is classified, based on the earliest NIHSS score, as no stroke symptoms (0), minor stroke (1–4), moderate stroke (5–15), moderate to severe stroke (16–20), and severe stroke (21–42).

The scale focuses on symptoms caused by anterior circulation stroke and under-represents posterior circulation and brainstem stroke. The NIHSS scores correlate with both degree of ischemic tissue damage and short- and long-term outcomes (criterion validity).

The NIHSS is the most frequently used stroke scale in clinical practice and clinical trials. It is well validated and has high inter-rater reliability. Online training is available through the National Institute of Neurological Disorders and Stroke, the National Stroke Association, and the American Stroke Association (see learn.heart.org/hihss.aspx). It is not, however, without limitations. Some of the items have poor reliability (facial palsy, ataxia, dysarthria and level of consciousness), and there is some redundancy in the items. A modified NIHSS, with fewer items and simpler grading, has higher reliability and validity than the standard NIHSS.[18-19]

## Neurocognitive Testing

Neurocognitive function is an ideal endpoint for clinical trials of neuroprotective interventions. Global measures of cognitive function yield a single test score. The single test score approach to measuring neurocognitive function is useful when evaluating the overall temporal course of a major neurocognitive disorder, such as the rate of decline or recovery. It also is appealing for research purposes because of the simplicity of statistical analysis of change in one test score rather than analysis of change in many test scores. Ideally, global measures of cognitive function that yield a single cognition endpoint should be applicable across a wide functional range (i.e., without floor and ceiling effects), sensitive to small changes in cognitive functioning, and relevant to a wide variety of pathologies (e.g., ischemic and hemorrhagic stroke, traumatic brain injury).

The single test score approach, however, lacks domain specificity and generally has low sensitivity to both mild changes in global cognitive function and modest changes that are restricted to a single domain. Multidomain neuropsychological testing does not have these limitations.

## The Montreal Cognitive Assessment

The MoCA is a cognitive screening test that assesses multiple cognitive domains: orientation to time and place, attention and working memory, short-term memory (learning and recall), visuospatial abilities (copying a geometric shape), language (naming and repetition), aspects of executive function, and abstract thinking.[20] The test and administration instructions are freely accessible (see www.mocatest.org). There are alternate forms designed for use in longitudinal settings and a basic form for use with subjects with limited education. It is available in many languages.

## Telephone Interview for Cognitive Status

The TICS is a brief, standardized cognitive test that was developed to be administered via telephone for situations where in-person cognitive screening is impractical.[21] It may also be administered face-to-face, and because it does not use visual stimuli it is also suitable for assessing cognitive function in individuals who are visually impaired or who are unable to read or write. The TICS correlates highly with the Mini-Mental State Examination (MMSE), has high test-retest reliability, and excellent sensitivity and specificity for the detection of cognitive impairment.

## Multidomain Neuropsychological Testing

Cognition is not a unitary phenomenon but rather is the net result of the integrated workings of multiple neural networks that govern distinct processes (e.g., attention, language, memory) that may be selectively affected. Thus, many cognitive outcomes studies employ combinations (batteries) of tests to assess multiple domains of cognitive function. There are, however, *many* tests that may be chosen.[22–23] Consequently, outcome studies utilizing test batteries vary widely in terms of the tests employed, which complicates comparison of outcomes across studies. Test score interpretation also poses challenges. Evaluation of cognitive change over time by serial cognitive testing must take into account measurement error due to normal test-retest variability because low or abnormal scores commonly occur in normal samples.[24–26]

## DISABILITY AND HANDICAP SCALES

Basic ADLs consist of self-care tasks that include functional mobility, toilet hygiene, bathing/showering, dressing, personal hygiene and grooming, and self-feeding. IADLs are higher-level functional abilities that are necessary for functioning within community settings. The ability to independently perform these activities normally is lost before basic ADLs. These activities include shopping, housekeeping, telephone communication, managing money, managing medications, and transportation. The Barthel index (BI) and the Lawton-Brody IADL Scale are the most widely used disability scales. Other measures of ADLs include the Katz Index of Independence in Activities of Daily Living, the Physical Self-Maintenance Scale (PSMS), and the Independent Living Scale (ILS).

## Activities of Daily Living Scales

### Barthel Index

The Barthel Index is a widely used measure of independence in performing 10 ADLs (Box 6.7).[27] Each activity is rated on an ordinal scale. A maximum score of 100 indicates independence in function in all 10 items, with no loss of function scored as 10 points, partial loss of independence as 5 points, and complete disability as 0 points for each item. Use of aids to be independent is allowed.

### Disability Rating Scale

The Disability Rating Scale (DRS) tracks recovery in moderate to severe TBI, from coma to reintegration into the community.[28–29] It is a 30-point continuous scale that

**Box 6.7** The Barthel Index

**SCORE**

**FEEDING**
- 0 = unable
- 5 = needs help cutting, spreading butter, etc., or requires modified diet
- 10 = independent

**BATHING**
- 0 = dependent
- 5 = independent (or in shower)

**GROOMING**
- 0 = needs to help with personal care
- 5 = independent face/hair/teeth/shaving (implements provided)

**DRESSING**
- 0 = dependent
- 5 = needs help but can do about half unaided
- 10 = independent (including buttons, zips, laces, etc.

**BOWELS**
- 0 = incontinent (or needs to be given enemas)
- 5 = occasional accident
- 10 = continent

**BLADDER**
- 0 = incontinent, or catheterized and unable to manage alone
- 5 = occasional accident
- 10 = continent

**TOILET USE**
- 0 = dependent
- 5 = needs some help, but can do something alone
- 10 = independent (on and off, dressing, wiping)

**TRANSFERS (BED TO CHAIR AND BACK)**
- 0 = unable, no sitting balance
- 5 = major help (one or two people, physical), can sit
- 10 = minor help (verbal or physical)
- 15 = independent

**MOBILITY (ON LEVEL SURFACES)**
- 0 = immobile or <50 yards
- 5 = wheelchair independent, including corners, >50 yards
- 10 = walks with help of one person (verbal or physical) >50 yards
- 15 = independent (but may use any aid; for example, stick) >50 yards

**STAIRS**
- 0 = unable
- 5 = needs help (verbal, physical, carrying aid)
- 10 = independent

_____ **TOTAL (0–100)**

**Copyright Information**

The Maryland State Medical Society holds the copyright for the Barthel Index. It may be used freely for non- commercial purposes with the following citation:

Mahoney FI, Barthel D. Functional evaluation: the Barthel Index.

*Maryland State Med J* 1965;14:56–61. Used with permission. Permission is required to modify the Barthel Index or to use it for commercial purposes.

evaluates eight areas of functioning in four categories: (1) arousability, awareness, and responsivity; (2) cognitive ability for self-care activities; (3) dependence on others; and (4) employability. Each area of functioning is rated on a scale of 0–3 or 0–5, with 0 representing no deficit or disability. The range of total DRS scores is from 0 to 29, with 0 indicating no disability, higher scores representing increasing disability, and scores in the range of 22 to 29 representing increasing degrees of vegetative state.

## Instrumental Activities of Daily Living Scales

### Lawton-Brody Instrumental Activities of Daily Living Scale

The Lawton-Brody Instrumental Activities of Daily Living (IADL) Scale assesses independence in ability to perform more complex IADLs necessary for functioning in community settings.[30] The scale comprises 8 items, each of which is rated on a 2-point scale (0–1), yielding a summary score ranging from 0 (low functioning) to 8 (high functioning) (see Box 6.8). IADLs are scored based on what an individual is *able* to do and not necessarily on what they are doing.

## HEALTH-RELATED QUALITY OF LIFE SCALES

HR-QOL refers to the impact that health status has on an individual's well-being. The purpose of HR-QOL measurement is to quantify the degree to which the medical condition or its treatment impacts the individual's life. Since it is from the patient's perspective, the patient makes the assessment. Thus, the instruments are self-report questionnaires. HR-QOL is also multidimensional and encompasses the impact of injury, disease, or disability on physical function, occupational function, psychological state, and social roles and interactions. These measurements can be used to assess changes over time and compare the effectiveness of different treatments within clinical trials.

HR-QOL questionnaires can be classified as assessing dimensions of life that are generally applicable to people (i.e., generic HR-QOL) or assessing variables that relate to a specific disease, injury, or disorder (condition-specific HR-QOL). Generic HR-QOL instruments are often used to supplement condition-specific QOL measures because they enable comparisons with other patient groups and the general population.

## The EuroQol Five-Dimension Scale

The EuroQol Five-Dimension Scale (EQ-5D) measures five dimensions of HR-QOL: mobility, self-care, usual activities, pain/discomfort, and anxiety/depression.[31] Each dimension is rated on a 5-point scale reflecting level of perceived problem, with the lowest score of 1 indicating the best health state and higher scores indicating more severe or frequent problems.

## Short Form Health Survey 36

The Short Form Health Survey 36 (SF-36) is a generic HR-QOL measure comprising 36 questions assessing eight domains: (1) vitality, (2) physical functioning, (3) bodily pain, (4) general health perceptions, (5) physical role functioning,

### Ability to Use Telephone

1 Operates telephone on own initiative; looks up and dials numbers
2 Dials a few well-known numbers
3 Answers telephone, but does not dial
4 Does not use telephone at all

### Shopping

1 Takes care of all shopping needs independently
2 Shops independently for small purchases
3 Needs to be accompanied on any shopping trip
4 Completely unable to shop

### Food Preparation

1 Plans, prepares, and serves adequate meals independently
2 Prepares adequate meals if supplied with ingredients
3 Heats and serves prepared meals or prepares meals but does not maintain adequate diet
4 Needs to have meals prepared and served

### Housekeeping

1 Maintains house alone with occasion assistance (heavy work)
2 Performs light daily tasks such as dishwashing, bed-making
3 Performs light daily tasks, but cannot maintain acceptable level of cleanliness
4 Needs help with all home maintenance tasks
5 Does not participate in any housekeeping tasks

### Laundry

1 Does personal laundry completely
2 Launders small items, rinses socks, stockings, etc.
3 All laundry must be done by others

### Mode of Transportation

1 Travels independently on public transportation or drives own car
2 Arranges own travel via taxi, but does not otherwise use public transportation
3 Travels on public transportation when assisted or accompanied by another
4 Travel limited to taxi or automobile with assistance of another
5 Does not travel at all

### Responsibility for Own Medications

1 Is responsible for taking medication in correct dosages at correct time
2 Takes responsibility if medication is prepared in advance in separate dosages
3 Is not capable of dispensing own medication

### Ability to Handle Finances

1 Manages financial matters independently (budgets, writes checks, pays rent and bills, goes to bank); collects and keeps track of income
2 Manages day-to-day purchases, but needs help with banking, major purchases, etc.
3 Incapable of handling money

_____ IADL SCORE (0–8)

**Source**: Lawton MP, Brody EM. Assessment of older people: self-maintaining and instrumental activities of daily living. *Gerontologist*. 1969;9:179–86.

(6) emotional role functioning, (7) social role functioning, and (8) mental health.[32] The scoring is norm-based. Higher scores reflect greater levels of health.

## The Stroke Specific Quality of Life Scale

The Stroke Specific Quality of Life Scale (SS-QOL) is an HR-QOL measure that is specific to patients with stroke (Box 6.9).[33-34] It comprises 49 items that are assessed on a 5-point scale (1–5), resulting in a summary score that ranges from 49 to 245, with higher scores indicating better function. It assesses 12 domains: energy, family roles, language, mobility, mood, personality, self-care, social roles, thinking, upper extremity function, vision, and work productivity.

## OUTCOME MEASURES RESOURCES

There are several resources that clinicians and clinical researchers may refer to when choosing outcome measures for and evaluating results of clinical neuroprotection trials. These resources provide comprehensive descriptions of the outcome measures, background information on validity and reliability, a reference list of published studies, and in many cases the rating forms. The *Handbook of Neurologic Rating Scales* is one such resource.[35] Online resources include the Center for Outcome Measurement in Brain Injury (COMBI) and the Rehabilitation Measures Database. The COMBI (http://www.tbims.org/combi/) provides outcome measures used for clinical and research purposes in the assessment and treatment of brain injuries. There are currently more than 25 instruments featured on the COMBI. The Rehabilitation Measures Database (http://www.rehabmeasures.org) is a compendium of measures for spinal cord injuries, traumatic brain injuries, and stroke.

## The NIH Toolbox for the Assessment of Neurological and Behavioral Function

The NIH Toolbox for the Assessment of Neurological and Behavioral Function is a computer-driven battery of 45 tests assessing cognitive, emotional, motor, and sensory function of individuals aged 3–85 (http://www.nihtoolbox.org). The NIH Toolbox was developed for the purpose of establishing a standard set of measures that can serve as a "common currency," allowing comparison of results both across studies and across the lifespan.[36-37] The Toolbox was launched in 2012, and its use in research has steadily increased over time. The NIH Toolbox was developed to facilitate wide adoption of this set of outcome measures and thereby advance the science of intervention and treatment efficacy evaluation.

The NIH Toolbox is easily administered and time efficient; the full battery of 45 tests can be completed in less than 2 hours. There is a Spanish version. The tests have high reliability. The normative sample is national (United States) and comprises thousands of people. The norms are age-based but can be refined further by ethnicity, education level, and gender. All Toolbox measures include the standard error of measurement, and many have values for minimally important difference. To ensure that those administering and interpreting the tests are trained properly, users must be preapproved to access the Toolbox's cognition measures.

Box 6.9 STROKE SPECIFIC QUALITY OF LIFE SCALE (SS-QOL)

Score each item according to the following key

1 Total help—Couldn't do it at all—Strongly agree
2 A lot of help—A lot of trouble—Moderately agree
3 Some help—Some trouble—Neither agree nor disagree
4 A little help—A little trouble—Moderately disagree
5 No help needed—No trouble at all—Strongly disagree

### Energy

1. I felt tired most of the time.
2. I had to stop and rest during the day.
3. I was too tired to do what I wanted to do.

### Family Roles

1. I didn't join in activities just for fun with my family.
2. I felt I was a burden to my family.
3. My physical condition interfered with my personal life.

### Language

1. Did you have trouble speaking? For example, get stuck, stutter, stammer, or slur your words?
2. Did you have trouble speaking clearly enough to use the telephone?
3. Did other people have trouble in understanding what you said?
4. Did you have trouble finding the word you wanted to say?
5. Did you have to repeat yourself so others could understand you?

### Mobility

1. Did you have trouble walking?
   (If patient can't walk, go to question 4 and score questions 2–3 as 1.)
2. Did you lose your balance when bending over to or reaching for something?
3. Did you have trouble climbing stairs?
4. Did you have to stop and rest more than you would like when walking or using a wheelchair?
5. Did you have trouble with standing?
6. Did you have trouble getting out of a chair?

### Mood

1. I was discouraged about my future.
2. I wasn't interested in other people or activities.
3. I felt withdrawn from other people.
4. I had little confidence in myself.
5. I was not interested in food.

### Personality

1. I was irritable.
2. I was inpatient with others.
3. My personality has changed.

### Self Care

1. Did you need help preparing food?
2. Did you need help eating? For example, cutting food or preparing food?
3. Did you need help getting dressed? For example, putting on socks or shoes, buttoning buttons, or zipping?
4. Did you need help taking a bath or a shower?
5. Did you need help to use the toilet?

### Social Roles

1. I didn't go out as often as I would like.
2. I did my hobbies and recreation for shorter periods of time than I would like.
3. I didn't see as many of my friends as I would like.
4. I had sex less often than I would like.
5. My physical condition interfered with my social life.

### Thinking

1. It was hard for me to concentrate.
2. I had trouble remembering things.
3. I had to write things down to remember them.

### Upper Extremity Function

1. Did you have trouble writing or typing?
2. Did you have trouble putting on socks?
3. Did you have trouble buttoning buttons?
4. Did you have trouble zipping a zipper?
5. Did you have trouble opening a jar?

### Vision

1. Did you have trouble seeing the television well enough to enjoy a show?
2. Did you have trouble reaching things because of poor eyesight?
3. Did you have trouble seeing things off to one side?

### Work/Productivity

1. Did you have trouble doing daily work around the house?
2. Did you have trouble finishing jobs that you started?
3. Did you have trouble doing the work you used to do?

_____ TOTAL SS-QOL SCORE (49–245)

The NIH Toolbox comprises four batteries assessing four domains of function. The Motor Battery assesses balance, dexterity, endurance, locomotion, and strength. The Sensation Battery assesses audition, olfaction, pain, taste, vestibular function, and vision. The Cognition Battery includes measures of executive function, attention, episodic memory, language, processing speed, and working memory.[38] The Emotional Health battery assesses psychological well-being, social relationships, stress and self-efficacy, and negative affect.

## CONCLUSION

Driven by the motivation to deliver improved care, neuroprotection for critical care and perioperative medicine is evolving from an empirically based art to an evidence-based science. This evolution rests on the objective and quantitative assessment of neurological and functional outcomes using standardized scales in controlled clinical trials and outcomes studies that test the efficacy of interventions in preventing or reversing neurological injury.

Over the years, there has been a proliferation of tools for measuring global outcome, neurological impairment, disability, handicap, and HR-QOL. The selection of appropriate clinical endpoints is a crucial step in clinical neuroprotection trial design. It requires careful consideration of the measure's reliability, whether it is a valid indicator of the construct that is under investigation, and whether it is responsive to changes in that construct.

This chapter describes some of the most popular outcome measures, most of which are in the public domain. All scales, however, have their weaknesses; thus, future research in clinical neuroprotection will include development of new and improved tools.

## REFERENCES

1. Roberts L, Counsell C. Assessment of clinical outcomes in acute stroke trials. *Stroke.* 1998;29(5):986–91.

2. Lyden PD, Lau GT. A critical appraisal of stroke evaluation and rating scales. *Stroke.* 1991;22(11):1345–52.

3. Friedman LM, Furberg CD, DeMets DL. *Fundamentals of clinical trials,* 3rd edition. New York: Mosby, 1995:21–6.

4. Hacke W, Kaste M, Fieschi C, et al. Intravenous thrombolysis with recombinant tissue plasminogen activator for acute hemispheric stroke. The European Cooperative Acute Stroke Study (ECASS). *JAMA.* 1995;274(13):1017–25.

5. Mendelow AD, Gregson BA, Rowan EN, Murray GD, Gholkar A, Mitchell PM; STICH II Investigators. Early surgery versus initial conservative treatment in patients with spontaneous supratentorial lobar intracerebral haematomas (STICH II): a randomised trial. *Lancet.* 2013;382(9890):397–408.

6. The National Institute of Neurological Disorders and Stroke rt-PA Stroke Study Group. Tissue plasminogen activator for acute ischemic stroke. *N Engl J Med.* 1995;333:1581–7.

7. Jennett B, Bond M. Assessment of outcome after severe brain damage. *Lancet.* 1975;1:480–4.

8. Wright, J. The Glasgow Outcome Scale. The Center for Outcome Measurement in Brain Injury. 2000. Available from: http://www.tbims.org/combi/gos

9. Teasdale GM, Pettigrew LE, Wilson JT, Murray G, Jennett B. Analyzing outcome of treatment of severe head injury: a review and update on advancing the use of the Glasgow Outcome Scale. *J Neurotrauma.* 1998;15(8):587–97.

10. Sander A. The Extended Glasgow Outcome Scale. The Center for Outcome Measurement in Brain Injury. 2002. Available from: http://www.tbims.org/combi/gose.

11. Wilson JTL, Pettigrew LEL, Teasdale GM. Structured interviews for the Glasgow Outcome Scale and the Extended Glasgow Outcome Scale: guidelines for their use. *J Neurotrauma.* 1998;15(8):573–85.

12. van Swieten JC, Koudstaal PJ, Visser MC, Schouten HG, van Gijn J. Interobserver agreement for the assessment of handicap in stroke patients. *Stroke.* 1988;19(5):604–7.

13. Saver JL, Filip B, Hamilton S, et al.; FAST-MAG Investigators and Coordinators. Improving the reliability of stroke disability grading in clinical trials and clinical practice: the Rankin Focused Assessment (RFA). *Stroke*. 2010;41(5): 992–5.

14. Patel N, Rao VA, Heilman-Espinoza ER, Lai R, Quesada RA, Flint AC. Simple and reliable determination of the modified Rankin Scale in neurosurgical and neurological patients: the mRS-9Q. *Neurosurgery*. 2012;71(5): 971–5; discussion 975.

15. Teasdale G, Jennett B. Assessment of coma and impaired consciousness. A practical scale. *Lancet*. 1974;2(7872):81–4.

16. Hagen C. Malkmus D. Durham E. Levels of cognitive function. In *Rehabilitation of the head injured adult: comprehensive physical management*. Professional staff of Rancho Los Amigos Hospital. Downey, CA: Rancho Los Amigos; 1979.

17. Brott T, Adams HP Jr, Olinger CP, et al. Measurements of acute cerebral infarction: a clinical examination scale. *Stroke*. 1989;20(7):864–70.

18. Lyden P, Lu M, Jackson C, et al. Underlying structure of the National Institutes of Health Stroke Scale: results of a factor analysis. NINDS tPA Stroke Trial Investigators. *Stroke*. 1999;30(11):2347–54.

19. Meyer BC, Lyden PD. The modified National Institutes of Health Stroke Scale: its time has come. *Int J Stroke*. 2009;4(4):267–73.

20. Nasreddine ZS, Phillips NA, Bédirian V, et al. The Montreal Cognitive Assessment, MoCA: a brief screening tool for mild cognitive impairment. *J Am Geriatr Soc*. 2005;53(4): 695–99.

21. Brandt J, Spencer M, Folstein M. The Telephone Interview for Cognitive Status. *Neuropsychiatry Neuropsychol Behav Neurol*. 1988;1:111–117.

22. Lezak MD, Howieson DB, Bigler ED, Tranel D. *Neuropsychological assessment*. 5th edition. New York: Oxford University Press; 2012.

23. Strauss EH, Sherman EMS, Spreen O. *A compendium of neuropsychological tests*, 3rd edition. Oxford: Oxford University Press; 2006.

24. Heilbronner RL, Sweet JJ, Attix DK, Krull KR, Henry GK, Hart RP. Official position of the American Academy of Clinical Neuropsychology on serial neuropsychological assessments: the utility and challenges of repeat test administrations in clinical and forensic contexts. *Clin Neuropsychol*. 2010;24(8):1267–78.

25. Binder LM, Iverson GL, Brooks BL. To err is human: "abnormal" neuropsychological scores and variability are common in healthy adults. *Arch Clin Neuropsychol*. 2009;24(1):31–46.

26. Brooks BL, Iverson GL. Comparing actual to estimated base rates of "abnormal" scores on neuropsychological test batteries: implications for interpretation. *Arch Clin Neuropsychol*. 2009;25(1):14–21.

27. Mahoney FI, Barthel D. Functional evaluation: the Barthel Index. *Md State Med J*. 1965;14:61–5.

28. Rappaport M, Hall KM, Hopkins HK, Belleza T, Cope DN. Disability rating scale for severe head trauma: coma to community. *Arch Phys Med Rehabil*. 1982;63(3):118–23.

29. Wright, J. The Disability Rating Scale. The Center for Outcome Measurement in Brain Injury; 2000. Available from: http://www.tbims.org/combi/drs

30. Lawton MP, Brody EM. Assessment of older people: self-maintaining and instrumental activities of daily living. *Gerontologist*. 1969;9(3):179–86.

31. EuroQol Group. EuroQol: a new facility for the measurement of health-related quality of life. *Health Policy*. 1990;16(3):199–208.

32. Ware JEJ, Kosinski M, Gandek B. *SF-36 health survey: manual and interpretation guide*. Lincoln: Quality Metric; 2001.

33. Williams LS, Weinberger M, Harris L, Biller J. Measuring quality of life in a way that is meaningful to stroke patients. *Neurology.* 1999;53(8):1839–43.

34. Williams LS, Weinberger M, Harris L, Clark DO, Biller J. Development of a stroke-specific quality of life scale. *Stroke.* 1999;30(7):1362–9.

35. Herndon RM. *Handbook of neurologic rating scales,* 2nd edition. New York: Demos Medical Publishing; 2006.

36. Hodes RJ, Insel TR, Landis SC; NIH Blueprint for Neuroscience Research. The NIH toolbox: setting a standard for biomedical research. *Neurology.* 2013;80(11 Suppl 3):S1.

37. Gershon RC, Wagster MV, Hendrie HC, Fox NA, Cook KF, Nowinski CJ. NIH toolbox for assessment of neurological and behavioral function. *Neurology.* 2013;80(11 Suppl 3):S2–6.

38. Weintraub S, Dikmen SS, Heaton RK, et al. Cognition assessment using the NIH Toolbox. *Neurology.* 2013;80(11 Supple 3):S54–64.

# 7 Assessment of Postoperative Cognitive Decline

Suzan Uysal and David L. Reich

## INTRODUCTION

As the clinical disciplines of anesthesiology and surgery have advanced, rates of surgery-related catastrophic brain injury have significantly declined. Brain protection, however, remains an important concern due to risk of a variety of adverse neurological outcomes including prolonged coma, stroke, seizures, delirium, and postoperative cognitive decline (POCD).[1] POCD, the focus of this chapter, is widely believed to reflect a relatively mild form of surgery-related brain injury that is not revealed by standard neurological examination but may nevertheless have significant functional impact on patients.

In response to this concern, researchers began using formal neurocognitive testing to study POCD in the 1980s in heart surgery patients. Early studies found very high incidences of cognitive decline, stimulating substantial interest among anesthesiologists and surgeons.[2–3] Since then, the many neurocognitive outcome studies that have been performed in this patient population have helped drive changes in clinical practice. More recently, there has been growing interest in POCD following major noncardiac surgical procedures.[4]

Over the past three decades, there have been many studies of POCD, and the field continues to be very active, with more than 50 papers published annually on the topic in each of the years from 2013 through 2016. The findings, however, are inconsistent with respect to incidence, etiology, prevention, and treatment. Consequently, the topic has become controversial, with some investigators viewing POCD as a hidden epidemic, while others question its societal and economic importance or doubt its existence.[5–7] There is consensus in the literature that variation in neurocognitive assessment methodologies underlies much of the inconsistency. We argue that this body of research also has been hampered by weak and flawed neurocognitive assessment methods.

This chapter provides a critical examination of assessment methods for studying POCD, with regard to (1) definition of the phenomenon, (2) the role of hypotheses regarding mechanisms and localization of neural injury, and (3) psychometric considerations for the design of POCD assessment protocols. Our goal is to inform clinicians and researchers about best practices of relevant neurocognitive assessment and the implications of these best practices to interpretation of the existing literature and design of future studies.

## DEFINITION OF POCD

POCD is not an established diagnostic entity, and there are no standard diagnostic criteria. Some studies have identified POCD as encompassing either a decline in cognitive test performance or a postoperative delirium. Some have identified declines in cognitive function that become apparent one or more years after surgery as POCD. Some have identified POCD on the basis of postoperative testing only. Some have even identified changes in event-related potentials as POCD.[8]

Most studies identify POCD on the basis of a pre- to postoperative decline in cognitive test performance. The oft-used terms "postoperative cognitive dysfunction" and "postoperative cognitive deficit," however, are misleading because the postoperative test scores do not necessarily reach the deficit range relative to normative data. Thus we prefer the term "postoperative cognitive decline" because it more accurately describes the entity reported by most studies.

We propose the following definition of POCD framed as a set of diagnostic criteria and discuss each of these criteria in the following sections. Postoperative cognitive decline is a pre- to postoperative decline in cognitive function that is:

1. a new-onset neurocognitive disorder or an exacerbation of a pre-existing neurocognitive disorder that is temporally related to surgery;
2. not wholly attributable to other conditions that were present prior to surgery; and
3. distinct from postoperative delirium.

### Identifying Pre- to Postoperative Cognitive Decline

The first criterion (new onset/exacerbation) is accurately assessed in research when neurocognitive function is measured both pre- and postoperatively and demonstrates declines within patients, rather than inferred from postoperative test score standings relative to normative sample data. This is crucial because surgical patients, especially cardiac and geriatric, often have cognitive deficits prior to surgery.[9–13] In the case of cardiac surgery patients, preoperative cognitive deficits may be a marker of occult cerebrovascular disease; they are associated with vascular risk factors, vascular health status, cerebral ischemic lesions, and reduced cerebral blood flow.[14–17]

There is no consensus on what constitutes clinically meaningful pre- to postoperative cognitive decline, thus a wide variety of methods have been used to operationally define POCD on the basis of test score change. Two of the most common methods are the percent change method and the standard deviation (SD) method. The percent change method expresses test score change (the pre- to postoperative difference score) relative to the pre-operative score for each test. Most studies have used a criterion of 20% or greater decline in raw test score. The SD method expresses test score change relative to the preoperative baseline sample SD for each test. Studies have commonly used the criterion of 1 SD or greater decline, but some studies have used 0.5 SD or 2 SD criteria. Since most studies yield multiple test scores, binary classification of patients as having or not having POCD usually also includes a criterion minimum number of test scores exhibiting the decline (e.g., 20% decline in 20% of the test scores, or 1 SD decline in two or more tests).

Several studies have demonstrated that applying different statistical definitions of POCD to the same patient data set results in markedly different incidences.[18–21] One study applied five different criteria to the same data set and found that the incidence of POCD at 6 weeks ranged from 1% to 34%.[20] Another study applied two common statistical definitions of POCD to data from a sample of 112 healthy, middle-aged volunteers *without surgery* and found a 14–28% incidence of decline from baseline to 3 months that met statistical criteria for "POCD."[21] These findings make the point that many statistical definitions of POCD are arbitrary and do not properly account for measurement error.

Statistical methods that incorporate information about test-retest reliability offer a more valid way to evaluate change and are better suited to longitudinal neurocognitive outcome studies. Reliable change index (RCI) and standardized regression-based (SRB) models take into account, to varying degrees, factors that contribute to test score change that are not treatment effects. These include measurement error, practice effects, regression to the mean, and other sources of systematic biases, such as baseline level of test performance, test-retest interval, effects of aging, and effects of neurological or medical conditions.[22] These methods are based on the distribution of test-retest difference scores in a matched normative data set. Thus, neurocognitive change scores for each patient and each test are interpreted *relative to the variability of the change scores in a normative sample.*

Since published normative test score change data often do not match important clinical study parameters that influence change, researchers usually must develop their own normative data set using an appropriately matched comparison sample and test-retest interval. The size of the normative sample must be sufficiently large to avoid spuriously low or high test-retest correlations, and the control sample should be matched to the patient sample on demographic factors (e.g., age, gender, education, preoperative level of intellectual function) and risk for cognitive decline.

## Distinguishing POCD from Pre-existing Cognitive Impairment

The second criterion, that cognitive decline is wholly attributable to preoperative conditions, is the most difficult to establish with certainty because research studies usually do not incorporate clinical history data in their analyses. Study findings are based on neurocognitive test data alone and therefore run the risk of identifying *any* pre- to postoperative decline as POCD, including common conditions such as Alzheimer's disease, vascular dementia, and alcohol-induced neurocognitive disorders.

Studies that exclude patients with preoperative Mini-Mental State Examination (MMSE) scores below the traditional cutscore of 24 for probable dementia do not avoid the problem of differentiating declines that are related to surgery versus a pre-existing, progressive neuropathological process. That cutscore has poor sensitivity (0.45) for detecting dementia in patients with more than 16 years of education and does not exclude patients with mild cognitive impairment, a dementia prodrome.[23]

Studies that examine whether patients with pre-existing cognitive impairment are more prone to POCD must compare the longitudinal cognitive trajectories of the surgical sample to a matched control sample. Without such a comparison, it is not possible to attribute cognitive decline to the surgery rather than the pre-existing condition. A study of 300 hip replacement surgery patients found that 32% of the sample was cognitively impaired pre-surgically (defined as at least two of seven test scores $\geq 2$ SDs below the normative mean) and that this subset of patients had a much higher rate of cognitive decline at 7 days, 3 months, and 12 months postoperatively.[24] A nonsurgical control sample also was studied to define normal test-retest variability over the study interval for the purpose of computing RCIs. The control group data, however, were not examined for incidence of cognitive impairment at baseline (i.e., similarity to the surgical sample for risk of cognitive decline) nor were rates of decline between control group subjects with versus without cognitive impairment at baseline.

## Distinguishing POCD Versus Postoperative Delirium

The third criterion requires that postoperative delirium be excluded as the underlying cause of neurocognitive test score decline. Delirium is characterized by (1) a core disturbance in attention (i.e., reduced ability to direct, focus, sustain, and shift attention) and awareness (reduced orientation to the environment), (2) an abrupt onset (over several hours to a few days) and fluctuating severity (over the course of a day), and (3) *additional* disturbances in cognition (e.g., memory, language, visuospatial ability, or perception).[25] Delirium is distinct from other neurocognitive disorders, and, by definition, other neurocognitive disorders do not occur exclusively in the context of delirium. We have previously detailed the differences between postoperative delirium and POCD.[26]

The distinction between delirium and POCD rests on the concept that neurocognitive processes are organized hierarchically, both functionally and anatomically. Subcortical processes of arousal and attention are at the lowest level; cortical processes, such as language, visuospatial cognition, and memory, are at intermediate levels; and prefrontal executive processes are at the highest level. High-level processes depend on the integrity of lower level processes, and approaches to neurocognitive assessment and test data interpretation must recognize this hierarchy. Attention is a fundamental cognitive process. A marked deficit in attention, as occurs in delirium, undermines higher level cognitive processes. In clinical practice, once a diagnosis of delirium is established on the basis of history, behavior, and very limited testing, further neurocognitive testing provides no additional information until after the delirium resolves. Low neurocognitive test scores in a patient with delirium do not reflect additional neurocognitive disorder; they simply reflect delirium.

Studies assessing cognitive function shortly after surgery in the absence of delirium assessment may overestimate the incidence of POCD, especially in patients who are prone to delirium (e.g., older patients). This likely was a shortcoming of many POCD studies that were conducted before the introduction of structured delirium assessment tools.

Studies that do assess both postoperative delirium and POCD shortly after surgery should not identify patients with the two conditions concurrently because this is inconsistent with the diagnostic criteria for neurocognitive disorders.[25] One study that exemplifies this error identified postoperative delirium in 12 patients on post-operative day 7.[27] Eight of those patients underwent cognitive testing on postoperative day 7, seven of whom were identified as having concurrent short-term POCD. The single patient who met study criteria for delirium but not POCD raises questions regarding the accuracy of delirium diagnosis in this patient, given that a gross disturbance in attention necessarily undermines higher cognitive functions.

The crucial reason to differentiate delirium from POCD is that delirium is typically reversible. In the context of surgery, precipitating causes for delirium include pharmacological agents (e.g., anesthetics, analgesics, sedatives), infection, acute metabolic disturbances (e.g., electrolyte abnormalities, anemia), organ failure (e.g., congestive heart failure, renal insufficiency), and hypoxemia. The incidence of postoperative delirium increases with procedural complexity/duration and patient vulnerabilities, such as frailty, comorbidities, and reduced cerebral reserve that occurs with prior stroke, dementia, and milder forms of cognitive impairment. Postoperative delirium may therefore be considered as a potential marker for pre-existing brain disease.

## PUTATIVE MECHANISMS UNDERLYING POCD

The ultimate goal of POCD assessment is to elucidate etiology in order to provide sound bases for prevention and intervention. Study design, including tests selection, therefore should be guided by hypotheses regarding the potential mechanisms and localization of neural injury posed by the surgical procedure.

In cardiac surgery, the cause of most major adverse neurological outcomes is ischemia due to embolization or hypoperfusion.[28–29] It is reasonable to hypothesize that milder forms of ischemia underlie POCD in this population. Emboli and microemboli are introduced into the cerebral circulation by cardiopulmonary bypass and surgical manipulations of atherosclerotic blood vessels during aortic cannulation and cross-clamping. Cerebral emboli generally pass along the superficial vascular tree as far as their size permit, and rarely follow the branches passing to deep brain structures. Emboli entering the anterior cerebral circulation most often enter the middle cerebral artery (MCA) rather than the anterior cerebral artery since the MCA is a direct extension of the internal carotid artery and carries the majority of anterior circulation blood flow. Small emboli and microemboli therefore will lodge in the most distal portions of the superficial branches of the middle and posterior cerebral arteries. Diffusion weighted magnetic resonance imaging (DW-MRI), an imaging modality that is particularly sensitive to acute ischemic injury, has provided evidence of new focal cerebral ischemic lesions in a high percentage (30–50%) of cardiac surgical patients.[30–32] The lesions are usually small, multiple, bilateral, supratentorial, and "clinically silent" (i.e., not associated with overt stroke). New ischemic lesions also occur in a substantial number of patients undergoing carotid artery surgery and coronary or cerebral-angiographic interventions.[33] Studies examining the relationship between intraoperative embolic load detected by transcranial Doppler ultrasound and cognitive outcome, however, have resulted in inconsistent findings.[34] Studies examining the relationship between new ischemic brain lesions on DW-MRI and cognitive outcome have also resulted in inconsistent findings.[35–37]

Cerebral hypoperfusion occurs with perfusion pressures that are below the limits of autoregulation, cerebral venous hypertension, and superior vena caval cannula malposition. The watershed regions are particularly vulnerable to hypotensive hypoperfusion injury. Hypoperfusion states may also occur when cerebral blood flow rate is insufficient to meet neuronal metabolic needs, as may occur during rewarming that occurs too rapidly or overshoots normothermia, and during the period of circulatory arrest for aortic arch surgery. Global cerebral ischemia, however, may result in localized injury because neuronal populations vary in their vulnerability. Regions of high vulnerability are the CA1 region of the hippocampus; neocortical layers 3, 5, and 6; and structures supplied by the distal branches of deep and superficial blood vessels (i.e., the deep cerebral white matter and the border zones between the major cerebral artery territories).

Noncardiac surgical procedures also carry risk of ischemia due to embolization or hypoperfusion. Orthopedic surgical procedures carry a risk of intraoperative cerebral embolism and microembolism, primarily by embolization of fat and bone marrow released into the circulation during operative manipulation of bone, and thromboembolism after tourniquet release. Surgical procedures performed in the beach chair position (e.g., arthroscopic shoulder and sinus surgery), especially when combined with induced hypotension, carry a risk of global cerebral hypoperfusion. Measuring intraoperative blood pressure at the level of the thigh may grossly underestimate arterial pressure at the Circle of Willis due to hydrostatic pressure differences. A prolonged period of arterial hypoxemia due to anatomical (congenital heart disease) or physiological (one-lung ventilation) reasons could also be a mechanism of injury.

There is emerging concern in the literature that anesthesia causes POCD by promoting Alzheimer's disease pathology.[38] Recent animal studies have shown that some general anesthetics may precipitate or exacerbate β-amyloid plaques, neurofibrillary tangles, and neuroinflammation.[39-40] The gap between the basic and clinical neuroscience, however, remains large. Epidemiological studies have found no relationship between history of exposure to surgery and anesthesia to the later development of Alzheimer's disease or dementia.[41-43]

## PSYCHOMETRIC CONSIDERATIONS IN POCD RESEARCH ASSESSMENTS
### Test Selection

As described earlier, in cardiac and thoracic aortic surgery the brain structures most likely to be affected are the cerebral cortex convexity, watershed areas of the cerebral cortex, deep cerebral white matter, and the CA1 field of the hippocampus. Thus POCD batteries designed to study cardiac and thoracic aortic surgery patients should emphasize tests of episodic memory, working memory, and cognitive processing speed because these functions are associated with the areas of highest vulnerability. Tests of episodic memory are essential because the hippocampus is a critical structure in the neural circuit subserving episodic memory.[44-45] Tests of working memory and processing speed are essential because these cognitive processes are prominently affected with lesions in the deep cerebral white matter. They are also prominently affected in subcortical small vessel ischemic vascular cognitive impairment and are expected to be sensitive to pre-existing occult cerebrovascular disease.[46]

The same logic that addresses putative mechanisms and localization of POCD within the context of cardiac and thoracic aortic surgery should also be applied to the design of test battery protocols to study POCD associated with noncardiac surgery. For example, cognitive outcome studies based on the hypothesis that anesthesia causes POCD by precipitating or exacerbating Alzheimer's neuropathology should feature tests that are sensitive indicators of that disease. Likewise for other potential etiologies, analogous considerations apply.

Cognition is not a unitary phenomenon, but rather is the net result of the integrated workings of multiple neural networks subserving distinct processes (e.g., attention, language, memory) that may be selectively affected by neural insults. Thus, there is no single test or test score that can fully describe a patient's neurocognitive status and no single test that can identify and characterize POCD. Global brief mental status tests such as the MMSE are useful clinically as screening tools to identify cases requiring further assessment, but scores in the normal range can be misleading as they do not necessarily reflect normal neurocognitive function. For example, it is not uncommon for patients with a high premorbid level of function and a significant but selective episodic memory disorder to obtain MMSE scores of 28–29 out of 30, which are within the normal range for the patient's age and educational background. Other drawbacks of the MMSE and the single test score approach are low sensitivity to mild changes in global cognitive function, low sensitivity to modest changes that are restricted to a single domain, and lack of domain specificity.

Many cognitive outcome studies employ combinations (batteries) of tests that assess multiple domains of function. Because there are many tests to choose from, there has been great variability in the tests employed in POCD studies.[47–48] Test batteries designed to assess POCD should be comprised of tests that are sensitive indicators of cerebral dysfunction. The tests should have established clinical validity; experimental measures and modifications of validated tests do not meet this standard. The tests should have high test-retest reliability. Several of the tests used in the International Study of Postoperative Cognitive Dysfunction (ISPOCD), a multicenter large-scale study of cognitive outcomes of noncardiac surgery, have test-retest correlations that have been identified as unacceptably low.[49] Finally, the tests should be suitable for repeated administration, having either small or nonexistent practice effects, or include alternate forms that minimize practice effects. We have previously reviewed the strengths and weaknesses of many specific tests that have been commonly used in cardiac surgery neurocognitive outcome studies.[50]

Test batteries to assess for POCD should always include tests of episodic memory because of all cognitive capacities it is the most vulnerable to disease, injury, and aging. In designing batteries for longitudinal studies, the selection of memory tests requires special consideration. Of memory tests, multitrial word list learning and memory tests with alternate forms of equivalent difficulty are optimal, with the alternate forms administered in a counterbalanced fashion across test sessions. Paragraph recall tests are less desirable because they usually do not have equivalent forms and are less sensitive indicators of memory disorder due to the facilitating effects of context and associative learning.[47] Multitrial word list learning and memory tests also have the advantage of yielding multiple test scores that reflect the memory subprocesses of encoding, storage, and retrieval. These subprocesses may be selectively affected by brain injury and disease, and the profile of test scores may be interpreted to infer the localization and nature of the underlying pathology.

Of word list learning and memory tests, some are better suited to POCD studies than others. The Rey Auditory Verbal Learning Test (RAVLT) has several weaknesses compared to other tests. Its six alternative forms, developed by different authors at different times, have not been shown to be of equivalent difficulty.[51] Because the test consists of 15 unrelated words presented over five trials, many patients become overwhelmed upon first hearing the list and obtain very low scores on Trial 1.[46] A further caution regarding word list memory tests is that immediate recall after a single presentation of a word list should not be used as a measure of episodic memory. This "immediate memory span" score actually reflects attention capacity, the same process that is assessed by Digit Span Forward tasks.[46] Such tasks are usually performed normally in patients with anterograde amnesia. The RAVLT Trial 1 parameter has proved to have poor sensitivity to primary memory deficits; it does not differentiate amnestic from nonamnestic groups.[52–53] This criticism also applies to the Postoperative Quality Recovery Scale (PQRS) cognitive domain scale verbal memory item because it is identical to the RAVLT Trial 1 in content and format.[54]

## Time of Testing

POCD studies rest on the comparison between preoperative and postoperative neurocognitive test data.[55] The ability to obtain baseline data, however, is limited by patient availability prior to surgery. Preoperative testing performed just prior to major surgery is suboptimal because preoperative anxiety may confound the neurocognitive test data. In ideal circumstances, therefore, preoperative neurocognitive testing should be performed at least 1 day in advance of surgery in an appropriate environment.

Postoperative testing should be performed with a sufficient delay following surgery to limit potential confounds caused by factors such as pain, sleep disturbance, and use of analgesics and sedatives. Studies testing for POCD prior to hospital discharge after major surgery typically find very high rates of cognitive decline that are transient and at least partly attributable to analgesia and acute postoperative conditions.[56–57] Motor limitations imposed by intravenous lines affect speed to perform timed tests requiring writing or other hand movements (e.g., Trail Making Test and the Grooved Pegboard Test).

The Statement of Consensus on Assessment of Neurobehavioral Outcomes After Cardiac Surgery recommended that at least one postoperative assessment be performed a minimum of 3 months following cardiac surgery to eliminate potential confounds.[58] Long-term studies beyond the first year pose difficulties in data interpretation, especially in the absence of age- and disease-matched control groups. With increasing time after surgery, test data may be increasingly confounded by the effects of aging, age-related brain disease, and new medical problems that may obscure the association between surgery and neurocognitive decline. Patients who are free of cognitive impairment at the time of surgery but at risk for future decline independent of surgery include those with preclinical Alzheimer's disease (i.e., Alzheimer's neuropathology but normal cognitive function), genetic risk for Alzheimer's disease, or vascular risk factors at mid-life.[59–62] This latter group includes elective cardiac surgery candidates who also have an increased rate of cerebrovascular disease preoperatively as evidenced by neuroimaging.[63–64]

## Serial Testing and Practice Effects

Evaluation of cognitive change over time by repeated testing poses some challenges.[65] First and foremost is the *practice effect*, an improvement in test scores that is due to previous exposure to the test rather than to change in the underlying ability that the test is designed to measure. Since POCD assessment depends on longitudinal testing, the tests employed must have high test-retest reliability, with minimal practice effects or alternate forms that are identical in format and equivalent in difficulty but differing in content. Use of alternate forms is especially important in memory testing, where large item-specific practice effects will occur if the material to be recalled is repeated across test sessions.

Alternate forms dampen practice effects due to content familiarity, but they do not control for procedural learning.[66–67] Tests in which examinees develop a test-taking strategy are subject to practice effects even with the use of alternate forms. Tests of problem-solving and reasoning that have a single solution are especially prone to practice effects because, once the patient discovers the solution, the test no longer measures problem-solving and reasoning ability.

Other factors that influence the risk of practice effects include the length of the testing interval, the number of test sessions, baseline level of test performance, and possible presence of compromised cognitive function. Shorter test intervals produce larger practice effects than do longer intervals. The practice effect from one test session to the next cannot be assumed to be uniform across multiple test sessions as the greatest gains usually occur in the early test sessions and then plateau. More capable patients tend to benefit from practice to a greater degree unless they attain a maximum or near maximum test score, in which case a ceiling effect limits the ability to detect a practice effect. Patients with compromised brain function do not always benefit from practice to the same degree as patients with fully normal brain function.[68] A frequently employed strategy to control for practice effects involves subtracting out the "average practice effect" measured in a normal age-matched control sample from the clinical sample under investigation. This strategy rests on the assumption that the practice effect is equivalent between control and clinical samples and the same for all subjects.

## CLINICAL ASSESSMENT OF POSTOPERATIVE COGNITIVE DECLINE

Patients who present with signs or symptoms of cognitive decline following nonneurological surgery should undergo formal clinical neuropsychological assessment. It is not uncommon for clinical neuropsychologists to receive referrals for clinical assessment of POCD. Examining neuropsychologists should approach such assessments recognizing that patients presenting with a history of cognitive decline following surgery can usually be classified as (1) those with POCD, (2) those with a cognitive disorder that has been misattributed to surgery and anesthesia, (3) those motivated by the potential for secondary gain (e.g., actively engaged in medical malpractice litigation or seeking disability benefits), or (4) those with subjective complaints of cognitive decline who voice concerns that anesthesia or surgery had harmed their brain but who have no objective evidence of deficit or decline. The concerns of this later group are often fueled by lay media and web postings, similar to patients in preoperative consultation who express such concerns.[69]

Clinical evaluations for possible POCD are usually based on postoperative test data only; preoperative neurocognitive test data are rarely available as a point of comparison. The aim of the assessment is to determine whether there is objective evidence of cognitive deficit or decline as evidenced by postoperative neurocognitive test scores that are interpreted relative to normative data and/or relative to the estimated level of premorbid function for the patient. Assessment procedures should include symptom and performance validity testing for feigned neuropsychological impairment, given the potential for secondary gain by compensation-seeking in this patient population.

The clinical history of the cognitive signs and symptoms must be consistent with the criteria for POCD described earlier in order to support a diagnosis of POCD. Specifically, the neurocognitive disorder must have an onset that is temporally related to surgery, is not wholly attributable to a pre-existing condition, and is not postoperative delirium.

With regard to onset and course, an abrupt decline in cognitive function that is temporally related to surgery and follows either a static or gradually improving course is consistent with POCD. A gradually progressive course of cognitive decline following surgery is not consistent with POCD. Multiple long-term neurocognitive outcome studies in cardiac surgical patients have observed progressive declines in cognitive test scores over the course of years following surgery, but they are usually attributable to progressive cerebrovascular disease rather than surgical intervention or cardiopulmonary bypass. Studies comparing patients who underwent cardiac surgery to patients with coronary artery disease (CAD) treated medically, patients with CAD treated with coronary angioplasty, and patients with comparable risk factors for CAD but no surgery or percutaneous interventions, demonstrate that cardiac surgical patients have progressive cognitive declines similar to these patient groups.[70-76] Similar studies in noncardiac surgical patients also have shown that long-term cognitive decline is not attributable to surgery or illness, but rather to pre-existing mild dementia.[77]

In order to exclude the possibility that the neurocognitive disorder is *wholly* attributable to other conditions that were present prior to surgery, the clinician must ascertain the presence of pre-existing neurological or systemic conditions that can explain the cognitive disorder. The presence of preoperative cognitive signs and symptoms is to be expected in a substantial number of cardiac surgical patients with CAD and vascular risk factors; cognitive status in aging is linked to cardiac and peripheral vascular health.[78-79] Baseline cognitive impairment is also present in a substantial number of geriatric surgical patients; population studies of community-living elders aged 70 years and older indicate a 14–18% prevalence rate for mild cognitive impairment (MCI), a neurocognitive condition that usually represents the prodrome of an ensuing dementia.[80] The presence of cognitive symptoms predating the surgery in question does not exclude the possibility of POCD. In fact, the presence of preoperative brain pathology, such as medial temporal lobe atrophy, white matter lesions, cerebral infarction, and cerebral hypoperfusion, is associated with increased risk for POCD.[81-87] Similarly, behavioral markers for probable brain pathology, such as alcohol abuse and cognitive impairment, are also associated with increased risk for POCD.[88-89]

The clinical history must also include information about any perioperative complications because these may increase the risk for POCD. It is especially important to inquire about postoperative delirium, which often is a flag for unrecognized or undiagnosed brain pathology that was present preoperatively. A study in patients who underwent total hip/knee replacement under spinal anesthesia found that patients with preoperative presence of biomarkers for Alzheimer's disease (low CSF Ab40/Tau and CSF Ab42/Tau ratios) had the highest incidence of delirium.[90] Cognitive impairment, dementia, and brain disease all predispose patients to developing delirium precipitated by any cause. Potential precipitating factors include an array of perioperative factors, especially anesthetic agents, analgesics, and other medications, but also surgical trauma, cerebral hypoxia, cerebral hypoperfusion, pain, and infection.[91–94] The precipitating causes of delirium are the same for patients with and without cerebral compromise, but the former group has a lower threshold of tolerance and a higher vulnerability for delirium. Since postoperative delirium may signal the presence of unrecognized pre-existing brain pathology and neurocognitive disorder, it is appropriate that patients who develop postoperative delirium should be referred for clinical neuropsychological assessment. Ideally, this should be performed after the delirium clears, after hospital discharge, and after recovery from surgery.

Examining neuropsychologists should recognize that some cases of POCD may consist of a very selective neurocognitive disorder due to a strategic infarct in a site that is critical for higher "cortical" functions. Such disorders include anterograde amnesia, a variety of executive function disorders, certain aphasic syndromes, communication disorders that are due to disconnection between language circuitry and sensory input (pure alexia, pure word deafness) or motor output (pure agraphia), selective disorders of perceptual processing or recognition (the various visual agnosias, prosopagnosia, achromatopsia, auditory agnosia, tactile agnosia), disorders of spatial attention (hemi-inattention, simultanagnosia), disorders of body schema (autotopagnosia, right-left confusion, finger agnosia), and a variety of callosal disconnection syndromes. Sites in which strategically localized infarctions may cause selective neurocognitive syndromes include hippocampus and/or components of the hippocampal memory circuit, specific cortical regions or their connections, lacunar infarcts in specific thalamic relay nuclei or basal ganglia, and watershed infarctions involving the border zones between the anterior cerebral artery and MCA, and/or the posterior cerebral artery and MCA.

When clinical evaluations for POCD reveal objective evidence of neurocognitive deficit or decline on postoperative testing, and the clinical history is consistent with POCD, further medical diagnostic investigation, especially by neuroimaging, is indicated.

## CONCLUSION

In summary, we propose a set of guidelines to aid researchers and clinicians in the assessment of POCD (Box 7.1). Clinical experience shows us that POCD is a real phenomenon, yet the research literature over the past 30 years has produced inconsistent findings, leading to controversy over whether the phenomenon is real. This is in large part due to widely varying neurocognitive assessment methods, as well as weak and flawed assessment methods and test data interpretation. Neurocognitive function is an ideal endpoint for clinical trials of neuroprotective interventions; however, there is no single endpoint measure or set of measures that has been well validated for and widely applied to studies of POCD. Neurocognitive test score interpretation poses challenges because variability in cognitive test performance and test scores is the norm and low or abnormal scores commonly occur in normal samples.[95–96]

The simple administration of a cognitive test protocol is not equivalent to *meaningful* measurement of cognition. Research teams studying cognitive outcomes therefore should include a clinical neuropsychologist as a full collaborator. Neuropsychologists have expertise in neurocognitive assessment, psychometrics, and diagnosis of neurocognitive disorders. Their training includes a doctoral degree, internship, and several years of postdoctoral fellowship (residency); additional competency may be demonstrated by board certification.[97] Failure to incorporate a neuropsychologist as a member of the

Box 7.1 Guidelines for Research and Clinical Assessments of POCD

- The definition of POCD should be consistent with established diagnostic criteria for neurocognitive disorders and exclude postoperative delirium.
- POCD test battery choice should be guided by specific hypotheses regarding putative mechanisms and localization of neural injury.
- POCD test batteries should be comprised of tests that have established clinical diagnostic validity, are sensitive indicators of cerebral dysfunction, have high test-retest reliability, and are suitable for repeated administration.
- Preoperative testing should be performed at least 1 day before surgery to limit confounding effects of anxiety on test scores.
- Postoperative testing should be performed well after surgery to limit confounding factors such as pain, analgesic and sedative effects, and sleep disturbance.
- The POCD research team should include a clinical neuropsychologist throughout the continuum of research.
- Patients who develop postoperative delirium, and patients who are identified as having POCD in research studies, should be referred for neurological and clinical neuropsychological examinations.
- For clinical assessments, a diagnosis of POCD rests on objective evidence of cognitive deficit or decline, in combination with a clinical history that is consistent with POCD.
- Clinical POCD assessments should include symptom and performance validity testing for feigned neuropsychological impairment.

neurocognitive outcomes research team increases the likelihood of poor study design, flawed data analysis, and flawed data interpretation. Furthermore, inclusion of neuropsychologists throughout the continuum of neurocognitive outcomes research is recommended for compliance with best practices and ethical guidelines regarding boundaries of competence and scope of practice.[98–99]

Neuropsychologists who are involved in POCD research, in addition to their specialty expertise, should be knowledgeable about POCD assessment and the potential mechanisms of cerebral injury associated with the specific surgery under investigation, as well as the mechanisms of cerebral compromise and the neurocognitive profile associated with the illness or injury leading to the need for surgical intervention.

In the effort to improve postoperative cognitive outcomes, especially in older patients, some have called for incorporating formal cognitive testing into the perioperative assessment to identify at-risk patients through closer collaboration among surgeons, anesthesiologists, and geriatricians.[5] Clinical neuropsychologists also should play a central role.

## REFERENCES

1. Eagle KA, Guyton RA, Davidoff R, et al. ACC/AHA guidelines for coronary artery bypass graft surgery: executive summary and recommendations: a report of the American College of Cardiology/American Heart Association task force on practice guidelines (Committee to revise the 1991 guidelines for coronary artery bypass graft surgery). *Circulation*. 1999;100(13):1464–80.

2. Shaw PJ, Bates D, Cartlidge NE, et al. Early intellectual dysfunction following coronary bypass surgery. *Q J Med*. 1986;58(225):59–68.

3. Shaw PJ, Bates D, Cartlidge NE, et al. Long-term intellectual dysfunction following coronary artery bypass graft surgery: a six month follow-up study. *Q J Med*. 1987;62(239):259–68.

4. Moller JT, Cluitmans P, Rasmussen LS, et al. Long-term postoperative cognitive dysfunction in the elderly ISPOCD1 study. ISPOCD investigators. International Study of Post-Operative Cognitive Dysfunction. *Lancet*. 1998;351(9106):857–61.

5. O' Brien H, Mohan H, Hare CO, Reynolds JV, Kenny RA. Mind over matter? The hidden epidemic of cognitive dysfunction in the older surgical patient. *Ann Surg*. 2017;265(4):677–91.

6. Avidan MS, Evers AS. Review of clinical evidence for persistent cognitive decline or incident dementia attributable to surgery or general anesthesia. *J Alzheimers Dis*. 2011;24(2):201–16.

7. Sanders RD. Persistent post-operative cognitive decline: naked truth, invisibility cloak or the "emperor's new clothes?" *J Alzheimers Dis*. 2011;24(2):217–20.

8. Mracek J, Holeckova I, Chytra I, Mork J, Stepanek D, Vesela P. The impact of general versus local anesthesia on early subclinical cognitive function following carotid endarterectomy evaluated using P3 event-related potentials. *Acta Neurochir (Wien)*. 2012;154(3):433–8.

9. Millar K, Asbury AJ, Murray GD. Pre-existing cognitive impairment as a factor influencing outcome after cardiac surgery. *Br J Anaesth*. 2001;86(1):63–7.

10. Rankin KP, Kochamba GS, Boone KB, Petitti DB, Buckwalter JG. Presurgical cognitive deficits in patients receiving coronary artery bypass graft surgery. *J Int Neuropsychol Soc*. 2003;9(6):913–24.

11. Rosengart TK, Sweet J, Finnin EB, et al. Neurocognitive functioning in patients undergoing coronary artery bypass graft surgery or percutaneous coronary intervention: evidence of impairment before intervention compared with normal controls. *Ann Thorac Surg*. 2005;80(4):1327–34; discussion 1334–5.

12. Ernest CS, Murphy BM, Worcester MU, et al. Cognitive function in candidates for coronary artery bypass graft surgery. *Ann Thorac Surg*. 2006;82(3):812–8.

13. Silbert BS, Scott DA, Evered LA, Lewis MS, Maruff PT. Preexisting cognitive impairment in patients scheduled for elective coronary artery bypass graft surgery. *Anesth Analg*. 2007;104(5):1023–8.

14. Maekawa K, Goto T, Baba T, Yoshitake A, Katahira K, Yamamoto T. Impaired cognition preceding cardiac surgery is related to cerebral ischemic lesions. *J Anesth*. 2011;25(3):330–6.

15. Moraca R, Lin E, Holmes JH 4th, et al. Impaired baseline regional cerebral perfusion in patients referred for coronary artery bypass. *J Thorac Cardiovasc Surg*. 2006;131(3):540–6.

16. Ernest CS, Elliott PC, Murphy BM, et al. Predictors of cognitive function in candidates for coronary artery bypass graft surgery. *J Int Neuropsychol Soc*. 2007;13(2):257–66.

17. Kidher E, Harling L, Sugden C, et al. Aortic stiffness is an indicator of cognitive dysfunction before and after aortic valve replacement for aortic stenosis. *Interact Cardiovasc Thorac Surg*. 2014;19(4):595–604.

18. Raymond PD, Hinton-Bayre AD, Radel M, Ray MJ, Marsh NA. Assessment of statistical change criteria used to define significant change in neuropsychological test performance following cardiac surgery. *Eur J Cardiothorac Surg*. 2006;29(1):82–8.

19. Lewis MS, Maruff P, Silbert BS, Evered LA, Scott DA. The sensitivity and specificity of three common statistical rules for the classification of post-operative cognitive

dysfunction following coronary artery bypass graft surgery. *Acta Anaesthesiol Scand.* 2006;50(1):50–7.

20. Mahanna EP, Blumenthal JA, White WD, Croughwell ND, Clancy CP, Smith LR, Newman MF. Defining neuropsychological dysfunction after coronary artery bypass grafting. *Ann Thorac Surg.* 1996;61(5):1342–7.

21. Keizer AM, Hijman R, Kalkman CJ, Kahn RS, van Dijk D. The incidence of cognitive decline after (not) undergoing coronary artery bypass grafting: the impact of a controlled definition. *Acta Anaesthesiol Scand.* 2005;49(9):1232–5.

22. Slick D. Psychometrics in neuropsychological assessment. In: Strauss E, Sherman EMS, Spreen O, editors. *A compendium of neuropsychological tests: administration, norms, and commentary.* 3rd ed. New York: Oxford University Press; 2006:24–28.

23. O'Bryant SE, Humphreys JD, Smith GE, et al. Detecting dementia with the Mini-Mental State Examination in highly educated individuals. *Arch Neurol.* 2008;65(7):963–7.

24. Silbert B, Evered L, Scott DA, et al. Preexisting cognitive impairment is associated with postoperative cognitive dysfunction after hip joint replacement surgery. *Anesthesiology.* 2015;122(6):1224–34.

25. American Psychiatric Association. *Diagnostic and statistical manual for mental disorders,* 5th edition (DSM-5). Washington, DC: American Psychiatric Press; 2013.

26. Silverstein JH, Timberger M, Reich DL, Uysal S. Central nervous system dysfunction after noncardiac surgery and anesthesia in the elderly. *Anesthesiology.* 2007;106(3):622–8.

27. Rudolph JL, Marcantonio ER, Culley DJ, et al. Delirium is associated with early postoperative cognitive dysfunction. *Anaesthesia.* 2008;63(9):941–7.

28. Hogue CW, Gottesman RF, Stearns J. Mechanisms of cerebral injury from cardiac surgery. *Crit Care Clin.* 2008;24(1):83–98.

29. Smith C. Neuropathology of brain injury in cardiac surgery. In: Bonser RS, Pagano D, Haverich A, editors. *Brain protection in cardiac surgery.* London: Springer-Verlag; 2011:37–44.

30. Bendszus M, Reents W, Franke D, et al. Brain damage after coronary artery bypass grafting. *Arch Neurol.* 2002;59(7):1090–5.

31. Floyd TF, Shah PN, Price CC, et al. Clinically silent cerebral ischemic events after cardiac surgery: their incidence, regional vascular occurrence, and procedural dependence. *Ann Thorac Surg.* 2006;81(6):2160–6.

32. Cook DJ, Huston J 3rd, Trenerry MR, Brown RD Jr, Zehr KJ, Sundt TM 3rd. Postcardiac surgical cognitive impairment in the aged using diffusion-weighted magnetic resonance imaging. *Ann Thorac Surg.* 2007;83(4):1389–95.

33. Bendszus M, Stoll G. Silent cerebral ischaemia: hidden fingerprints of invasive medical procedures. *Lancet Neurol.* 2006;5(4):364–72.

34. Patel N, Minhas JS, Chung EM. Intraoperative embolization and cognitive decline after cardiac surgery: a systematic review. *Semin Cardiothorac Vasc Anesth.* 2016;20(3):225–31.

35. Patel N, Minhas JS, Chung EM. The presence of new MRI lesions and cognitive decline after cardiac surgery: a systematic review. *J Card Surg.* 2015;30(11):808–12.

36. Nah HW, Lee JW, Chung CH, et al. New brain infarcts on magnetic resonance imaging after coronary artery bypass graft surgery: lesion patterns, mechanism, and predictors. *Ann Neurol.* 2014;76(3):347–55.

37. Sun X, Lindsay J, Monsein LH, Hill PC, Corso PJ. Silent brain injury after cardiac surgery: a review: cognitive dysfunction and magnetic resonance imaging diffusion-weighted imaging findings. *J Am Coll Cardiol.* 2012;60(9):791–7.

38. Bilotta F, Qeva E, Matot I. Anesthesia and cognitive disorders: a systematic review of the clinical evidence. *Expert Rev Neurother.* 2016;16(11):1311–20.

39. Whittington RA, Bretteville A, Dickler MF, Planel E. Anesthesia and tau pathology. *Prog Neuropsychopharmacol Biol Psychiatry.* 2013;47:147–55.

40. Xie Z, Xu Z. General anesthetics and β-amyloid protein. *Prog Neuropsychopharmacol Biol Psychiatry.* 2013;47:140–6.

41. Seitz DP, Reimer CL, Siddiqui N. A review of epidemiological evidence for general anesthesia as a risk factor for Alzheimer's disease. *Prog Neuropsychopharmacol Biol Psychiatry.* 2013;47:122–7.

42. Knopman DS, Petersen RC, Cha RH, Edland SD, Rocca WA. Coronary artery bypass grafting is not a risk factor for dementia or Alzheimer disease. *Neurology.* 2005;65(7):986–90.

43. Sprung J, Jankowski CJ, Roberts RO, et al. Anesthesia and incident dementia: a population-based, nested, case-control study. *Mayo Clin Proc.* 2013;88(6):552–61.

44. Zola-Morgan S, Squire LR, Amaral DG. Human amnesia and the medial temporal region: enduring memory impairment following a bilateral lesion limited to field CA1 of the hippocampus. *J Neurosci.* 1986;6(10):2950–67.

45. Rempel-Clower NL, Zola SM, Squire LR, Amaral DG. Three cases of enduring memory impairment after bilateral damage limited to the hippocampal formation. *J Neurosci.* 1996;16(16):5233–55.

46. Raz N, Rodrigue KM, Kennedy KM, Acker JD. Vascular health and longitudinal changes in brain and cognition in middle-aged and older adults. *Neuropsychology.* 2007;21(2):149–57.

47. Lezak MD, Howieson DB, Bigler ED, Tranel D. *Neuropsychological assessment.* 5th ed. New York: Oxford University Press; 2012.

48. Strauss EH., Sherman EMS, Spreen O. *A compendium of neuropsychological tests,* 3rd ed. Oxford: Oxford University Press; 2006.

49. Lowe C, Rabbitt P. Test/re-test reliability of the CANTAB and ISPOCD neuropsychological batteries: theoretical and practical issues. Cambridge Neuropsychological Test Automated Battery. International Study of Post-Operative Cognitive Dysfunction. *Neuropsychologia.* 1998;36(9):915–23.

50. Uysal S, Reich DL. Neurocognitive outcomes of cardiac surgery. *J Cardiothorac Vasc Anesth.* 2013;27(5):958–71.

51. Hawkins KA, Dean D, Pearlson GD. Alternative forms of the Rey Auditory Verbal Learning Test: a review. *Behav Neurol.* 2004;15(3-4):99–107.

52. Mungas D. Differential clinical sensitivity of specific parameters of the Rey Auditory-Verbal Learning Test. *J Consult Clin Psychol.* 1983;51(6):848–55.

53. Schmidt M. *Rey Auditory Verbal Learning Test: A handbook.* Los Angeles: Western Psychological Services; 1996.

54. Royse CF, Newman S, Chung F, et al. Development and feasibility of a scale to assess postoperative recovery: the post-operative quality recovery scale. *Anesthesiology.* 2010;113(4):892–905.

55. Selnes OA, Zeger SL. Coronary artery bypass grafting baseline cognitive assessment: essential not optional. *Ann Thorac Surg.* 2007;83(2):374–6.

56. Wang Y, Sands LP, Vaurio L, Mullen EA, Leung JM. The effects of postoperative pain and its management on postoperative cognitive dysfunction. *Am J Geriatr Psychiatry.* 2007;15(1):50–9.

57. Zywiel MG, Prabhu A, Perruccio AV, Gandhi R. The influence of anesthesia and pain management on cognitive dysfunction after joint arthroplasty: a systematic review. *Clin Orthop Relat Res.* 2014;472(5):1453–66.

58. Murkin JM, Newman SP, Stump DA, Blumenthal JA. Statement of consensus on assessment of neurobehavioral outcomes after cardiac surgery. *Ann Thorac Surg.* 1995;59(5):1289–95.

59. Bennett DA, Wilson RS, Boyle PA, Buchman AS, Schneider JA. Relation of neuropathology to cognition in persons without cognitive impairment. *Ann Neurol.* 2012;72(4):599–609.

60. Knopman D, Boland LL, Mosley T, et al.; Atherosclerosis Risk in Communities (ARIC) Study Investigators. Cardiovascular risk factors and cognitive decline in middle-aged adults. *Neurology.* 2001;56(1):42–8.

61. Knopman DS, Mosley TH, Catellier DJ, Coker LH. Fourteen-year longitudinal study of vascular risk factors, APOE genotype, and cognition: the ARIC MRI study. *Alzheimers Dement.* 2009;5(3):207–14.

62. Evered LA, Silbert BS, Scott DA, Maruff P, Ames D. Prevalence of dementia 7.5 years after coronary artery bypass graft surgery. *Anesthesiology.* 2016;125(1):62–71.

63. Maekawa K, Goto T, Baba T, Yoshitake A, Morishita S, Koshiji T. Abnormalities in the brain before elective cardiac surgery detected by diffusion-weighted magnetic resonance imaging. *Ann Thorac Surg.* 2008;86(5):1563–9.

64. Nakamura Y, Kawachi K, Imagawa H, et al. The prevalence and severity of cerebrovascular disease in patients undergoing cardiovascular surgery. *Ann Thorac Cardiovasc Surg.* 2004;10(2):81–4.

65. Heilbronner RL, Sweet JJ, Attix DK, Krull KR, Henry GK, Hart RP. Official position of the American Academy of Clinical Neuropsychology on serial neuropsychological assessments: the utility and challenges of repeat test administrations in clinical and forensic contexts. *Clin Neuropsychol.* 2010;24(8):1267–78.

66. Benedict RH, Zgaljardic DJ. Practice effects during repeated administrations of memory tests with and without alternate forms. *J Clin Exp Neuropsychol.* 1998;20(3):339–52.

67. Beglinger LJ, Gaydos B, Tangphao-Daniels O, et al. Practice effects and the use of alternate forms in serial neuropsychological testing. *Arch Clin Neuropsychol.* 2005;20(4):517–29.

68. Wilson BA, Watson PC, Baddeley AD, Emslie H, Evans JJ. Improvement or simply practice? The effects of twenty repeated assessments on people with and without brain injury. *J Int Neuropsychol Soc.* 2000;6(4):469–79.

69. Thaler A, Siry R, Cai L, Garcia PS, Chen L, Liu R. Memory loss, Alzheimer's disease and general anesthesia: a preoperative concern. *J Anesth Clin Res.* 2012;3(2):pii: 1000192.

70. Selnes OA, Grega MA, Borowicz LM Jr, Royall RM, McKhann GM, Baumgartner WA. Cognitive changes with coronary artery disease: a prospective study of coronary artery bypass graft patients and nonsurgical controls. *Ann Thorac Surg.* 2003;75(5):1377–84; discussion 1384–6.

71. Selnes OA, Grega MA, Borowicz LM Jr, Barry S, Zeger S, Baumgartner WA, McKhann GM. Cognitive outcomes three years after coronary artery bypass surgery: a comparison of on-pump coronary artery bypass graft surgery and nonsurgical controls. *Ann Thorac Surg.* 2005;79(4):1201–9.

72. McKhann GM, Grega MA, Borowicz LM Jr, et al. Is there cognitive decline 1 year after CABG? Comparison with surgical and nonsurgical controls. *Neurology.* 2005;65(7):991–9.

73. Selnes OA, Grega MA, Bailey MM, et al. Cognition 6 years after surgical or medical therapy for coronary artery disease. *Ann Neurol.* 2008;63(5):581–90.

74. Sweet JJ, Finnin E, Wolfe PL, et al. Absence of cognitive decline one year after coronary bypass surgery: comparison to nonsurgical and healthy controls. *Ann Thorac Surg.* 2008;85(5):1571–8.

75. Selnes OA, Grega MA, Bailey MM, et al. Do management strategies for coronary artery disease influence 6-year cognitive outcomes? *Ann Thorac Surg.* 2009;88(2):445–54.

76. van Dijk D, Spoor M, Hijman R, et al.; Octopus Study Group. Cognitive and cardiac outcomes 5 years after off-pump vs on-pump coronary artery bypass graft surgery. *JAMA.* 2007;297(7):701–8.

77. Avidan MS, Searleman AC, Storandt M, et al. Long-term cognitive decline in older subjects was not attributable to noncardiac surgery or major illness. *Anesthesiology.* 2009;111(5):964–70.

78. Elwood PC, Pickering J, Bayer A, Gallacher JE. Vascular disease and cognitive function in older men in the Caerphilly cohort. *Age Ageing.* 2002;31(1):43–8.

79. Gauthier CJ, Lefort M, Mekary S, et al. Hearts and minds: linking vascular rigidity and aerobic fitness with cognitive aging. *Neurobiol Aging.* 2015;36(1):304–14.

80. Petersen RC, Roberts RO, Knopman DS, et al. Mild cognitive impairment: ten years later. *Arch Neurol.* 2009;66(12):1447–55.

81. Maekawa K, Baba T, Otomo S, Morishita S, Tamura N. Low pre-existing gray matter volume in the medial temporal lobe and white matter lesions are associated with postoperative cognitive dysfunction after cardiac surgery. *PLoS One.* 2014;9(1):e87375.

82. Price CC, Tanner JJ, Schmalfuss I, et al. A pilot study evaluating presurgery neuroanatomical biomarkers for postoperative cognitive decline after total knee arthroplasty in older adults. *Anesthesiology.* 2014;120(3):601–13.

83. Chen MH, Liao Y, Rong PF, Hu R, Lin GX, Ouyang W. Hippocampal volume reduction in elderly patients at risk for postoperative cognitive dysfunction. *J Anesth.* 2013;27(4):487–92.

84. Messerotti Benvenuti S, Zanatta P, Valfre C, Polesel E, Palomba D. Preliminary evidence for reduced preoperative cerebral blood flow velocity as a risk factor for cognitive decline three months after cardiac surgery: an extension study. *Perfusion.* 2012;27(6):486–92.

85. Messerotti Benvenuti S, Zanatta P, Longo C, Mazzarolo AP, Palomba D. Preoperative cerebral hypoperfusion in the left, not in the right, hemisphere is associated with cognitive decline after cardiac surgery. *Psychosom Med.* 2012;74(1):73–80.

86. Goto T, Baba T, Honma K, et al. Magnetic resonance imaging findings and postoperative neurologic dysfunction in elderly patients undergoing coronary artery bypass grafting. *Ann Thorac Surg.* 2001;72(1):137–42.

87. Lund C, Sundet K, Tennoe B, et al. Cerebral ischemic injury and cognitive impairment after off-pump and on-pump coronary artery bypass grafting surgery. *Ann Thorac Surg.* 2005;80(6):2126–31.

88. Bekker A, Lee C, de Santi S, et al. Does mild cognitive impairment increase the risk of developing postoperative cognitive dysfunction? *Am J Surg.* 2010;199(6):782–8.

89. Hudetz JA, Iqbal Z, Gandhi SD, et al. Postoperative cognitive dysfunction in older patients with a history of alcohol abuse. *Anesthesiology.* 2007;106(3):423–30.

90. Xie Z, Swain CA, Ward SA, et al. Preoperative cerebrospinal fluid beta-amyloid/tau ratio and postoperative delirium. *Ann Clin Transl Neurol.* 2014;1(5):319–28.

91. Inouye SK. Delirium in older persons. *N Engl J Med.* 2006;354(11):1157–65.

92. Inouye SK, Westendorp RG, Saczynski JS. Delirium in elderly people. *Lancet.* 2014;383(9920):911–22.

93. Whitlock EL, Vannucci A, Avidan MS. Postoperative delirium. *Minerva Anestesiol.* 2011;77(4):448–56.

94. Rudolph JL, Jones RN, Rasmussen LS, Silverstein JH, Inouye SK, Marcantonio ER. Independent vascular and cognitive risk factors for postoperative delirium. *Am J Med.* 2007;120(9):807–13.

95. Binder LM, Iverson GL, Brooks BL. To err is human: "abnormal" neuropsychological scores and variability are common in healthy adults. *Arch Clin Neuropsychol.* 2009;24:31–46.

96. Brooks BL, Iverson GL. Comparing actual to estimated base rates of "abnormal" scores on neuropsychological test batteries: implications for interpretation. *Arch Clin Neuropsychol.* 2009;25:14–21.

97. American Academy of Clinical Neuropsychology. American Academy of Clinical Neuropsychology (AACN) practice guidelines for neuropsychological assessment and consultation. *Clin Neuropsychol.* 2007;21(2):209–31.

98. Turner SM, DeMers ST, Fox HR, Reed G. APA's guidelines for test user qualifications: an executive summary. *Am Psychol* 2001 56:1099–113.

99. American Psychological Association. Ethical principles of psychologists and code of conduct. *Am Psychol.* 2002;57:1060–73.

# PART III
# NEUROPROTECTION IN CRITICAL CARE

# 8 Neuroprotection for Traumatic Brain Injury

Jonathan J. Ratcliff and David W. Wright

## GENERAL CONSIDERATIONS

Traumatic brain injury (TBI) is a heterogeneous and clinically complex global health problem that worldwide affects approximately 10 million people annually.[1] In the United States alone, TBI leads to nearly 300,000 hospital admissions, resulting in 80,000 permanently disabled survivors and more than 50,000 deaths every year.[2] With more than 5 million US residents and another 7 million Europeans living with TBI-related disability, the individual and societal burdens are profound.[3-4] In the United States, falls account for the majority of TBI (35%), followed by motor vehicle collisions, blunt impact, and assaults.[5] Less commonly, penetrating trauma is the cause of TBI.

TBI is a disorder that encompasses diverse pathological conditions, each with a unique presentation, progression, treatment, and prognosis. To add to the complexity, most patients present with a combination of pathologies that make it exceedingly difficult to characterize a particular phenotype. Hence, TBI can be categorized in a variety of ways: by clinical severity, mechanism of injury, radiographic appearance, distribution of injury, or pathology. Despite tremendous clinical heterogeneity, TBI is fundamentally the product of a force that results in tissue strain, deformation, and structural injury to the brain.

The force transmitted to the brain often results in specific hemorrhage patterns that may be rapidly characterized with computed tomography (CT); this represents the primary injury. These radiographic patterns are associated with different clinical manifestations depending on the volume of the hemorrhage and the region affected. Contusions are the most common form of bleeding after TBI. This type of lesion is frequently observed in the orbitofrontal and inferior temporal lobe regions. Patients with contusions predominantly have depressed level of consciousness and limited focal weakness but may experience rapid deterioration associated with hemorrhage expansion and edema within the first 72 hours.

Traumatic subarachnoid hemorrhage (SAH) is associated with increased mortality regardless of volume, but with larger volumes mortality may increase two-fold. In addition to headache and depressed level of consciousness, posttraumatic SAH can result in obstructive hydrocephalus or delayed cerebral vasospasm (although the latter occurs much less often after traumatic SAH than after aneurysmal SAH).[6] Traumatic intraventricular hemorrhage is uncommon but, when present, is associated with worse outcomes.

Diffuse axonal injury (DAI) is a common mechanism of injury and cause of long-term disability after TBI. Clinically, patients with severe forms of DAI often have depressed mental status that is beyond what would be expected on the basis of findings on brain imaging. CT imaging may reveal small punctate hemorrhagic foci that arise from axonal shearing. Magnetic resonance imaging (MRI) is much more sensitive for detecting DAI than is CT. Axonal-shearing injury tends to be most severe in specific brain regions that are anatomically predisposed to maximal stress from rotational forces. Macroscopic tissue tears, best visualized by MRI, tend to occur in midline structures, including the dorsolateral midbrain and pons, posterior corpus callosum, parasagittal white matter, periventricular regions, and internal capsule. Microscopic damage occurs more diffusely, as manifested by axonal retraction bulbs throughout the white matter of the cerebral hemispheres. Small hemorrhages, known as gliding contusions, are sometimes associated with focal-shearing lesions (Figure 8.1).

Extra-axial hematomas are common following TBI, and clinical presentation varies greatly. Epidural hematomas may present with focal findings or depressed mental status secondary to compression of the brain and cerebral herniation. On CT imaging, epidural hematomas are elliptical and convex and are limited by the skull suture lines. Because epidural hematomas often reflect arterial bleeding, these hemorrhages require urgent surgery. Underlying brain tissue is often preserved if the hematoma can be evacuated prior to development of secondary injury. Patients

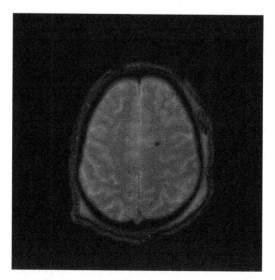

FIGURE 8.1 Gradient echo (GRE) sequence during magnetic resonance imaging (MRI) reveals several small foci of hemorrhage near the vertex. These findings are seen following diffuse axonal injury (DAI). Image courtesy of Jason Allen, MD, Assistant Professor, Department of Radiology, Emory University.

with epidural hematomas therefore may do well and recover completely if treated aggressively with surgical evacuation and medical management. Subdural hematomas also produce symptoms ranging from local compression to herniation. They are commonly seen in the elderly due to bleeding from the bridging veins that become increasingly vulnerable with aging and associated cerebral atrophy. On CT imaging, subdural hematomas are crescent shaped and may expand over the entire hemisphere. Unlike epidural hematomas, which almost always present acutely, the age of the blood in subdural hematoma may be acute, subacute, or chronic.

The initial injuries to neurons, glial cells, astrocytes, and the neurovascular bundle lead to cellular necrosis, edema, hemorrhage, and compression of neural structures. Within only a few moments following the initial injury, systemic and cellular secondary injury processes begin. Hypotension and hypoxia exacerbate these cellular and metabolic responses to traumatic injury. The ensuing cascade of events extends the magnitude of the neurologic injury; mitigation of these progressive events is the central tenet of TBI critical care treatments.

## MECHANISMS OF AND RISKS FOR NEUROLOGICAL INJURY

The secondary injury that ensues after TBI provides an opportunity for neuroprotection. Prevention and reversal of secondary injury should be the focus of care from the pre-hospital environment, to the emergency department, to the perioperative and critical care arenas. Effective neuroprotection, however, requires an understanding of the mechanisms of secondary injury at the cellular level.

In addition to systemic hypotension and hypoxia, intracranial hypertension, fever, hyper- or hypoglycemia, acidosis, hyper- or hypocapnia, cerebral vasospasm, and coagulopathy can also exacerbate secondary injury after TBI.[7-8] These clinical events can initiate and propagate cellular mechanisms of secondary injury, including neuronal depolarization, glutamate excitotoxicity, lipid peroxidation, increase in proinflammatory proteins, blood–brain barrier (BBB) disruption, mitochondrial dysfunction, brain glucose utilization disruption, generation of nitric oxide and oxygen free radicals, metabolic mismatch, and disturbance of ionic homeostasis.[9-10]

### Hypoxemia

Multiple investigations have demonstrated that hypoxemia ($SpO_2$ < 90% or $PaO_2$ < 60 mm Hg) is associated with increased risk of poor outcome after TBI in a dose-dependent fashion.[7,11-12] Therefore, observation and correction of hypoxemia is essential.

### Hypotension

Hypotension is associated with poor outcome largely due to hypoxic-ischemic injury. Historically defined as systolic blood pressure (SBP) of lower than 90 mm Hg or mean arterial pressure (MAP) of lower than 65 mm Hg, hypotension is common among TBI patients and is often due to extracranial injuries in multisystem trauma patients. A dose-dependent relationship exists between the severity and duration of hypotension and outcome following TBI; thus, rapid recognition and correction of this condition is a priority.[7,11-13] The updated Brain Trauma Foundation guidelines recommend that SBP be maintained greater than 100 mm Hg for those aged 50–69 years.[14] Patients between the ages of 15–49 years and those 70 years or older should have an SBP target of 110 mm Hg or greater. The most prudent strategy is to achieve normal hemodynamic parameters until resuscitation may be directed with more sophisticated monitoring.

## Intracranial Hypertension

Management of intracranial hypertension is a mainstay of critical care for TBI.[15] Intracranial hypertension is frequently the result of mass lesions (hemorrhage) and edema (both local and diffuse). Edema can be cytotoxic (due to loss of cellular membrane integrity) and/or vasogenic (due to breakdown of the BBB). Intracranial pressure (ICP) in the adult patient is thought to be pathologic when greater than 20 mm Hg; the extent and duration that ICP exceeds this level is associated with increased mortality and morbidity in a dose-dependent fashion.[16–17] Routine invasive monitoring is required to recognize and guide treatment of elevated ICP.

## MONITORING FOR NEUROLOGIC INJURY
### Clinical Assessment

Detailed and frequent monitoring is a defining feature of the ICU management of a TBI patient. The sequential neurologic examination performed by clinicians at the bedside is the foundation for physiologic monitoring in the ICU and is essential to understanding the clinical situation and optimizing care.[18] The exam should focus on assessing the level of consciousness, as with the Glasgow Coma Scale (GCS) or Full Outline of UnResponsiveness (FOUR) score, as well as brainstem reflexes. Performed serially, the clinical examination is a specific tool for detecting clinical deterioration. Observation of an evolving or deteriorating exam, however, may be confounded by treatments employed to prevent secondary injury, such as sedation. A deteriorating exam may also be a late sign of irreversible damage from progressive secondary injury that has already occurred.

The GCS is the most frequently used clinical scale for assessing severity of injury, with injury severity stratified as mild (GCS 13–15), moderate (GCS 9–12), and severe (GCS 3–8).[19–20] It is also used to prognosticate and to monitor for neurological improvement and deterioration. The principal advantage of the GCS is that it is easy to perform and is reproducible. It is, however, limited in the evaluation of brainstem integrity. It is also limited in evaluation of the intubated patient since intubation precludes assessment of verbal responsiveness.

The FOUR score is a coma grading scale that was developed to overcome limitations of the GCS.[21] It assesses four parameters: eye response, motor response, brainstem reflexes (pupillary reflexes, corneal reflexes, and cough), and respiration pattern. The FOUR score is particularly advantageous over the GCS in the intubated patient because there is no verbal component, and therefore complete assessments may be performed. It also allows for delineation of herniation syndromes.[21] The GCS, however, remains useful in the emergency setting because it may be calculated after a rapid evaluation and is highly reliable across the spectrum of care providers.

The goal of continuous physiologic monitoring is to identify antecedent physiologic variables that predict clinical deterioration, rapidly identify emerging crises, and validate appropriate responses to therapy. Cardiac and pulmonary ICU physiologic monitoring, including blood pressure, heart rate and rhythm, respiratory rate, end-tidal $CO_2$, and pulse oximetry, is the minimum standard of care for the severe TBI patient. Use of minimally invasive and noninvasive technologies for cardiac output monitoring are on the rise, but utility and accuracy have not been fully determined.

Recently, there has been a focused effort to develop and validate neurophysiologic monitors. The goal is to provide clinicians with specific physiologic targets to mitigate the risk of otherwise occult progressive secondary injury. ICP monitors, continuous electroencephalography (cEEG), and transcranial Doppler (TCD) are routinely deployed for TBI patients. Cerebral metabolism monitoring with microdialysis, cerebral oxygenation, and noninvasive cerebral blood flow (CBF) monitoring are also being used in many trauma centers.

## Intracranial Pressure Monitoring

The recently updated Brain Trauma Foundation guidelines recommend ICP monitoring for all salvageable TBI patients with an abnormal CT scan and a GCS score of 3–8.[14] Intraventricular pressure monitoring remains the preferred method for ICP monitoring, primarily because it provides a more accurate assessment of pressure and allows for therapeutic drainage of cerebrospinal fluid. Parenchymal ICP monitors may also be used, especially if the ventricles are effaced or when continuous monitoring is needed.

Observational studies examining the merits of ICP monitoring have produced mixed results. Patients with elevated ICP have worse outcomes, and ICP monitoring provides a tool to guide treatment. The relationship between ICP monitoring and improvement in patient outcome after TBI is not clear. In some observational studies, ICP monitoring has been associated with prolonged mechanical ventilation and worse functional outcome, whereas other studies have indicated benefit.[22–28] These observational studies, however, often had flaws inherent to their design, such as patient selection bias in which sicker patients received an ICP monitor.

To evaluate the benefit of ICP monitoring, a multicenter clinical trial was conducted in Latin America that compared protocols for ICP management with and without invasive ICP monitoring.[29] The study found that there was no difference in the primary functional outcome, although the ICP-monitored group required fewer brain-specific therapies and had a shorter ICU length of stay. This study highlights the need to further explore treatment thresholds and existing management options for elevated ICP.

## Transcranial Doppler

TCD is a noninvasive method that utilizes ultrasound waves to measure CBF velocity in the large intracranial vessels. The clinical utility of TCD in the setting of TBI remains under investigation, but routine monitoring in this population is growing. TCD can help identify vasospasm and critical intracranial hypertension. TCD has been suggested as a noninvasive method for monitoring ICP through use of the pulsatility index (PI), but evidence to support routine use for this purpose is limited and demonstrated mixed results.[30–32] cEEG combines EEG with video recording captured over an extended period of time (typically a minimum of 24 hours) to monitor for secondary brain injury and neurologic deterioration. The Critical Care Continuous EEG Task Force of the American Clinical Neurophysiology Society has developed expert consensus recommendations for the use of cEEG.[33] cEEG is advised for the diagnosis of nonconvulsive seizures, nonconvulsive status epilepticus (NCSE), and other paroxysmal events. One in three adult, comatose, severe TBI patients monitored with cEEG experience seizures, which are typically nonconvulsive. It is widely believed that these seizures cause secondary injury, although there are no level 1 data showing that anticonvulsant therapy given to eliminate nonconvulsive seizure activity after TBI improves outcome.

In the treatment of TBI patients with refractory intracranial hypertension, continuous high-dose sedation is often used to reduce cerebral metabolic demand.[34] It can be a clinical challenge, however, to judge when an optimal level of sedation has been achieved. cEEG and its derivatives, such as bispectral index (BIS) monitoring, may be used to guide sedation by targeting an EEG response (e.g., EEG continuous delta or burst-suppression, or a BIS level between 40 and 60), hence minimizing the risk of under- or over-sedation.[35]

## Brain Multimodality Monitoring

Over the past 10 years, multimodal neuromonitoring following brain injury has become increasingly complex. Several variables related to the pathophysiology of TBI have been identified as promising targets for goal-directed therapy. This has resulted in increasingly widespread adoption of these tools, but questions remain regarding optimal therapeutic strategies that result in positive clinical outcomes. A reasonable conclusion is that the science of neuromonitoring is in a learning phase and that continued development of these technologically sophisticated monitors, which provide real-time insight into cerebral physiology and associated therapeutic protocols, require ongoing clinical investigation.

## Cerebral Metabolism

Microdialysis (MD) is an invasive laboratory device that samples brain tissue vulnerable to secondary injury and analyzes the local biochemistry. Multiple assays are available to measure the dialysate for concentrations of glucose, lactate, and pyruvate, among other metabolic parameters. It has been suggested that MD can identify cerebral metabolic crisis.[36] *Metabolic crisis* is defined clinically by an elevation in the lactate/pyruvate ratio (LPR >40) with concurrent brain tissue hypoglycemia of less than 0.4 μmol/L, which can only be observed with continuous MD.[37] Two clinical manifestations of metabolic crisis have been identified. Type I metabolic crisis is characterized by elevated LPR and low tissue oxygen and is believed to result from a deficiency of energy substrates. Type II metabolic crisis is characterized by elevated LPR and normal tissue oxygen concentrations and is believed to be due to severe mitochondrial dysfunction.[37] Several observational studies have linked metabolic crisis with worse outcome.

Despite the monitoring capabilities of MD and the intuitive relationship between metabolic crisis and poor outcome, interventions that correct MD-derived biomarkers and improve outcome remain elusive.[37] In one clinical trial, aggressive maintenance of CPP and control of ICP failed to improve oxidative metabolism or normalize biomarkers of metabolic crisis.[36] Furthermore, it has been suggested that active treatment of ischemia may result in local hyperoxia without improving oxygen utilization and reducing free-radical formation, which could result in further damage to severely crippled mitochondria.[38] MD has a role in the critical care of the TBI patient and enhances understanding of the cerebral physiology, but therapeutic protocols require further delineation.

## Cerebral Oxygenation

Cerebral oxygenation is a function of oxygen content of the blood and cerebral perfusion. Monitoring of cerebral oxygenation may be performed using jugular venous bulb oximetry ($SjvO_2$), direct brain tissue oxygen tension measurement ($PbtO_2$), near-infrared spectroscopy (NIRS), and oxygen-15 positron emission tomography (PET). Both low $PbtO_2$ and low $SjvO_2$ respond favorably to hyperoxia, CPP augmentation, and blood transfusion. The most frequently utilized modalities are $SjvO_2$, which measures global cerebral oxygenation, and $PbtO_2$, which measures focal cerebral oxygenation using an invasive probe. A $PbtO_2$ value of less than 15 mm Hg is considered a threshold for focal cerebral ischemia, whereas cerebral compromise occurs with a $PbtO_2$ of less than 20 mm Hg.[39–40] An $SjvO_2$ of less than 50–55% is the threshold associated with worsened outcome.[14,39]

Although deficient brain tissue oxygenation has been associated with poor outcome following TBI, it is unclear if treating and avoiding low cerebral oxygen improves outcomes.[39,41] There have been reports suggesting that goal-directed ICP/CPP plus $PbtO_2$ therapy results in superior clinical outcome compared to ICP/CPP-directed therapy alone.[42–43] However, there also are reports demonstrating no clinically significant benefit.[43] Future phase III clinical trials will address the potential benefit that $PbtO_2$ therapy adds to ICP/CPP goal-directed therapy.

Despite the absence of robust clinical outcome data, $PbtO_2$ use is increasing in the critical care of TBI patients. There is, however, debate as to whether the monitor should be placed remotely or adjacent to the region of injury. The view that $PbtO_2$ is merely a marker of ischemia is probably overly simplistic and likely reflects a complex interplay of oxygen delivery, demand, and utilization.[41]

## Optimal Cerebral Perfusion Pressure

Modern critical care of the TBI patient requires maintaining optimal cerebral perfusion and limiting intracranial hypertension. By definition, optimal CPP is the pressure at which an adequate supply of blood and oxygen is delivered to the tissue to meet metabolic demand. There is skepticism that the common goal of maintaining a CPP 60–70 mm Hg is applicable across the spectrum of TBI and that it may result in either hypo- or hyperperfusion in certain patients.[44–45] Disruption of autoregulation after TBI, patient age, and pre-injury arterial hypertension likely influence optimal CPP for individual patients, supporting the theory of a personalized approach to CPP management.[45]

In 2002, Steiner and colleagues reported a method for estimating optimal CPP using the pressure reactivity index (PRx), a representation of cerebrovascular pressure reactivity.[46] PRx is measured by calculating the correlation coefficients from the averaged values of 10-second epochs of arterial blood pressure and ICP over a moving 5-minute window. Negative or zero values of PRx suggest appropriate cerebrovascular reactivity and are a surrogate marker for intact cerebrovascular autoregulation. Optimal CPP can be estimated by graphing PRx against CPP, with optimal CPP at the bottom of a U-shaped curve where PRx is most negative. Steiner and colleagues demonstrated that when observed CPP was close to the derived optimal CPP, patients had improved outcomes.[46–47]

Aries and colleagues presented an algorithm for automated and continuous updating of optimal CPP derived from 4-hour time windows.[47] In an effort to validate this algorithm, they evaluated the association between clinical deviation from calculated optimal CPP and clinical outcome in a retrospective analysis. Clinical deviation from optimal CPP was associated with worse outcome.[47] Although promising, CPP optimization using real-time PRx calculation has yet to be adopted as a routine clinical practice.

## NEUROPROTECTION STRATEGIES
### Controlling Intracranial Hypertension

ICP control after TBI is a multistep process, with increasingly invasive and higher risk strategies that are employed should early stage interventions fail to produce the desired effect. Intracranial hypertension may act negatively on the brain in two ways. The pressure exerts mechanical forces on the brain that could result in cerebral herniation, which can be fatal. Additionally, elevated ICP opposes CBF, which is primarily driven by the CPP (defined as MAP − ICP). CBF reductions result in decreased oxygen and glucose delivery, which in turn can exacerbate ischemic and metabolic injury.

### Cerebral Blood Volume Manipulation

Basic strategies to control ICP include proper patient positioning to ensure adequate venous drainage, elevating the head of the bed to 30–45 degrees, and keeping the neck straight to optimize jugular venous drainage to prevent cerebral venous congestion. Theoretically, minimizing usage of internal jugular venous catheters should prevent internal jugular thrombosis. Additionally, close monitoring should be directed toward the effects of positive end expiratory pressure (PEEP) on venous drainage and resulting ICP. PEEP should be minimized to provide sufficient support to prevent atelectasis and maintain oxygenation; in otherwise healthy lungs, 5 cm $H_2O$ generally is sufficient for this purpose. As PEEP increases, so does intrathoracic pressure, leading to increased central venous pressure (CVP). Increased CVP acts as resistance to cerebral venous drainage and results in cerebral venous congestion. PEEP titration of the TBI patient should be performed with care and in conjunction with neuromonitoring.

Cerebral blood volume (CBV) may also be managed by reducing intracranial CBF. Arterial blood flow may be manipulated using several strategies, including hyperventilation, sedation, and optimizing SBP. Strategies that decrease ICP also have the potential to increase ischemic injury if CBF is critically reduced. $PbtO_2$ is a reliable way to ensure that hyperventilation or blood pressure reduction is not resulting in reduced oxygen delivery.

Hyperventilation leads to a decrease in blood $CO_2$ content that induces cerebral vasoconstriction, decreased CBF, and decreased CBV, resulting in lower ICP. During routine care of the TBI patient, partial pressure of carbon dioxide $(PCO_2)$ should be kept in the normal (eucapnic) range between 35 and 40 mm Hg. Severe vasoconstriction that leads to ischemia and worsening outcome can occur when the $PCO_2$ is 25 mm Hg or less and therefore should be avoided unless concurrent invasive monitoring of jugular venous bulb oximetry or brain tissue oxygenation is employed.[14]

## Hyperosmolar Therapy

The brain parenchyma is composed of large quantities of water; therefore, brain volume may be altered by changing the brain water content. Hyperosmolar agents create an osmotic gradient for water to move from the parenchyma to the intravascular space across the BBB. The effectiveness of hyperosmolar therapy is predicated upon an intact BBB that limits the movement of the osmotic agent from the blood into the parenchyma. Mannitol and hypertonic saline are the two most commonly used therapies. Recent meta-analyses suggest that hypertonic saline may improve ICP control relative to mannitol, though this remains controversial.[48–49]

## Sedation

Sedatives and analgesics may reduce ICP by multiple mechanisms. First, they induce a reduction in cerebral metabolic rate and consequently CBF, leading to a parallel decrease in CBV. This decrease in CBV leads to a reduction in intracranial volume and lower ICP. Second, sedation and analgesia reduce pain and agitation. When poorly controlled, pain and agitation result in increased sympathetic tone, leading to arterial hypertension and an associated ICP surge. Third, analgesia improves tolerance of the endotracheal tube and, by reducing agitation and coughing, avoids increases in intrathoracic pressure, which can reduce jugular venous outflow and raise ICP.

Substantial data are lacking to guide optimal sedative choice. As a general rule, patients in ICP crisis should be sedated to a quiet, motionless state. Propofol, fentanyl, remifentanil, and midazolam, alone or in various combinations, are most often used for this purpose. When maximal intervention has failed to control ICP, neuromuscular blockade, or barbiturate anesthesia with pentobarbital, often titrated to burst suppression on cEEG, may be used.

## Surgical Decompression

Surgical decompression is effective in controlling ICP. The Decompressive Craniectomy in Diffuse TBI (DECRA) trial evaluated the potential clinical benefit of craniectomy following TBI by comparing early bifrontotemporal-parietal craniectomy to medical management.[50] While surgical decompression resulted in better ICP control, there was no observed clinical benefit with respect to mortality, and functional outcomes were actually worse in the surgical arm of the study. Conversely, in the RESCUEicp trial, delayed (1–12 hours) decompressive craniectomy significantly reduced mortality, but at the cost of increasing the numbers of survivors with moderate or severe disability.[51] The efficacy of surgical decompression for TBI patients remains controversial, and the decision to perform this procedure should be made on an individual basis, involving patients and families in the decision-making process.

## Corticosteroids

Corticosteroids are commonly used to treat ICP elevations related to vasogenic edema arising from mass lesions such as tumors; they are not, however, recommended for ICP management following TBI. The multicenter CRASH trial demonstrated that corticosteroids increase mortality in TBI patients.[52]

## Coagulopathy Reversal

It is estimated that one-third of TBI patients have signs of coagulopathy, which is associated with worsened outcome through microvascular thrombosis and hemorrhage expansion.[8] While the etiology of TBI-related coagulopathy is incompletely understood, leading hypotheses suggest a consumptive coagulopathy similar to disseminated intravascular coagulation (DIC), platelet dysfunction, and activation of protein C pathways secondary to hypoperfusion.[53-54]

A clinical trial comparing prophylactic fresh frozen plasma to normal saline following TBI found that fresh frozen plasma was associated with adverse effects, including increased incidence of delayed intracranial hematomas and higher mortality.[55] Use of blood and blood products carries inherent risk and therefore should be used judiciously to target normal clotting function (INR ≤1.4). Functional viscoelastic assays of whole blood coagulation, such as thromboelastography (TEG) and rotational thromboelastometry (ROTEM), can allow for individualized transfusion therapy and have been increasingly adopted for clinical use.[8] The benefit of viscoelastic-guided coagulopathy reversal after TBI requires prospective evaluation, but it appears to hold promise in maximizing the benefit of coagulopathy reversal while minimizing unnecessary blood product administration, thereby reducing associated risk and limiting use of finite resources.

## Hyperglycemia

Disturbed brain glucose metabolism is a complication of severe TBI as well as an independent risk factor for poor outcome.[56] Observations that persistent hyperglycemia is associated with worsened outcome led investigators to conduct a clinical trial evaluating strict glucose control.[57] In this small phase II trial, however, strict glucose control had no clinical benefit. Further investigation has demonstrated that strict glucose control increased episodes of cerebral hypoglycemia identified with cerebral microdialysis.[57-58] Increased glucose variability also appears to have a significant and negative relationship with TBI outcome.[59] As a general rule, serum glucose should be kept to 120–180 mg/dL, with careful avoidance of hypoglycemic episodes and dramatic variation.

## Anemia

Anemia following TBI is common and associated with poor outcome. It has been suggested that secondary brain injury may be propagated by decreased cerebral oxygen delivery associated with anemia. Observational data have demonstrated improved cerebral oxygenation after transfusion. To determine the best transfusion strategy following TBI, Robertson and colleagues conducted a 6-year, 200-subject randomized clinical trial comparing erythropoietin to placebo, and a liberal transfusion strategy (target Hgb ≥10 g/dL) to a restrictive transfusion trigger (target Hgb ≥7 g/dL).[60] This study showed no benefit of erythropoietin over placebo, and no clinical benefit with a more liberal transfusion strategy of greater than 10 g/dL. The liberal transfusion strategy did, however, lead to increased thromboembolic events compared to the restrictive transfusion strategy. These data are consistent with a subgroup analysis of the Transfusion Requirements in Critical Care Trial, which also failed to demonstrate an advantage of liberal transfusion goals.[61] Given these data, there is no conclusive evidence to support an Hgb transfusion trigger of 7 g/dL or higher during the immediate ICU course following TBI.

## Temperature Management

Observational studies have demonstrated an association between hyperthermia and worse outcome after TBI. Both the magnitude and duration of hyperthermia, without regard to etiology, are related to outcome, suggesting a dose–response relationship.[62] Evidence demonstrating favorable outcomes with fever prevention or control, however, is lacking. Nevertheless, it is prudent to control temperature aggressively, either with antipyretics or surface cooling, to maintain normothermia.

Although hypothermia appears to improve intracranial hypertension, there is not an established clinical benefit to this approach.[63] The European Study of Therapeutic Hypothermia for Intracranial Pressure Reduction after Traumatic Brain Injury (EuroTherm) demonstrated worse outcome in the hypothermia cohort.[64] Critics of the trial have observed that early hypothermia was instituted before other common ICP control measures and that, therefore, the trial results have limited applicability given the current common practice of using hypothermia as a late-stage intervention. Hypothermia for neuroprotection after TBI has failed to show benefit except in patients undergoing craniotomy for hematoma evacuation. The HypOthermia for Patients requiring Evacuation of Subdural Hematoma (HOPES) multicenter clinical trial will specifically address the question of benefit in this craniotomy cohort.

## Pharmacologic Neuroprotection after TBI

Despite an unprecedented and focused research effort over the past two decades to discover and develop a novel pharmacologic neuroprotective agent, no such agent has been identified. Progesterone, a neurosteroid, has been found to have a multipotent neuroprotective effect in more than 300 preclinical TBI studies. When tested in two well-designed and well-conducted phase III clinical trials, however, progesterone did not result in improved clinical outcome.[65–66]

## IMPLICATIONS FOR CLINICAL PRACTICE

TBI is a common clinically diverse entity resulting in tissue disruption and neuronal injury from mechanical forces transmitted to the brain. The presentation and clinical characteristics can vary depending on the location and clinical severity of the injury. Treatment decisions are often guided by the observed neurologic injury on clinical examination and neuroimaging (i.e., extra-axial hemorrhage, parenchymal contusions, or diffuse axonal injury).

While no single pharmacological agent has been shown to improve outcomes following TBI, it is clear that compliance with guidelines and the use of ICU protocols has improved outcomes dramatically. From 1970 to 1990, TBI-related mortality has dropped approximately 9% per decade.[67] This reduction in mortality can be attributed to improved general critical care and the identification, prevention, and aggressive treatment of secondary neurologic injury that may result from hypoxia, hypotension, intracranial hypertension, and cerebral hypoperfusion.

The current approach to neuroprotection for the TBI patient may be best characterized as targeting normal physiologic parameters that minimize secondary injury, creating a milieu in which the injured brain may have an opportunity to recover. This may be accomplished by maintaining normal cerebral perfusion pressure, oxygen delivery, ICP, volume status, and temperature, as well as promoting adequate nutrition. Titration of CPP and ICP should be performed in a manner that minimizes physiologic extremes and should be personalized to the individual patient.

## FUTURE DIRECTIONS

In spite of the history of negative clinical trials, there is reason to believe that clinical care and understanding of this disease process will soon improve. To further advance the care of the TBI patient, investigators and clinicians alike will need to focus on developing methods for identifying injury progression before the injury becomes irreversible, while developing and evaluating protocols for responding to identified stressors that a patient may be experiencing within the context of the patient's own milieu—that is, goal-directed personalized neurocritical care. This will be accomplished through a deepening understanding of the phenotype of a particular patient and injury pattern, improved neuroimaging and physiological monitoring, and developing appropriate protocols for responding to a variety of deranged physiologic and clinical variables. Research to accomplish these goals is currently ongoing and in various stages of development. As phenotyping, monitoring, and response to these derived physiologic variables are improved, it is expected that novel pharmacologic agents will continue to be developed and evaluated.

## REFERENCES

1. Hyder AA, Wunderlich CA, Puvanachandra P, et al. The impact of traumatic brain injuries: a global perspective. *NeuroRehabilitation.* 2007;22(5):341–53.
2. Rutland-Brown W, Langlois JA, Thomas KE, et al. Incidence of traumatic brain injury in the United States, 2003. *J Head Trauma Rehabil.* 2006;21(6):544–8.
3. Thurman DJ, Alverson C, Dunn KA, et al. Traumatic brain injury in the United States: a public health perspective. *J Head Trauma Rehabil.* 1999;14(6):602–15.
4. Tagliaferri F, Compagnone C, Korsic M, et al. A systematic review of brain injury epidemiology in Europe. *Acta Neurochir (Wien).* 2006;148(3):255–68; discussion 268.
5. Faul M, Xu L, Wald MM, et al. Traumatic Brain in the United States: emergency department visits, hospitalizations and deaths 2002–2006. http://www.cdc.gov/traumaticbraininjury/pdf/blue_book.pdf. 2010; Date Accessed: January 5, 2016.
6. Perrein A, Petry L, Reis A, et al. Cerebral vasospasm after traumatic brain injury: an update. *Minerva Anestesiol.* 2015;81(11):1219–28.
7. McHugh GS, Engel DC, Butcher I, et al. Prognostic value of secondary insults in traumatic brain injury: results from the IMPACT study. *J Neurotrauma.* 2007;24(2):287–93.

8. Laroche M, Kutcher ME, Huang MC, et al. Coagulopathy after traumatic brain injury. *Neurosurgery.* 2012;70(6):1334–45.

9. Corps KN, Roth TL, McGavern DB. Inflammation and neuroprotection in traumatic brain injury. *JAMA Neurol.* 2015;72(3):355–62.

10. Kochanek PM, Jackson TC, Ferguson NM, et al. Emerging therapies in traumatic brain injury. *Semin Neurol.* 2015;35(1):83–100.

11. Chesnut RM, Marshall LF, Klauber MR, et al. The role of secondary brain injury in determining outcome from severe head injury. *J Trauma.* 1993;34(2):216–22.

12. Manley G, Knudson MM, Morabito D, et al. Hypotension, hypoxia, and head injury: frequency, duration, and consequences. *Arch Surg.* 2001;136(10):1118–23.

13. Jeremitsky E, Omert L, Dunham CM, et al. Harbingers of poor outcome the day after severe brain injury: hypothermia, hypoxia, and hypoperfusion. *J Trauma.* 2003;54(2):312–9.

14. Carney N, Totten AM, O'Reilly C, et al. Guidelines for the management of severe traumatic brain injury, 4th edition. *Neurosurgery,* 2016;80(1):6–15.

15. Bratton SL, Chestnut RM, Ghajar J, et al. Guidelines for the management of severe traumatic brain injury. I. Blood pressure and oxygenation. *J Neurotrauma.* 2007;24 Suppl 1:S7–13.

16. Mangat HS. Severe traumatic brain injury. *Continuum (Minneap Minn).* 2012; 18(3):532–46.

17. Narayan RK, Greenberg RP, Miller JD, et al. Improved confidence of outcome prediction in severe head injury. A comparative analysis of the clinical examination, multimodality evoked potentials, CT scanning, and intracranial pressure. *J Neurosurg.* 1981;54(6):751–62.

18. Le Roux P. Intracranial pressure after the BEST TRIP trial: a call for more monitoring. *Curr Opin Crit Care.* 2014;20(2):141–7.

19. Teasdale G, Jennett B. Assessment of coma and impaired consciousness. A practical scale. *Lancet.* 1974;2(7872):81–4.

20. Teasdale G, Jennett B. Assessment and prognosis of coma after head injury. *Acta Neurochir (Wien).* 1976;34(1-4):45–55.

21. Wijdicks EF, Bamlet WR, Maramattom BV, et al. Validation of a new coma scale: the FOUR score. *Ann Neurol.* 2005;58(4):585–93.

22. Cremer OL, van Dijk GW, van Wensen E, et al. Effect of intracranial pressure monitoring and targeted intensive care on functional outcome after severe head injury. *Crit Care Med.* 2005;33(10):2207–13.

23. Griesdale DE, McEwen J, Kurth T, et al. External ventricular drains and mortality in patients with severe traumatic brain injury. *Can J Neurol Sci.* 2010;37(1):43–8.

24. Shafi S, Diaz-Arrastia R, Madden C, et al. Intracranial pressure monitoring in brain-injured patients is associated with worsening of survival. *J Trauma.* 2008;64(2):335–40.

25. Howells T, Elf K, Jones PA, et al. Pressure reactivity as a guide in the treatment of cerebral perfusion pressure in patients with brain trauma. *J Neurosurg.* 2005;102(2):311–7.

26. Lane PL, Skoretz TG, Doig G, et al. Intracranial pressure monitoring and outcomes after traumatic brain injury. *Can J Surg.* 2000;43(6):442–8.

27. Agrawal D, Raghavendran K, Schaubel DE, et al. A propensity score analysis of the impact of invasive intracranial pressure monitoring on outcomes after severe traumatic brain injury. *J Neurotrauma,* 2015;33(9):853–8.

28. Stein SC, Georgoff P, Meghan S, et al. Relationship of aggressive monitoring and treatment to improved outcomes in severe traumatic brain injury. *J Neurosurg.* 2010;112(5):1105–12.

29. Chesnut RM, Temkin N, Carney N, et al. A trial of intracranial-pressure monitoring in traumatic brain injury. *N Engl J Med.* 2012;367(26):2471–81.

30. Ragauskas A, Daubaris G, Dziugys A, et al. Innovative non-invasive method for absolute intracranial pressure measurement without calibration. *Acta Neurochir Suppl.* 2005;95:357–61.

31. Bellner J, Romner B, Reinstrup P, et al. Transcranial Doppler sonography pulsatility index (PI) reflects intracranial pressure (ICP). *Surg Neurol.* 2004;62(1):45–51; discussion 51.

32. Zweifel C, Czosnyka M, Carrera E, et al. Reliability of the blood flow velocity pulsatility index for assessment of intracranial and cerebral perfusion pressures in head-injured patients. *Neurosurgery.* 2012;71(4):853–61.

33. Herman ST, Abend NS, Bleck TP, et al. Consensus statement on continuous EEG in critically ill adults and children, part I: indications. *J Clin Neurophysiol.* 2015;32(2):87–95.

34. Roberts I, Sydenham E. Barbiturates for acute traumatic brain injury. *Cochrane Database Syst Rev.* 2012;12:Cd000033.

35. Sessler CN, Grap MJ, Ramsay MA. Evaluating and monitoring analgesia and sedation in the intensive care unit. *Crit Care.* 2008;12 Suppl 3:S2.

36. Stein NR, McArthur DL, Etchepare M, et al. Early cerebral metabolic crisis after TBI influences outcome despite adequate hemodynamic resuscitation. *Neurocrit Care.* 2012;17(1):49–57.

37. Carre E, Ogier M, Boret H, et al. Metabolic crisis in severely head-injured patients: is ischemia just the tip of the iceberg? *Front Neurol.* 2013;4:146.

38. Diringer MN. Hyperoxia: good or bad for the injured brain? *Curr Opin Crit Care.* 2008;14(2):167–71.

39. Bratton SL, Chestnut RM, Ghajar J, et al. Guidelines for the management of severe traumatic brain injury. X. Brain oxygen monitoring and thresholds. *J Neurotrauma.* 2007;24 Suppl 1:S65–70.

40. Nangunoori R, Maloney-Wilensky E, Stiefel M, et al. Brain tissue oxygen-based therapy and outcome after severe traumatic brain injury: a systematic literature review. *Neurocrit Care.* 2012;17(1):131–8.

41. Lazaridis C, Andrews CM. Brain tissue oxygenation, lactate-pyruvate ratio, and cerebrovascular pressure reactivity monitoring in severe traumatic brain injury: systematic review and viewpoint. *Neurocrit Care.* 2014;21(2):345–55.

42. Lin CM, Lin MC, Huang SJ, et al. A prospective randomized study of brain tissue oxygen pressure-guided management in moderate and severe traumatic brain injury patients. *Biomed Res Int.* 2015;2015:529580.

43. Green JA, Pellegrini DC, Vanderkolk WE, et al. Goal directed brain tissue oxygen monitoring versus conventional management in traumatic brain injury: an analysis of in hospital recovery. *Neurocrit Care.* 2013;18(1):20–5.

44. Vespa P. What is the optimal threshold for cerebral perfusion pressure following traumatic brain injury? *Neurosurg Focus.* 2003;15(6):E4.

45. White H, Venkatesh B. Cerebral perfusion pressure in neurotrauma: a review. *Anesth Analg.* 2008;107(3):979–88.

46. Steiner LA, Czosnyka M, Piechnik SK, et al. Continuous monitoring of cerebrovascular pressure reactivity allows determination of optimal cerebral perfusion pressure in patients with traumatic brain injury. *Crit Care Med.* 2002;30(4):733–8.

47. Aries MJ, Czosnyka M, Budohoski KP, et al. Continuous determination of optimal cerebral perfusion pressure in traumatic brain injury. *Crit Care Med.* 2012;40(8):2456–63.

48. Li M, Chen T, Chen SD, et al. Comparison of equimolar doses of mannitol and hypertonic saline for the treatment of elevated intracranial pressure after traumatic brain injury: a systematic review and meta-analysis. *Medicine (Baltimore).* 2015;94(17):e736.

49. Diringer MN. New trends in hyperosmolar therapy? *Curr Opin Crit Care.* 2013;19(2):77–82.

50. Cooper DJ, Rosenfeld JV, Murray L, et al. Decompressive craniectomy in diffuse traumatic brain injury. *N Engl J Med.* 2011;364(16):1493–502.

51. Hutchinson PJ, Kolias AG, Timofeev IS, et al. Trial of decompressive craniectomy for traumatic intracranial hypertension. *N Engl J Med.* 2016;375(12):1119–30.

52. Roberts I, Yates D, Sandercock P, et al. Effect of intravenous corticosteroids on death within 14 days in 10008 adults with clinically significant head injury (MRC CRASH trial): randomised placebo-controlled trial. *Lancet.* 2004;364(9442):1321–8.

53. Stein SC, Smith DH. Coagulopathy in traumatic brain injury. *Neurocrit Care.* 2004;1(4):479–88.

54. Harhangi BS, Kompanje EJ, Leebeek FW, et al. Coagulation disorders after traumatic brain injury. *Acta Neurochir (Wien).* 2008;150(2):165–75; discussion 175.

55. Etemadrezaie H, Baharvahdat H, Shariati Z, et al. The effect of fresh frozen plasma in severe closed head injury. *Clin Neurol Neurosurg.* 2007;109(2):166–71.

56. Salim A, Hadjizacharia P, Dubose J, et al. Persistent hyperglycemia in severe traumatic brain injury: an independent predictor of outcome. *Am Surg.* 2009;75(1):25–9.

57. Coester A, Neumann CR, Schmidt MI. Intensive insulin therapy in severe traumatic brain injury: a randomized trial. *J Trauma.* 2010;68(4):904–11.

58. Oddo M, Schmidt JM, Carrera E, et al. Impact of tight glycemic control on cerebral glucose metabolism after severe brain injury: a microdialysis study. *Crit Care Med.* 2008;36(12):3233–8.

59. Matsushima K, Peng M, Velasco C, et al. Glucose variability negatively impacts long-term functional outcome in patients with traumatic brain injury. *J Crit Care.* 2012;27(2):125–31.

60. Robertson CS, Hannay HJ, Yamal JM, et al. Effect of erythropoietin and transfusion threshold on neurological recovery after traumatic brain injury: a randomized clinical trial. *JAMA.* 2014;312(1):36–47.

61. Hebert PC, Wells G, Blajchman MA, et al. A multicenter, randomized, controlled clinical trial of transfusion requirements in critical care. Transfusion Requirements in Critical Care Investigators, Canadian Critical Care Trials Group. *N Engl J Med.* 1999;340(6):409–17.

62. Li J, Jiang JY. Chinese Head Trauma Data Bank: effect of hyperthermia on the outcome of acute head trauma patients. *J Neurotrauma.* 2012;29(1):96–100.

63. Jiang JY, Xu W, Li WP, et al. Effect of long-term mild hypothermia or short-term mild hypothermia on outcome of patients with severe traumatic brain injury. *J Cereb Blood Flow Metab.* 2006;26(6):771–6.

64. Andrews PJ, Sinclair HL, Rodriguez A, et al. Hypothermia for intracranial hypertension after traumatic brain injury. *N Engl J Med.* 2015;373(25):2403–12.

65. Wright DW, Yeatts SD, Silbergleit R, et al. Very early administration of progesterone for acute traumatic brain injury. *N Engl J Med.* 2014;371(26):2457–66.

66. Skolnick BE, Maas AI, Narayan RK et al. A clinical trial of progesterone for severe traumatic brain injury. *N Engl J Med.* 2014;371(26):2467–76.

67. Stein SC, Georgoff P, Meghan S, et al. 150 years of treating severe traumatic brain injury: a systematic review of progress in mortality. *J Neurotrauma.* 2010;27(7):1343–53.

# 9 Neuroprotection for Cardiac Arrest

Joseph H. Pitcher and David B. Seder

## GENERAL CONSIDERATIONS

Cardiac arrest is a catastrophic event with persistently high mortality. In 1953, a report of 1,200 cases of in-hospital cardiac arrest treated with cardiopulmonary resuscitation (CPR) found that return of spontaneous circulation (ROSC) was achieved in 56% of patients, but, of those patients, only 28% survived more than a few days.[1] The authors suggested that with earlier resuscitation the survival rate would improve to 50% in the next few years. Since that time, CPR and cardiac arrest care have become more sophisticated and neurological outcomes have improved, but few if any centers have met these predictions sixty years later. In patients who achieve ROSC, survival to hospital discharge after out-of-hospital cardiac arrest (OHCA) and in-hospital cardiac arrest remains low, at 29% and 22%, respectively, although some centers publish rates of up to 56%, depending on the case mix and severity of illness.[2] The Institute of Medicine has recently addressed the urgent need to improve cardiac arrest care by calling for increased public health, hospital, and research efforts over the next 10 years.

This chapter will discuss mechanisms of neurological injury after cardiac arrest, tools to measure and monitor the extent of brain injury, interventions to protect the brain from reperfusion injury and improve outcomes, and areas of investigation likely to improve survival from cardiac arrest in the future.

## MECHANISMS OF AND RISKS FOR NEUROLOGICAL INJURY

Neurological injury following cardiac arrest can be separated into three general phases: (1) intra-arrest ischemic injury; (2) immediate reperfusion injury, beginning from ROSC and lasting approximately 20 minutes; and (3) delayed postreperfusion injury, beginning several hours after ROSC, peaking at 12–24 hours, and continuing for up to 5 days. At a systemic level, a distinct post–cardiac arrest syndrome includes varying levels of brain injury, circulatory dysfunction, and multiorgan ischemia-reperfusion injury and dysfunction. These conditions must be diagnosed and managed, as well as the underlying cause of the initial arrest (i.e., pulmonary embolism, asthma, myocardial infarction, cardiac arrhythmia).

## Intra-Arrest Cerebral Ischemic Injury

Neuronal cells are particularly sensitive to ischemia, and brain injury is the leading cause of death following successful resuscitation from cardiac arrest.[3] In the intra-arrest phase, cellular anoxia causes depletion of adenosine triphosphate (ATP) and failure of multiple energy processes, which leads to depolarization of the plasma membrane.[4] The longer the period of ischemic depolarization, the more likely that neuronal cells will die either by early necrosis or delayed apoptosis, even if reperfusion occurs. Neuronal susceptibility, however, is not uniform, and an absolute temporal threshold beyond which functional recovery cannot be obtained has never been determined.

Highly vulnerable neuronal populations are located in the hippocampus, cerebellum, striatum and cerebral cortex, but magnetic resonance imaging (MRI) and autopsy studies suggest that postresuscitation ischemic injuries may also involve deep gray matter structures and the cortical white matter tracts at end-vascular distributions (see Figure 9.1).[5-7] After depolarization, glutamate is released into the extracellular space, where accumulation results in excessive and sustained activation of the α-amino-3-hydroxy-5-methyl-4-isoxazolepropionic acid (AMPA), kainate

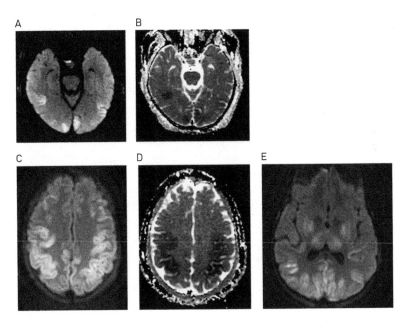

FIGURE 9.1 Patterns of brain injury after cardiac arrest seen on magnetic resonance imaging. A, B. Patient 1 exhibits moderate injury limited to patchy cortical injury in the temporal and occipital lobes, seen on diffusion weighted imaging (DWI) and with apparent diffusion coefficient (ADC) correlate. C, D, E. Patient 2 exhibits severe diffuse cortical injury in the frontal, parietal, and occipital lobes seen on DWI and with an ADC correlate. There is also deep injury involving the thalamus and putamen bilaterally. This patient's progressive electroencephalogram (EEG) findings are shown in Figure 9.2.

(KA), and N-methyl-D-aspartate (NMDA) receptors.[8] Sustained NMDA receptor activation results in rapid neuronal injury and death, whereas AMPA and KA receptor-mediated injury occurs more slowly, requiring hours of sustained activation. NMDA receptor activation increases intracellular calcium by multiple mechanisms that in turn increase the generation of superoxide free radical species.

## POSTRESUSCITATION NEUROLOGICAL INJURY

In the immediate reperfusion phase, the cascade of injury initiated during the ischemic period is amplified. Oxygen free radical formation increases with restoration of blood flow, and intracellular calcium continues to rise. After a certain threshold of intracellular calcium is reached, mitochondria take up the excess calcium, leading to devastating effects on the mitochondria that include opening of mitochondrial permeability transition pores (PTP), generation and accumulation of reactive oxygen species, and release of cytochrome c.[4,8] Opening of PTP appears to be a major contributor to programmed neuronal cell death. Once released from the mitochondria, cytochrome c activates a cascade of proteolytic enzymes that triggers apoptosis.[8] In the delayed reperfusion phase, the slower AMPA and KA receptors are activated, resulting in the influx of sodium and a massive influx of intracellular calcium, causing further activation of injury pathways.

Globally, post–cardiac arrest brain injury is characterized by variable levels of impaired autoregulation of cerebral blood flow, impaired oxygen extraction, cerebral edema, and seizure activity.[9–11] Electron microscopy shows capillary beds full of platelet plugs, sludged red blood cells, and endothelial flaps that increase cerebral vascular resistance and prevent oxygen delivery to injured tissues.[12] An initial hyperemic response follows ROSC, and then a period of increased cerebral vascular resistance, decreased cerebral blood flow, and impaired cerebral oxygenation extraction. In patients with severe brain injury seizures are common, and they potentiate injury by drastically increasing oxygen consumption and glutamate levels.[13] Late cerebral edema after cardiac arrest results from diffuse ischemic injury and peaks at 48–72 hours, though this peak depends on the timing of rewarming. One study found intracranial pressure (ICP) of greater than 25 mm Hg in 21% of patients at 24 hours and 26% at 48 hours after cardiac arrest.[9]

Even in the absence of myocardial infarction, variable postresuscitation cardiac dysfunction may develop within minutes of ROSC.[14] Unless an infarction is present, cardiac function reaches a nadir approximately 8 hours after resuscitation, improves at 24 hours, and normalizes at 48 hours. Cardiac index, left ventricular systolic function, and diastolic function are impaired despite normal coronary blood flow, suggesting myocardial stunning. This transient cardiomyopathy is due to the combined effects of coronary hypoperfusion, chest compressions, defibrillations and epinephrine administration.

The whole-body ischemia of cardiac arrest followed by reperfusion causes relative adrenal suppression and generalized endothelial activation. Relative adrenal suppression, defined by a response to corticotrophin stimulation of less than 9 μg/dL, occurs in up to 52% of patients in the first 12–24 hours after cardiac arrest and may be associated with an increase in shock-related mortality.[15] Endothelial activation results in increased vascular permeability, release of pro-inflammatory cytokines, a pro-coagulant state, and changes in vascular tone, causing a sepsis-like syndrome.[16] Inflammatory cytokines are found at increased levels in the blood within 3 hours following cardiac arrest and contribute to multiple organ dysfunction. Gut ischemia and increased vascular permeability allow the translocation of bacteria and endotoxins, which are elevated within the first 48 hours after cardiac arrest. The post-arrest inflammatory milieu leaves the immune system tolerant to endotoxin, which can be protective against an overwhelming inflammatory response, but this immunosuppressive state increases the risk of infection.

The combination of transient cardiomyopathy, increased inflammation, elevated cerebrovascular resistance, and increased ICP combine to result in increased risk for cerebral ischemia in the postresuscitation period. Ischemia is a major contributor to secondary injury after cardiac arrest and must be avoided.

## Risks for Neurological Injury

Multiple pre-arrest, intra-arrest, and post-arrest factors contribute to mortality and poor functional outcome after cardiac arrest. Pre-arrest risk factors for poor outcome include older age, diabetes, hypertension, chronic respiratory disease, active cancer, chronic kidney disease, and poor premorbid performance status.[17–20] Intra-arrest factors that are associated with improved outcome include the initial heart rhythm (i.e., ventricular fibrillation or tachycardia as opposed to the nonshockable rhythms), shorter time to ROSC, and bystander CPR. Post-arrest factors for poor outcome include hypotension, hypoxia, hyperoxia, dyscarbia, hyperglycemia, seizures, and fever. Modification of post-arrest risk factors may reduce secondary injury and are thus important treatment targets.

## Hypotension

Hypotension after resuscitation from cardiac arrest is associated with increased mortality and worse neurological outcome. Patients with impaired cerebral autoregulation after cardiac arrest are at risk for further neurological injury, even with "normal" blood pressures. The optimal blood pressure after cardiac arrest is controversial. Several studies have shown an association of mean arterial pressures (MAP) of 90–100 mm Hg with improved survival and neurological outcomes.[21] Others suggest no advantage when the MAP is greater than 65–70 mm Hg.[22]

Targeted temperature management (TTM) may restore cerebral autoregulation, making it difficult to compare the findings of recent studies of patients who received TTM to those of earlier studies in which few or no patients received TTM. Impaired cerebral autoregulation occurs in 35% of patients treated with TTM, compared to 72–100% of those who are not.[10–11,13] In one study, patients with impaired cerebral autoregulation were more likely to have chronic hypertension and had a higher mortality rate.[23] The data also suggested that, in patients with impaired cerebral autoregulation, a mean arterial pressure of 85–105 mm Hg was necessary to ensure adequate cerebral blood flow.

It is also unclear how long higher blood pressures should be maintained in this patient population. Early studies in patients resuscitated from cardiac arrest who were not treated with TTM showed impaired autoregulation for up to 72 hours.[10] It is unclear, however, whether impaired autoregulation resolves more rapidly in patients treated with TTM. Some studies suggest that higher blood pressures in the first 6 hours may be the most beneficial.[21–22] A small physiologic study, however, found that increasing the MAP from 70 mm Hg to 90 mm Hg for 30 minutes in comatose patients who were resuscitated from OHCA and treated with TTM did not change cerebral oxygen saturations at $17 \pm 5$ hours post–cardiac arrest.[24]

Another study showed continued impairment of autoregulation at 24 hours.[23] A study of postresuscitation care in animals showed a profound neurological benefit when investigators induced a MAP of 140 mm Hg for 4 hours after a cardiac arrest.[25] Induced hypertension after cardiac arrest, however, has not been tested in humans.

Optimal blood pressure after cardiac arrest is most likely not a "one-size-fits all" phenomenon and should be tailored to each individual, although how to do so is complex. Most neurointensivists prefer a higher MAP target, up to 85–100 mm Hg, but patients with anterior myocardial infarctions or recurrent arrhythmias may suffer harm by increased afterload and arrhythmia-provoking vasopressors, making a risk–benefit analysis necessary. Certainly, hypotension must be avoided, and, ultimately, the correct blood pressure targets will depend on the severity of the brain injury, the amount of time elapsed since cardiac arrest, whether or not the patient is treated with TTM, whether or not the patient has impaired cerebral autoregulation, and possibly the partial pressure of arterial carbon dioxide ($PaCO_2$). While a MAP greater than 65 mm Hg may be sufficient for the majority of patients, this target may be insufficient for more than a third of patients who require a MAP of 85 mm Hg or more to maintain adequate cerebral perfusion pressure. In the future, neuromonitoring devices that measure cerebral oxygen saturation, cerebral blood flow, or brain metabolism may be the key to identifying individual treatment targets.

## Hyperoxia and Hypoxia

Both hypoxia and hyperoxia can worsen reperfusion injury and contribute to secondary brain injury. Hypoxia decreases oxygen delivery to the brain, increases the risk of ischemia, and is associated with worse neurological outcomes. The deleterious effects of hypoxia on cerebral function and neuronal metabolism are well established and reviewed in Chapter 1.

Hyperoxia worsens reperfusion injury by increasing free radical production and can also cause cerebral vasoconstriction and provoke seizures.[26] Multiple animal studies have confirmed that hyperoxia after cardiac arrest, compared to normoxia, results in greater neurological deficit and more histological evidence of neuronal damage.[27] Even short periods of hyperoxia can have harmful effects. Dogs exposed to 100% oxygen for 1 hour after cardiac arrest, compared to those in which rapid titration within the first 12 minutes targeted an oxygen saturation of 94–96%, had worse neurological outcomes and more degenerating neurons within the hippocampus.

Only one small, randomized prospective trial evaluated the effects of hyperoxia in humans with cardiac arrest.[28] In this study, 28 patients were randomized to receive either 30% or 100% fraction of inspired oxygen ($FiO_2$) immediately after ROSC for 1 hour, initiated by a mobile intensive care unit. Patients were then admitted to the hospital and treated with standard care. The groups did not differ with respect to neurological outcome, survival to hospital discharge, or neurological biomarkers, but this is not surprising given the small number of patients studied. In the subset of patients who did not undergo TTM, however, hyperoxia treatment was associated with higher serum neuron-specific enolase levels at 24 hours, suggesting greater neuronal injury.

Multiple retrospective reviews have considered hyperoxia after cardiac arrest. Most studies agree that a partial pressure of arterial oxygen ($PaO_2$) of greater than 300 mm Hg is harmful and associated with increased risk of mortality, worse neurological outcome, and lower likelihood of being discharged as functionally independent.[19,29-30] There are a few studies that did not find an association of outcome with hyperoxia, however, these studies had lower mean $PaO_2$ values and a lower rate of severe hyperoxia than earlier studies, potentially reducing the deleterious effect of hyperoxia.[17,20]

Less severe hyperoxia may be harmful as well. One study found that for each 100 mm Hg increase in $PaO_2$, there was a 24% increase in risk of mortality.[30] Another study found that a mean $PaO_2$ of 117–134 mm Hg in the first 24 hours after cardiac arrest was associated with improved neurological outcome, compared to higher and lower values.[19] The duration of exposure to hyperoxia may also be important. One study found that for each hour of exposure to a $PaO_2$ of greater than 300 mm Hg occurring within 24 hours of cardiac arrest, there was a decreased survival with an odds ratio (OR) of 0.83 per hour.[29]

In conclusion, the majority of animal and human studies indicate that hyperoxia is harmful in the context of post–cardiac arrest treatment. In light of current evidence, it is prudent to use the strategy of rapid titration to a normal physiologic goal (e.g., pulse oximetry of 94–99%) and the use of ventilator protocols to reduce exposure to severe hyperoxia.

## Hypercapnia and Hypocapnia

The response of cerebral blood flow to the $PaCO_2$ is preserved after cardiac arrest except in the most severe brain injuries.[24] Hypocapnia causes cerebrovascular constriction, which decreases blood flow and increases the risk of cerebral ischemia. Several retrospective studies have shown that cardiac arrest patients with a $PaCO_2$ of less than 30–35 mm Hg within the first 24 hours had worse neurological outcomes and increased mortality.[19,31]

Hypercapnia causes cerebrovascular dilation and increases cerebral blood flow but can also increase cerebral blood volume, leading to cerebral edema and elevated ICP. These effects may be attenuated by TTM therapy.[32] Laboratory studies of ischemia-reperfusion injury after cardiac arrest suggest that mild hypercapnia may confer neuroprotection by decreasing glutamate secretion, increasing cerebral glucose utilization, and lowering cerebral lactate levels.[33] The clinical data regarding mild hypercapnia, however, are still preliminary. One study found that $PaCO_2$ levels of greater than 50 mm Hg in the first 24 hours were associated with worse neurological outcomes.[34] Two larger studies showed that $PaCO_2$ values of greater than 45 mm Hg in the first 24 hours were associated with better neurological outcomes and an increased rate of survival to hospital discharge.[20,31] One study found that the odds of good outcome increased as the time spent with a $PaCO_2$ above 45 mm Hg increased.[20] Further evidence supporting the beneficial effects of hypercapnia is provided by a physiologic study using jugular bulb oximetry, noninvasive cerebral oxygen monitoring, and cerebral microdialysis to assess cerebral ischemia after cardiac arrest.[35] This study found that increasing the $PaCO_2$ from 38 mm Hg to 45 mm Hg improved cerebral oxygen saturations and decreased cerebral lactate levels compared to normocapnia, suggesting that hypercapnia improved coupling of cerebral blood flow and neuronal metabolic demands.

In summary, the majority of laboratory and clinical studies indicate that a $PaCO_2$ of 35–50 mm Hg in the postresuscitation period is associated with improved outcomes compared to hypocapnia. Some studies suggest an additional benefit of TTM in the setting of hypercapnia in that it may limit cerebral edema. A clinical trial of mild hypercapnia with therapeutic hypothermia after cardiac arrest will help clarify the optimal target.

## Hyperglycemia and Hypoglycemia

In animal models, hyperglycemia prior to or during cardiac arrest has been shown to increase hypoxic-ischemic brain damage by worsening intracellular acidosis, increasing free radical formation, increasing mitochondrial damage, increasing extracellular glutamate levels, and disrupting the blood–brain barrier (BBB).[36] Laboratory studies have also shown that insulin attenuates neuronal injury due to cardiac arrest.[37] Clinical studies have demonstrated an inverse relationship between hyperglycemia early after cardiac arrest and survival.[18] However, some question whether hyperglycemia may simply be a marker of prolonged CPR, since throughout resuscitation, catecholamine levels increase and lead to greater hyperglycemia.[38]

Less is known about the effects of hyperglycemia after reperfusion, or if treatment of hyperglycemia reduces reperfusion injury. Multiple retrospective studies have found that lower blood glucose values (67–143 mg/dL) at 12, 24, and 48 hours are associated with better neurological outcomes compared to higher values (>144–193 mg/dL).[39–40] A single randomized clinical trial compared strict (72–108 mg/dL) to moderate (108–144 mg/dL) glucose control over a 48-hour interval after OHCA.[41] The strict glucose control group had significantly more episodes of hypoglycemia (30–54 mg/dL) compared to the moderate glucose control group (18% vs. 2%), but there was no difference in 30-day mortality. It is important to note, however, that while this study did not show improved outcomes with "strict" versus "moderate" glucose control, none of the patients experienced episodes of severe hypoglycemia. At this time, there are no published prospective studies comparing moderate glucose control to more lenient control of 144–180 mg/dL. One retrospective study found that blood glucose values of 116–143 mg/dL at 12 hours after ROSC were associated with improved neurological outcomes compared to both higher and lower values.[40]

While these studies suggest that lower blood glucose values within the normal range are associated with better neurological outcomes, the optimal range is not well defined. Current guidelines suggest targeting a blood glucose in higher normoglycemic to mildly hyperglycemic ranges not to exceed 144–180 mg/dL, citing concerns for the harmful effects of hypoglycemia.[42] Lower targets appear to be feasible, but clinicians must monitor closely for hypoglycemia.

## Seizures

Seizures and/or myoclonus occur in 10–40% of patients who remain comatose after cardiac arrest.[13] Estimates of their frequency are quite variable because diagnostic criteria for postanoxic status epilepticus are problematic, with weak inter-rater reliability.[43] Seizures increase cerebral metabolism by up to 300%, leading to depletion of ATP, lactate accumulation, and increased glutamate release.[44] In animal models, seizures lasting longer than 25–30 minutes cause selective neuronal necrosis in the cerebral cortex, hippocampus, cerebellum, and thalamus, many of the same regions that are most vulnerable to anoxic-ischemic injury.[5] In multiple animal models of ischemic brain injury, antiepileptic therapy is neuroprotective.[45]

While treatment of post–cardiac arrest seizures by antiepileptic drugs has not been shown to improve neurological outcome in humans, it can prevent increases in cerebral metabolism and thereby possibly limit secondary neuronal injury (see Figure 9.2). An increasing number of case reports document survival and recovery with aggressive treatment of postanoxic seizures.[46] Conversely, patients with

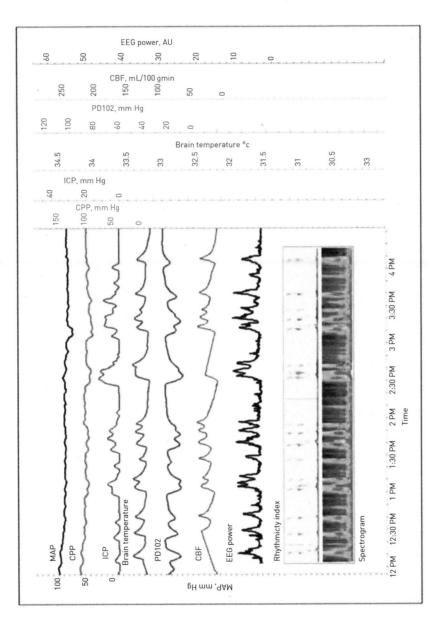

FIGURE 9.2  Note that when nonconvulsive seizures occur, there are increases in electroencephalogram (EEG) power, rhythmicity, and spectrographic power, brain temperature, and intracranial pressure and decreases in brain oxygen content and cerebral perfusion pressure suggesting cerebral metabolic distress. CBF, cerebral blood flow; CPP, cerebral perfusion pressure; EEG, electroencephalography; MAP, mean arterial pressure; PbtO₂, brain tissue oxygen content.

Adapted from Ko SB, Ortega-Gutierrez S, Choi HA, et al. Status epilepticus-induced hyperemia and brain tissue hypoxia after cardiac arrest. *Archives of Neurology.* 2011;68(10):1323–6.

untreated seizure activity after cardiac arrest usually remain comatose and almost always die.[47] Continuous electroencephalography (EEG) monitoring is therefore recommended in major guidelines for neuromonitoring and prognostication after cardiac arrest.[42]

## Fever

Fever has been associated with increased neuronal injury and unfavorable neurological outcome after cardiac arrest.[48] Phenomena associated with fever and neuronal injury include increased extracellular glutamate, increased oxygen free radicals, depletion of adenosine triphosphate levels, and presence of proteins involved in apoptosis.[49] Conversely, temperatures of lower than 37.8°C in the first 24 hours are associated with improved neurological outcomes.[18] Most experts suggest that fevers be suppressed for 24–72 hours with advanced cooling technology after the initial cooling period of TTM.

## MONITORING FOR NEUROLOGICAL INJURY
### Monitoring for Acute Brain Injury

It is imperative to make an early and accurate assessment of brain injury after a cardiac arrest event. This assessment will and should influence care. Crucial neurological questions that can be answered by neurological assessment and neuromonitoring include:

1. What is the severity of the brain injury?
2. Is convulsive or nonconvulsive seizure activity present?
3. Is ongoing brain ischemia present?
4. Is there a concurrent primary neurological process, such as aneurysmal subarachnoid hemorrhage?
5. Is the patient in the process of becoming brain dead?

Early stratification of brain injury severity after a cardiac arrest is necessary to improve the efficiency and effectiveness of care but should not be confused with prognostication. Early assessment of brain injury severity does not reliably predict neurological recovery and, since therapeutic decisions made in this period actively influence prognosis, should not be used to determine if life support should be discontinued. It is appropriate to categorize the severity of brain injury after cardiac arrest as "mild," "moderate," "severe," or "catastrophic" based on the duration of ischemia, depth of coma, and EEG performed within the first 6 hours of postresuscitation care. Such stratification helps clinicians determine which interventions, such as urgent coronary angiography or extracorporeal membrane oxygenation (ECMO), are most likely to influence outcome and to advocate for more aggressive treatments where warranted.

Early assessment of brain injury following resuscitation should routinely include determination of the "no-flow" (arrest without CPR) and "low-flow" (CPR) intervals, neurological examination findings after CPR, computed tomography (CT), and processed or raw EEG (see Figures 9.3 and 9.4). We discuss the interpretation of these findings in Table 9.1.

Competently handled, stratification of brain injury severity after a cardiac arrest event facilitates informed decisions regarding patient care, allowing clinicians and families to triage patients to the most appropriate treatment pathways. Assessment of brain injury severity after an arrest, however, is difficult, confusing, and imprecise. There are many potential confounders in a changing landscape of evidence

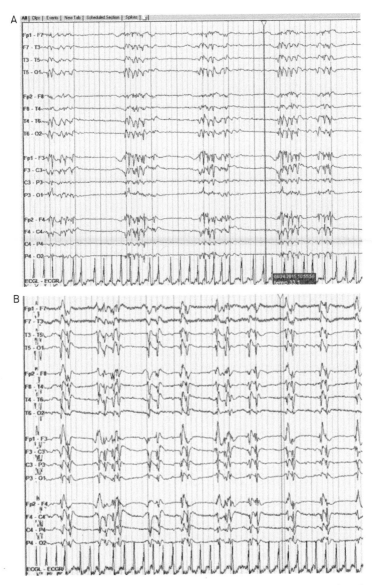

FIGURE 9.3 Patterns of brain injury after cardiac arrest seen on electroencephalogram (EEG).
A, B, C. A severely brain-injured patient during hypothermia who demonstrates evolution of EEG activity at 2 hours from a "suppression-burst" pattern to a "PLEDs plus" pattern at 11 hours and relentless epileptiform activity at 23 hours after return of spontaneous circulation (ROSC).
D. A mildly brain injured patient shows continuous, reactive background without epileptiform bursts at 5 hours after ROSC.

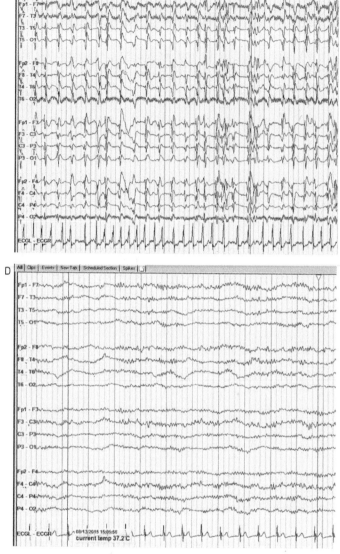

FIGURE 9.3 Continued

after decades of widely cited, low-quality publications that no longer reflect the current standard of care. Inappropriately early or incompetent assessment of brain injury severity results in incorrect triage and may adversely affect outcomes, including mortality rates. Clinicians must remember that the large quantities of sedating medications routinely administered during TTM can dramatically affect prognostication, and that outcomes with delayed prognostication after TTM are far better than those of the pre-TTM era (prior to 2002).[50]

While some patients recover quickly after cardiac arrest or after rewarming and require no specific testing, others remain comatose yet have the potential to awaken. Delayed awakening is especially common with large doses of sedation, analgesia, and antiepileptic drugs that were administered during hypothermia or in the setting

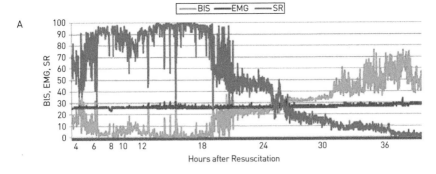

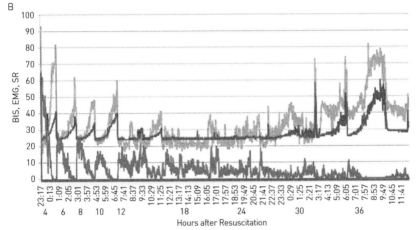

FIGURE 9.4 Patterns of brain injury after cardiac arrest seen on the bispectral index (BIS) monitor. A. Patient 1 exhibits very low BIS at 6 hours after cardiac arrest with a high suppression ratio—a pattern commonly seen with severe brain injury. There is no evidence of shivering, which also suggests severe injury.[114] This is the same patient in Figure 9.1 panels C, D, E. Note the discrimination is clear early after the arrest but is lost around 18 hours, correlating to an increase in epileptiform activity (corresponds to Patient 1, Figures 9.1 and 9.3). B. Patient 2 exhibits BIS that remains ≥20 and a suppression ratio near 0—a pattern consistent with a mild brain injury. Note electromyelogram (EMG) increases (*red line* trending up) with shivering when intermittent vecuronium is metabolized, with its confounding effects on the BIS and SR, and then returning to a flat EMG baseline with neuromuscular blockade.

of renal and/or hepatic dysfunction.[50–51] Clinicians must exercise extreme caution in predicting outcomes in such patients.

Multiple modes of testing have been used for prognostication, but most are insensitive and each carries a risk of falsely predicting a poor outcome. Additionally, studies involving prognosis are prone to a "self-fulfilling prophecy" in which decisions to withdraw life-sustaining therapy are made based on the very prognostic markers they are examining. This can cause overestimation of the specificity of the tests. For this reason, a multimodal approach to prognostication is necessary to accurately predict outcomes after cardiac arrest.[52] Table 9.2 summarizes the optimal timing of testing, sensitivity, and false-positive rate of the most supported modalities for predicting outcomes in cardiac arrest patients who have been treated with TTM, and these should only be applied to such patients.

**Table 9.1** Very Early (Within 6 Hours of ROSC) Assessment of Brain Injury Severity After Cardiac Arrest

| Modality | Interpretation/ Association with Severity of Brain Injury | Confounders | Utility | Data Quality | Refs |
|---|---|---|---|---|---|
| No-flow interval | • <2 minutes: Mild<br>• 3–8 minutes: Mild-Moderate<br>• >8 minutes: Moderate-Severe | • Unwitnessed arrests<br>• Diabetes | Moderate | Low | 101 |
| Total ischemic time (no-flow + low flow) | • >25 minutes: Severe<br>• <25 minutes: Mild-Moderate | • Unwitnessed<br>• CPR quality | Low | Low | 102 |
| Motor exam after resuscitation | • GCS motor subscore 4+: Mild<br>• GCS≥5: Mild-Moderate<br>• GCS 3-4: Moderate-Severe | • Sedation, NMB, seizures | Moderate | Low | 103 |
| CT findings at the time of ICU admission | • GWR<1.1: Catastrophic<br>• GWR<1.2: Mod/Severe<br>• SAH: Get CT angiogram and neurosurgery consultation | Scan quality and interpretation | Moderate | Low | 104 |
| EEG background | • Nonreactive: Severe<br>• Isoelectric: Severe/catastrophic<br>• Low-voltage: Unreliable<br>• Suppression-burst: Severe<br>• Reactive: Mild/Moderate<br>• Continuous: Mild/Moderate | Sedation, seizures and epileptiform activity, timing, technique, interobserver variability in interpretation | High | Moderate+ | 105, 106 |
| Processed EEG (in a patient that received NMB) | • Initial BIS 0: catastrophic<br>• Initial BIS <10: Severe<br>• Initial BIS 11–20: Moderate<br>• Initial BIS >20: Mild | Sedation, modality, seizures and epileptiform activity, timing of assessment | High | Moderate | 107 |

*(continued)*

Table 9.1 Continued

161

Neuroprotection for Cardiac Arrest

| Modality | Interpretation/ Association with Severity of Brain Injury | Confounders | Utility | Data Quality | Refs |
|---|---|---|---|---|---|
| Seizures | • SR6 > 80%: Catastrophic<br>• SR6 40–80%: Severe<br>• SR6 10–40%: Moderate<br>• SR6 <10%: Mild<br>• Early Severe myoclonus *with* EEG correlate: Severe<br>• Frequent PEDs or seizures arising from a suppressed background: Severe | Sedation, EEG interpretation | Moderate | Moderate | 105 |

*BIS*, bispectral index, measured in a chemically paralyzed patient as soon as possible after ROSC (median 4.5 hours); *CPR*, cardiopulmonary resuscitation; *CT*, computed tomography; *GCS*, Glasgow Coma Scale; *GWR*, gray to white matter ratio (Hounsfield units); *EEG*, electroencephalography; *ICU*, intensive care unit; *No-flow interval*, from arrest to onset of cardiopulmonary resuscitation; *NMB*, neuromuscular blockade; *PEDs*, periodic epileptiform discharges; *ROSC*, return of spontaneous circulation; *SAH*, subarachnoid hemorrhage; *SR6*, the suppression ratio (% of each 63 second EEG epoch that is isoelectric), at 6 hours after ROSC.

## Neurological Testing

The neurological examination is an important part of assessing prognosis. Findings that have been used for prognostication include the absence of a pupillary light reflex bilaterally, the absence of a corneal reflex, a Glasgow Coma Scale (GCS) motor response less than 3, the presence of myoclonus, and the presence of status myoclonus (continuous, repetitive myoclonic jerks lasting >30 minutes).[53] These findings are influenced by sedation, paralytics, hypothermia, and metabolic abnormalities. For this reason, the neurological examination is most accurate and only has prognostic value when performed after rewarming and more than 72 hours after discontinuing sedation.[42]

## Electroencephalography

EEG findings that have been associated with poor outcome include EEG that is nonreactive to external stimuli, burst-suppression, status epilepticus, low voltage output (<10 μV), and generalized periodic epileptiform discharges (GPEDs).[53] Studies examining EEG predictors of poor outcome have resulted in inconsistent findings, likely due to methodological variations in whether TTM was employed, when the EEG was performed (i.e., during TTM or after rewarming), variability of interpretation of EEG findings between neurologists, and technical differences

**Table 9.2** Modes of Prognostication with Sensitivity and False Positive Rates

| Modality | Timing | Value | Sensitivity | False Positive Rate | References |
|---|---|---|---|---|---|
| Pupillary light response | >72 hours | Absent | 20% | 1% | 108, 109 |
| Corneal reflex | >72 hours | Absent | 26% | 4% | 108, 109 |
| GCS motor response | >72 hours | <3 | 60% | 11% | 108, 109 |
| Myoclonus with EEG correlate | Variable | Present | Variable | 2% | 109, 110 |
| Myoclonus without EEG correlate | Variable | Present | 54% | 5–15% | 110 |
| EEG | After rewarming | Burst-suppression | Variable | 0% | 111 |
| | >72 hours | Nonreactive | Variable | <1% | 109 |
| SSEP | During TTM or after rewarming | Nonreactive bilateral N20 | 28–42% | <1% | 106, 108 |
| NSE | 24–72 hours | >33 µg/L | 50–84% | 22% | 50, 56, 108 |
| Qualitative MRI | 25–192 hours | Cortex score >27 | 60% | <1% | 112 |
| Quantitative MRI | 3–5 days | ADC <650 × 10$^{-6}$ in >10% of brain volume | 72% | 9% | 113 |
| Quantitative MRI | 3–5 days | ADC <650 × 19$^{-6}$ in >22% brain volume | 52% | <1% | 113 |

ADC, apparent diffusion coefficient; DWI, diffusion weighted imaging; EEG, electroencephalogram; GCS, Glasgow Coma Scale; MRI, magnetic resonance imaging; NSE, neuron-specific enolase; SSEP, somatosensory evoked potential.

among studies. EEG that is nonreactive to external stimuli after 72 hours and presence of a burst-suppression pattern after rewarming are the most established EEG predictors of poor outcome.[42]

## Evoked Potentials

Somatosensory evoked potentials (SSEPs) reflect the functional integrity of the somatosensory pathways, and the N20 wave component reflects arrival of the signal at the primary somatosensory cortex (described in Chapter 5). The absence of bilateral N20 waves in the SSEP beyond 3 days post-arrest and well after rewarming is a strong predictor of poor neurological outcome, indicating little to no chance of recovery from coma. SSEP is the prognostic marker most likely to influence a physician's decision to withdraw life-sustaining therapy; however, it can result in false-positive findings (i.e., N20 potentials are present bilaterally, but the patient still fails to recover).[54–55] Interpretation of SSEP may be confounded by high doses of sedative/hypnotics and hypothermia and should be performed in the absence of these conditions.

## Biomarkers

Neuron-specific enolase (NSE) and S-100B have been the most commonly studied biomarkers in brain injury research. NSE is a protein involved in glucose metabolism and is mainly found in neuronal and neuroendocrine cells. S-100B is a protein that is found in brain astrocytes. There is wide variability in cutoff values for both of these biomarkers when used to identify a poor prognosis. This may be due to a number of factors, including whether the patient was treated with TTM, the timing of blood sampling, differences in analytical methods among labs and assays, and differences in sampling techniques. A level of greater than 33 μg/L was considered indicative of poor outcome in the pre-TTM era, whereas subsequent studies have pointed to a level of greater than 80 μg/L after cooling.[56] While serum biomarkers can help support a good or poor prognosis, they are interpreted in conjunction with other modalities when establishing the prognosis after a cardiac arrest.

## Other Modalities

Qualitative and quantitative MRI, CT, and the bispectral index (BIS) have also been studied as prognostic modalities. Although the results of these studies have been promising, more studies are needed to confirm their sensitivity and false-positive rates.

## Monitoring For Secondary Brain Injury

### Electroencephalography

Seizures are common after cardiac arrest, with most seizures occurring during or after rewarming.[57] It is nearly impossible to diagnose seizures after cardiac arrest based on clinical examination alone due to the high frequency of nonconvulsive seizure-like movements, neuromuscular blockade, and shivering.[58] Continuous EEG monitoring is an important tool to identify seizure activity early in the post-arrest period in order to prevent further neurological injury. Neuromuscular blockade is frequently required to eliminate muscle artifact from the EEG and identify seizures. Continuous EEG monitoring is a key part of multimodal prognostication for patients who remain comatose.[42]

### Bispectral Index Monitoring

The BIS is a quantitative reformulation of raw EEG activity that measures the level of consciousness on a scale ranging from 0 (isoelectric EEG) to 100 (awake patient). Post–cardiac arrest care includes the use of neuromuscular blockade and concomitant sedation to ensure a lack of awareness. Targeting sedation to a BIS of 40–60 can help decrease the incidence of awareness during TTM.[59] The BIS monitor also presents the suppression ratio (SR), the percent of each 63-second epoch that is isoelectric. The SR is useful to determine the severity of brain injury at a very early time point and identify patients who might potentially benefit from early invasive interventions, such as cardiac catheterization for myocardial revascularization.[60] BIS monitors may also identify potential seizure activity, prompting further investigation with EEG.[61] BIS and other processed EEG modalities are simple to use and promising tools for postresuscitation triage. Their routine application in postresuscitation care, however, is not yet established and is hampered by the proprietary nature of the technology.

## Jugular Bulb Oximetry

After cardiac arrest, the loss of cerebral autoregulation can cause insufficient blood flow to areas of the brain. The cerebral metabolic rate of consumption of oxygen ($CMRO_2$) is also altered due to a number of factors including mitochondrial dysfunction, seizures, sedation, and neuronal cell death.[10] Jugular oximetry utilizes a small catheter with its tip placed at the internal jugular bulb to help identify insufficient oxygen delivery to the brain after cardiac arrest. Jugular oximetry is sensitive to changes in cerebral blood flow and may also identify patients with severe neurological injury.[10,35] Similar to a mixed venous oxygen saturation in the systemic circulation, insufficient blood flow causes increased oxygen extraction by cerebral tissue, leading to a decrease in jugular venous oxygen saturation ($SjVO_2$). An $SjVO_2$ of less than 55% or a calculated cerebral extraction of oxygen ($CEO_2$) of greater than 20–40% reflects an imbalance of cerebral blood flow to oxygen consumption and suggests the need to augment cerebral blood flow.

## Near-Infrared Spectroscopy

Near-infrared spectroscopy (NIRS) is a noninvasive monitoring tool that estimates regional cerebral tissue oxygen saturation ($rSO_2$) using near-infrared light sensors that are placed over the frontal lobes bilaterally.[62] This device continuously measures the balance between oxygen delivery and uptake within the frontal lobes, promptly alerts clinicians to cerebral hypoperfusion states, and may be useful in determining optimal blood pressures after cardiac arrest. The normal range of NIRS-derived $rSO_2$ values is 60–80%. By calculating the running correlation coefficient between $rSO_2$ values and mean arterial blood pressure, a cerebral oximeter index ($C_{ox}$) can be derived. A $C_{ox}$ of −1 to 0 suggests that blood pressure is coupled to CBF, and a value approaching 1 suggests insufficient blood pressure.[63] Although promising, further research is needed before NIRS can be widely recommended for use after cardiac arrest.

## NEUROPROTECTION STRATEGIES
## Physiologic Interventions

### Therapeutic Hypothermia

Multiple animal models have firmly established that hypothermia after cardiac arrest improves neurological outcomes.[25,64–67] Laboratory studies have also provided data regarding basic parameters for TTM, such as optimal time to initiate therapy, optimal duration of therapy, and optimal temperature. TTM has been shown to have the greatest neuroprotective effect when initiated during or soon after cardiac arrest (<2 hours), but there is some evidence that it may be beneficial if initiated within 6 hours of arrest.[64–65] Longer durations of TTM may be more protective than shorter durations. Experimental studies have shown less neurological injury with 24 versus 12 hours of TTM, and 48 hours versus no TTM; yet no studies have compared 24- versus 48-hour or longer intervals. Longer durations of TTM, however, also increase the risk of adverse effects from hypothermia (described later).[64,66] Cooling to a target of 32–36°C has been most studied. This range results in improved performance and decreased neurological deficits in comparison to both lower and higher temperatures, and it has fewer complications than lower temperatures.[67]

TTM attenuates neurological injury by reducing the cerebral metabolic rate, preventing the accumulation and release of extracellular glutamate, decreasing calcium influx through AMPA channels, inhibiting the apoptosis pathway, decreasing the post–cardiac arrest inflammatory state, and decreasing BBB disruption and its consequent cerebral edema.[68] However, hypothermia also has adverse effects, such as hyperkalemia with rewarming, mildly increased risk of bleeding due to platelet dysfunction, hyperglycemia, increased risk of infection, and increased risk of bradycardia and ventricular arrhythmias.[69]

The initial studies of hypothermia in post–cardiac arrest patients showed promising results compared to historical controls. A study of 22 patients treated after OHCA with TTM to 33°C for 12 hours found improved neurological outcomes, reduced mortality, and no significant adverse effects of hypothermia.[70] Another study of 13 OHCA patients treated with TTM to 33–34°C, initiated within 2 hours of ROSC and treated for 48 hours, found a trend toward improved neurological outcome but an increased risk of pneumonia.[71] A third study of 27 patients with OHCA and an initial rhythm of ventricular fibrillation (VF), treated with TTM to 33°C for 24 hours, found improved neurological outcomes at 6 months and no difference in adverse events.[72]

The first randomized controlled trial of hypothermia in cardiac arrest patients performed in 2002 examined 275 patients who had a witnessed OHCA of cardiac origin and received CPR within 5–15 minutes of the event but remained comatose.[73] Patients were randomized to normothermia (37.5°C) versus TTM to 32–34°C for 24 hours. The median time to ROSC was 22 minutes, and the median time to achieve target temperature was 8 hours. The TTM treatment group had a significantly higher incidence of good neurological outcomes as defined by Cerebral Performance Category (CPC) scores of 1–2 indicating survival with no, minimal, or moderate disability (55% vs. 39%), and a significantly lower incidence of 6-month mortality (41% vs. 55%). There was no difference in complication rates between the two groups. A smaller study of 77 patients with coma after resuscitation from OHCA of cardiac origin also showed improved outcomes with TTM.[74] Patients were randomized to normothermia versus TTM to 32–34°C initiated within 2 hours after the return of spontaneous circulation and maintained for 12 hours. Therapeutic hypothermia was associated with a significantly higher rate of discharge to home or a rehabilitation facility, but no significant difference in mortality.

A multicenter randomized trial investigated the optimal target temperature in 950 survivors of OHCA by comparing TTM to 33°C versus 36°C.[75] Hypothermia was maintained for 36 hours and, thereafter, body temperature was maintained below 37°C with fever control measures until 72 hours after cardiac arrest. This study found no significant difference in mortality or 6-month neurological outcome, as evaluated by CPC and modified Rankin scores. The authors hypothesized that hypothermia itself may not be as important as the absence of fever. In other words, whereas 33°C and 36°C may not result in significantly different outcomes, both of these temperatures may be superior to the mean temperatures exceeding 37.5°C experienced by the control patients in earlier studies. Another point of debate is that the patient samples studied have been heterogeneous and that the risks and benefits of TTM may differ across patient subgroups.

Most experts and practice guidelines interpret the available data as a strong mandate to perform TTM after OHCA. The decision to target 33°C versus 36°C may depend on individual patient factors and local clinical practice. For instance, a patient with cerebral edema may benefit from a targeted temperature of 33°C, whereas a patient with shock or at risk for cardiac ischemia complications might benefit from targeting to 36°C. No randomized clinical trials have evaluated the use of therapeutic hypothermia exclusively in patients with an initial rhythm of pulseless elective activity (PEA) or asystole. In a retrospective review from a large registry in France, TTM was not associated with an improvement in neurological outcome in patients with initial rhythm of PEA/asystole, while a recent US analysis showed benefit in nonshockable rhythms.[76–77]

## Percutaneous Coronary Intervention

Myocardial infarction is a frequent cause of cardiac arrest, with a reported incidence of up to 38%.[78] During percutaneous coronary intervention (PCI), concurrent treatment with TTM is safe and feasible. Multiple retrospective studies have reported improved survival and neurological outcomes in patients with OHCA and electrocardiographic (ECG) findings of an ST-elevation myocardial infarction (STEMI) or a new left bundle branch block (LBBB) treated with PCI.[79] A few cohort studies have also found high rates of significant coronary lesions in patients with nonischemic ECG patterns with no other obvious cause of cardiac arrest.[80] This incidence is especially high in patients who have an initial ventricular fibrillation/ventricular tachycardia (VF/VT) rhythm. When early PCI was performed in these patients, they had similarly improved survival rates and neurological outcomes to the patients treated with PCI after STEMI. Clinicians should have a low threshold for early cardiac catheterization in patients who present with STEMI, a new LBBB, an initial rhythm of VF/VT, or when a cardiac cause of cardiac arrest cannot be excluded.

## Pharmacologic Interventions

For the most part, attempts to reduce hypoxic-ischemic reperfusion injury after cardiac arrest with pharmacologic neuroprotection have been disappointing.

## Magnesium

Magnesium, a competitive NMDA receptor antagonist that inhibits calcium entry into the cell via voltage-gated calcium channels, acts as a vasodilator of the peripheral and cerebral circulation, and lowers the temperature threshold for shivering. Studies of magnesium in animal models of cerebral ischemic injury have yielded conflicting results.[81] Some studies have found that magnesium was neuroprotective only when combined with mild hypothermia and that the combination of magnesium and hypothermia was more efficacious than hypothermia alone.[82]

Few clinical trials have evaluated the use of magnesium sulfate after cardiac arrest. In a study of 300 OHCA patients randomized to placebo, intravenous diazepam

(2 mg IV), intravenous magnesium sulfate, or both diazepam and magnesium sulfate administered immediately after cardiac arrest, magnesium was shown to be safe but was not associated with improved neurological outcome at 3 months.[83] To date, no clinical studies have evaluated the use of magnesium sulfate in combination with mild hypothermia. In healthy volunteers, intravenous magnesium sulfate during induction of hypothermia did improve patient comfort, reduced the time to achieve target temperature, and decreased the temperature threshold for shivering.[84] For this reason, many centers have incorporated magnesium infusion into their TTM shiver control protocols.

## Thiopental

Thiopental is an ultra–short-acting barbiturate that decreases cerebral metabolism, decreases cerebral edema, prevents seizures, and inhibits activation of AMPA receptors.[85] Studies examining its potential neurological benefits after cardiac arrest in animal models have yielded conflicting results.[85–86] Early studies in cardiac arrest patients showed that thiopental loading up to 30 mg/kg over 30 minutes after cardiac arrest was feasible, but dosing and rate of administration were often limited by hypotension and decreased cardiac function.[87] An initial pilot study using thiopental after cardiac arrest showed an increase in mortality in the first 6 hours in patients who had ischemic heart disease compared to historical controls, but an improved neurological outcome among patients who did not have ischemic heart disease or hemodynamic instability prior to drug administration.[88] A randomized controlled trial of thiopental 30 mg/kg administered 10–50 minutes after ROSC compared to standard therapy found no statistical difference in 30-day mortality or neurological outcome.[89] Furthermore, patients treated with thiopental had more hypotension (60% vs. 29%) and required more vasopressor support.

## Coenzyme Q

Coenzyme Q is a cofactor in the electron transport chain that acts as an antioxidant within the mitochondria. After cardiac arrest, coenzyme Q may prevent mitochondria from signaling the cell to undergo apoptosis by supporting ATP production, reducing reactive oxygen species, and stabilizing the mitochondrial membrane. In animal models of ischemia-reperfusion injury, treatment with coenzyme Q is neuroprotective.[90] An observational, prospective study in humans showed that cardiac arrest was associated with a low coenzyme Q level at 24 hours and that lower coenzyme Q levels were associated with worse neurological outcomes and survival.[91] In a pilot study, coenzyme Q plus TTM was compared to TTM alone.[92] Both groups received TTM for 24 hours at 35°C, and the coenzyme Q group was given a loading dose of 250 mg followed by 5 days of 150 mg three times daily. The coenzyme Q group had an improved 3-month survival, but no statistically significant improvement in neurological outcome. S-100B levels at 24 hours were decreased in the coenzyme Q group. Coenzyme Q is currently the only pharmacologic therapy tested in combination with TTM in humans.

## Corticosteroids

Corticosteroids have a wide range of physiological effects with potential benefits after cardiac arrest, including anti-inflammatory properties and enhancement of the vasopressor effects of catecholamines, but they may also decrease insulin sensitivity and impair the immune response to infection.[93] Two retrospective studies evaluated the effect of corticosteroids after cardiac arrest. In the first study, 232 of 458 consecutive patients received high-dose dexamethasone after OHCA for a median of 3.4 days.[94] Corticosteroids were not associated with an improved outcome. A second study evaluated 262 patients within a randomized controlled trial for thiopental after cardiac arrest; dexamethasone or methylprednisolone was optional based on the physicians' clinical judgment.[95] There were no differences in survival or neurological recovery between patients treated with low-, medium-, or high-dose corticosteroids in the first 8 hours after ROSC compared to patients who were not treated with corticosteroids.

## IMPLICATIONS FOR CLINICAL PRACTICE

Guidelines for postresuscitation cardiac arrest care were updated in 2015 by the American Heart Association (AHA).[42] Optimization of ventilation and oxygenation is recommended immediately after resuscitation. Respirations should be started at 10 breaths/minute with a goal end-tidal $CO_2$ ($EtCO_2$) of 30–40 mm Hg. A high concentration of oxygen is administered until an accurate oxyhemoglobin concentration or arterial blood gas is obtained. Once accurate measurements are obtained, the oxygen concentration should be titrated to the lowest possible $FiO_2$ to maintain oxyhemoglobin saturation of greater than 94%, and the $PaCO_2$ should be titrated to 35–45 mm Hg. These guidelines recommend treating hypotension with a goal MAP of greater than 65 mm Hg and an SBP of higher than 90 mm Hg with intravenous fluids and vasopressors, as needed. A 12-lead ECG is obtained as soon as possible. Emergent coronary angiography should be performed on any patient with evidence of a STEMI and considered in any patient in whom an acute MI is suspected as the etiology of cardiac arrest. TTM between 32°C and 36°C is recommended in all cardiac arrest patients who do not respond to verbal commands after ROSC regardless of initial rhythm, and TTM should be maintained for at least 24 hours. Initiation of TTM in the pre-hospital setting is not recommended. Once feasible, EEG should be performed regularly or continuously in comatose patients to identify seizures or status epilepticus, in which case antiepileptic therapy should be considered. Fevers of higher than 37.7°C should be actively prevented for up to 72 hours after the initial cooling period. The guidelines recommend a blood glucose target of 144–180 mg/dL, citing a lack of data supporting lower targets and concerns for harm from inadvertent hypoglycemia. The routine use of additional pharmacologic therapy, such as coenzyme Q10, in patients treated with therapeutic hypothermia is uncertain.

Prognostication is an essential part of cardiac arrest care. The AHA 2015 guidelines recommend using modes of prognostication that have a false-positive rate (i.e., test implies a poor prognosis but the patient recovers) approaching 0%.[42] This should occur no earlier than 72 hours after cardiac arrest and should be delayed much longer if the physical examination is confounded by hypothermia, sedation, or paralytic medications, except in individual circumstances that include terminal underlying disease, brain herniation, or other clearly nonsurvivable situations.

In post–cardiac arrest patients treated with TTM, consideration of the following prognosticators is recommended:

1. The absence of pupillary light reflexes more than 72 hours post-arrest;
2. Status myoclonus in the first 72–120 hours;

3. The absence of EEG reactivity to external stimuli more than 72 hours post-arrest;
4. Persistent burst suppression after rewarming;
5. Bilateral absence of the N20 SSEP wave 72 hours post-arrest and after rewarming; and
6. Extensive restricted diffusion on brain MRI at 2–6 days after cardiac arrest.

Isolated use of NSE and S-100B blood markers is not recommended for prediction of a poor neurological outcome. High values at 48 and 72 hours support the prognosis of a poor neurological outcome, whereas low NSE values (<20 ug/L) are reassuring.

## FUTURE DIRECTIONS

The future of neuroprotection after cardiac arrest will be based on a sophisticated analysis of the type and severity of injuries suffered by an individual patient, application of neuromonitoring that allows continuous titration of therapies, and establishment of effective therapies that create a neuroprotective milieu. Although this may seem a distant reality, rapid advances in neuromonitoring and neuroprotection and increased cardiac arrest research are likely to yield improvements in the foreseeable future.[2] One therapy likely to be part of this regimen is determination of the most appropriate dose (depth and duration) of TTM. Certain analyses have suggested either harm or benefit to subgroups of cardiac arrest patients treated with hypothermia as opposed to normothermia, and it is likely that the correct temperature target depends on the individual patient's pathophysiology.[96–97] Such a determination may require very early and accurate determination of the severity of the brain injury, assessment of systemic injuries, and an informed application of the correct dose of hypothermic therapy for optimal neuroprotection. Most clinicians agree it is unlikely that patients with mild and severe brain injuries require the same types therapy, so accurate classification is of great importance. Processed EEG is one of the most promising modalities for this purpose, and animal models suggest such a determination could be made with reasonable accuracy as early as 30–60 minutes after resuscitation.[98]

Early cerebral blood flow augmentation intended to open thrombosed and damaged microcapillary beds is another promising approach that has shown great promise in an animal model of aggressive early blood flow augmentation.[25] Such an approach is more difficult in humans with diseased hearts, and such a trial would require safe methods of blood flow augmentation combined with continuous neurological assessment to prevent breakthrough cerebral edema and ICP elevation. After cardiac arrest, patients with higher blood pressures tend to do better than patients with lower blood pressures.[21] Some investigators have suggested initiating "goal-directed" hemodynamic augmentation after cardiac arrest, but, at this time, this approach remains speculative.

Aggressive early management of postanoxic seizures may minimize secondary injury.[99] Furthermore, certain antiepileptic drugs may have neuroprotective properties after cardiac arrest that are independent of their effects on seizure activity.[100]

It has been established that mitochondrial injury results in persistently impaired mitochondrial function in cortical and hippocampal neurons after resuscitation from cardiac arrest, and this is strongly associated with activation of apoptotic pathways. Mitochondrial protective agents, including coenzyme Q and other synthetic agents, remain under investigation.

# REFERENCES

1. Stephenson HE, Reid C, Hinton JW. Some common denominators in 1200 cases of cardiac arrest. *Ann Surgery.* 1953;137:731–4.

2. Committee on the Treatment of Cardiac Arrest: Current Status and Future Directions; Board on Health Sciences Policy; Institute of Medicine. In-Hospital Cardiac Arrest and Post-Arrest Care. In: Graham R, McCoy MA, Schultz AM, eds. *Strategies to improve cardiac arrest survival: a time to act.* Washington, DC: 2015:243–314.

3. Laver S, Farrow C, Turner D, Nolan J. Mode of death after admission to an intensive care unit following cardiac arrest. *Intensive Care Med.* 2004;30(11):2126–8.

4. Neumar RW. Molecular mechanisms of ischemic neuronal injury. *Ann Emerg Med.* 2000;36(5):483–506.

5. Pulsinelli WA. Selective neuronal vulnerability: morphological and molecular characteristics. *Prog Brain Res.* 1985;63:29–37.

6. Jarnum H, Knutsson L, Rundgren M, et al. Diffusion and perfusion MRI of the brain in comatose patients treated with mild hypothermia after cardiac arrest: a prospective observational study. *Resuscitation.* 2009;80(4):425–30.

7. Cronberg T, Rundgren M, Westhall E, et al. Neuron-specific enolase correlates with other prognostic markers after cardiac arrest. *Neurology.* 2011;77(7):623–30.

8. Kostandy BB. The role of glutamate in neuronal ischemic injury: the role of spark in fire. *Neurol Sci.* 2012;33(2):223–37.

9. Gueugniaud PY, Garcia-Darennes F, Gaussorgues P, Bancalari G, Petit P, Robert D. Prognostic significance of early intracranial and cerebral perfusion pressures in post-cardiac arrest anoxic coma. *Intensive Care Med.* 1991;17(7):392–8.

10. Lemiale V, Huet O, Vigue B, et al. Changes in cerebral blood flow and oxygen extraction during post-resuscitation syndrome. *Resuscitation.* 2008;76(1):17–24.

11. Sundgreen C, Larsen FS, Herzog TM, Knudsen GM, Boesgaard S, Aldershvile J. Autoregulation of cerebral blood flow in patients resuscitated from cardiac arrest. *Stroke.* 2001;32(1):128–32.

12. Krep H, Bottiger BW, Bock C, et al. Time course of circulatory and metabolic recovery of cat brain after cardiac arrest assessed by perfusion- and diffusion-weighted imaging and MR-spectroscopy. *Resuscitation.* 2003;58(3):337–48.

13. Krumholz A, Stern BJ, Weiss HD. Outcome from coma after cardiopulmonary resuscitation: relation to seizures and myoclonus. *Neurology.* 1988;38(3):401–5.

14. Laurent I, Monchi M, Chiche JD, et al. Reversible myocardial dysfunction in survivors of out-of-hospital cardiac arrest. *J Am Coll Cardiol.* 2002;40(12):2110–6.

15. Kim JJ, Lim YS, Shin JH, et al. Relative adrenal insufficiency after cardiac arrest: impact on postresuscitation disease outcome. *Am J Emerg Med.* 2006;24(6):684–8.

16. Adrie C, Adib-Conquy M, Laurent I, et al. Successful cardiopulmonary resuscitation after cardiac arrest as a "sepsis-like" syndrome. *Circulation.* 2002;106(5):562–8.

17. Bellomo R, Bailey M, Eastwood GM, et al. Arterial hyperoxia and in-hospital mortality after resuscitation from cardiac arrest. *Crit Care.* 2011;15(2):R90.

18. Langhelle A, Tyvold SS, Lexow K, Hapnes SA, Sunde K, Steen PA. In-hospital factors associated with improved outcome after out-of-hospital cardiac arrest. A comparison between four regions in Norway. *Resuscitation.* 2003;56(3):247–63.

19. Lee BK, Jeung KW, Lee HY, et al. Association between mean arterial blood gas tension and outcome in cardiac arrest patients treated with therapeutic hypothermia. *Am J Emerg Med.* 2014;32(1):55–60.

20. Vaahersalo J, Bendel S, Reinikainen M, et al. Arterial blood gas tensions after resuscitation from out-of-hospital cardiac arrest: associations with long-term neurologic outcome. *Crit Care Med.* 2014;42(6):1463–70.

21. Beylin ME, Perman SM, Abella BS, et al. Higher mean arterial pressure with or without vasoactive agents is associated with increased survival and better neurological outcomes in comatose survivors of cardiac arrest. *Intensive Care Med.* 2013;39(11):1981–8.

22. Kilgannon JH, Roberts BW, Jones AE, et al. Arterial blood pressure and neurologic outcome after resuscitation from cardiac arrest. *Crit Care Med.* 2014;42(9):2083–91.

23. Ameloot K, Genbrugge C, Meex I, et al. An observational near-infrared spectroscopy study on cerebral autoregulation in post-cardiac arrest patients: time to drop 'one-size-fits-all' hemodynamic targets? *Resuscitation.* 2015;90:121–6.

24. Bouzat P, Suys T, Sala N, Oddo M. Effect of moderate hyperventilation and induced hypertension on cerebral tissue oxygenation after cardiac arrest and therapeutic hypothermia. *Resuscitation.* 2013;84(11):1540–5.

25. Safar P, Xiao F, Radovsky A, et al. Improved cerebral resuscitation from cardiac arrest in dogs with mild hypothermia plus blood flow promotion. *Stroke.* 1996;27(1):105–13.

26. Floyd TF, Clark JM, Gelfand R, et al. Independent cerebral vasoconstrictive effects of hyperoxia and accompanying arterial hypocapnia at 1 ATA. *J Appl Physiol.* 2003;95(6):2453–61.

27. Balan IS, Fiskum G, Hazelton J, Cotto-Cumba C, Rosenthal RE. Oximetry-guided reoxygenation improves neurological outcome after experimental cardiac arrest. *Stroke.* 2006;37(12):3008–13.

28. Kuisma M, Boyd J, Voipio V, Alaspaa A, Roine RO, Rosenberg P. Comparison of 30 and the 100% inspired oxygen concentrations during early post-resuscitation period: a randomised controlled pilot study. *Resuscitation.* 2006;69(2):199–206.

29. Elmer J, Scutella M, Pullalarevu R, et al. The association between hyperoxia and patient outcomes after cardiac arrest: analysis of a high-resolution database. *Intensive Care Med.* 2015;41(1):49–57.

30. Kilgannon JH, Jones AE, Parrillo JE, et al. Relationship between supranormal oxygen tension and outcome after resuscitation from cardiac arrest. *Circulation.* 2011;123(23):2717–22.

31. Schneider AG, Eastwood GM, Bellomo R, et al. Arterial carbon dioxide tension and outcome in patients admitted to the intensive care unit after cardiac arrest. *Resuscitation.* 2013;84(7):927–34.

32. Shiozaki T, Sugimoto H, Taneda M, et al. Effect of mild hypothermia on uncontrollable intracranial hypertension after severe head injury. *J Neurosurg.* 1993;79(3):363–8.

33. Vannucci RC, Brucklacher RM, Vannucci SJ. Effect of carbon dioxide on cerebral metabolism during hypoxia-ischemia in the immature rat. *Pediatr Res.* 1997;42(1):24–9.

34. Roberts BW, Kilgannon JH, Chansky ME, Mittal N, Wooden J, Trzeciak S. Association between postresuscitation partial pressure of arterial carbon dioxide and neurological outcome in patients with post-cardiac arrest syndrome. *Circulation.* 2013;127(21):2107–13.

35. Pynnonen L, Falkenbach P, Kamarainen A, Lonnrot K, Yli-Hankala A, Tenhunen J. Therapeutic hypothermia after cardiac arrest - cerebral perfusion and metabolism during upper and lower threshold normocapnia. *Resuscitation.* 2011;82(9):1174–9.

36. Lin B, Ginsberg MD, Busto R. Hyperglycemic exacerbation of neuronal damage following forebrain ischemia: microglial, astrocytic and endothelial alterations. *Acta Neuropathol.* 1998;96(6):610–20.

37. Wass CT, Scheithauer BW, Bronk JT, Wilson RM, Lanier WL. Insulin treatment of corticosteroid-associated hyperglycemia and its effect on outcome after forebrain ischemia in rats. *Anesthesiology.* 1996;84(3):644–51.

38. Longstreth WT Jr., Diehr P, Cobb LA, Hanson RW, Blair AD. Neurologic outcome and blood glucose levels during out-of-hospital cardiopulmonary resuscitation. *Neurology.* 1986;36(9):1186–91.

39. Daviaud F, Dumas F, Demars N, et al. Blood glucose level and outcome after cardiac arrest: insights from a large registry in the hypothermia era. *Intensive Care Med.* 2014;40(6):855–62.

40. Losert H, Sterz F, Roine RO, et al. Strict normoglycaemic blood glucose levels in the therapeutic management of patients within 12h after cardiac arrest might not be necessary. *Resuscitation.* 2008;76(2):214–20.

41. Oksanen T, Skrifvars MB, Varpula T, et al. Strict versus moderate glucose control after resuscitation from ventricular fibrillation. *Intensive Care Med.* 2007;33(12):2093–2100.

42. Callaway CW, Donnino MW, Fink EL, et al. Part 8: post-cardiac arrest care: 2015 American Heart Association guidelines update for cardiopulmonary resuscitation and emergency cardiovascular care. *Circulation.* 2015;132(18 Suppl 2):S465–82.

43. Beniczky S, Hirsch LJ, Kaplan PW, et al. Unified EEG terminology and criteria for non-convulsive status epilepticus. *Epilepsia.* 2013;54 Suppl 6:28–9.

44. Ingvar M. Cerebral blood flow and metabolic rate during seizures. Relationship to epileptic brain damage. *Ann N Y Acad Sci.* 1986;462:194–206.

45. Taft WC, Clifton GL, Blair RE, DeLorenzo RJ. Phenytoin protects against ischemia-produced neuronal cell death. *Brain Res.* 1989;483(1):143–8.

46. Rossetti AO, Oddo M, Liaudet L, Kaplan PW. Predictors of awakening from postanoxic status epilepticus after therapeutic hypothermia. *Neurology.* 2009;72(8):744–9.

47. Wijdicks EF, Hijdra A, Young GB, Bassetti CL, Wiebe S. Quality Standards Subcommittee of the American Academy of N. Practice parameter: prediction of outcome in comatose survivors after cardiopulmonary resuscitation (an evidence-based review): report of the Quality Standards Subcommittee of the American Academy of Neurology. *Neurology.* 2006;67(2):203–10.

48. Zeiner A, Holzer M, Sterz F, et al. Hyperthermia after cardiac arrest is associated with an unfavorable neurologic outcome. *Arch Intern Med.* 2001;161(16):2007–12.

49. Ginsberg MD, Sternau LL, Globus MY, Dietrich WD, Busto R. Therapeutic modulation of brain temperature: relevance to ischemic brain injury. *Cerebrovasc Brain Metabol Rev.* 1992;4(3):189–225.

50. Samaniego EA, Mlynash M, Caulfield AF, Eyngorn I, Wijman CA. Sedation confounds outcome prediction in cardiac arrest survivors treated with hypothermia. *Neurocrit Care.* 2011;15(1):113–9.

51. May TL, Seder DB, Fraser GL, Stone P, McCrum B, Riker RR. Moderate-dose sedation and analgesia during targeted temperature management after cardiac arrest. *Neurocrit Care.* 2015;22(1):105–11.

52. Sandroni C, Cariou A, Cavallaro F, et al. Prognostication in comatose survivors of cardiac arrest: an advisory statement from the European Resuscitation Council and the European Society of Intensive Care Medicine. *Resuscitation.* 2014;85(12):1779–89.

53. Sandroni C, Cavallaro F, Callaway CW, et al. Predictors of poor neurological outcome in adult comatose survivors of cardiac arrest: a systematic review and meta-analysis. Part 2: patients treated with therapeutic hypothermia. *Resuscitation.* 2013;84(10):1324–38.

54. Geocadin RG, Buitrago MM, Torbey MT, Chandra-Strobos N, Williams MA, Kaplan PW. Neurologic prognosis and withdrawal of life support after resuscitation from cardiac arrest. *Neurology.* 2006;67(1):105–8.

55. Leithner C, Ploner CJ, Hasper D, Storm C. Does hypothermia influence the predictive value of bilateral absent N20 after cardiac arrest? *Neurology.* 2010;74(12):965–9.

56. Steffen IG, Hasper D, Ploner CJ, et al. Mild therapeutic hypothermia alters neuron specific enolase as an outcome predictor after resuscitation: 97 prospective hypothermia patients compared to 133 historical non-hypothermia patients. *Crit Care.* 2010;14(2):R69.

57. Mani R, Schmitt SE, Mazer M, Putt ME, Gaieski DF. The frequency and timing of epileptiform activity on continuous electroencephalogram in comatose post-cardiac arrest syndrome patients treated with therapeutic hypothermia. *Resuscitation.* 2012;83(7):840–7.

58. Legriel S, Bruneel F, Sediri H, et al. Early EEG monitoring for detecting postanoxic status epilepticus during therapeutic hypothermia: a pilot study. *Neurocrit Care.* 2009;11(3):338–44.

59. Myles PS, Leslie K, McNeil J, Forbes A, Chan MT. Bispectral index monitoring to prevent awareness during anaesthesia: the B-Aware randomised controlled trial. *Lancet.* 2004;363(9423):1757–63.

60. Seder DB, Dziodzio J, Smith KA, et al. Feasibility of bispectral index monitoring to guide early post-resuscitation cardiac arrest triage. *Resuscitation.* 2014;85(8):1030–6.

61. Bousselmi R, Lebbi A, Ferjani M. Bispectral index changes during generalised tonic-clonic seizures. *Anaesthesia.* 2013;68(10):1084–5.

62. Murkin JM, Arango M. Near-infrared spectroscopy as an index of brain and tissue oxygenation. *Br J Anaesth.* 2009;103 Suppl 1:i3–13.

63. Joshi B, Brady K, Lee J, et al. Impaired autoregulation of cerebral blood flow during rewarming from hypothermic cardiopulmonary bypass and its potential association with stroke. *Anesth Analg.* 2010;110(2):321–8.

64. Colbourne F, Corbett D. Delayed and prolonged post-ischemic hypothermia is neuroprotective in the gerbil. *Brain Res.* 1994;654(2):265–72.

65. Preston E, Webster J. A two-hour window for hypothermic modulation of early events that impact delayed opening of the rat blood-brain barrier after ischemia. *Acta Neuropathol.* 2004;108(5):406–12.

66. Colbourne F, Li H, Buchan AM. Indefatigable CA1 sector neuroprotection with mild hypothermia induced 6 hours after severe forebrain ischemia in rats. *J Cerebral Blood Flow Metabol.* 1999;19(7):742–9.

67. Weinrauch V, Safar P, Tisherman S, Kuboyama K, Radovsky A. Beneficial effect of mild hypothermia and detrimental effect of deep hypothermia after cardiac arrest in dogs. *Stroke.* 1992;23(10):1454–62.

68. Liu L, Yenari MA. Therapeutic hypothermia: neuroprotective mechanisms. *Front Biosci.* 2007;12:816–25.

69. Nielsen N, Hovdenes J, Nilsson F, et al. Outcome, timing and adverse events in therapeutic hypothermia after out-of-hospital cardiac arrest. *Acta Anaesthesiol Scand.* 2009;53(7):926–34.

70. Bernard SA, Jones BM, Horne MK. Clinical trial of induced hypothermia in comatose survivors of out-of-hospital cardiac arrest. *Ann Emerg Med.* 1997;30(2):146–53.

71. Yanagawa Y, Ishihara S, Norio H, et al. Preliminary clinical outcome study of mild resuscitative hypothermia after out-of-hospital cardiopulmonary arrest. *Resuscitation.* 1998;39(1-2):61–6.

72. Zeiner A, Holzer M, Sterz F, et al. Mild resuscitative hypothermia to improve neurological outcome after cardiac arrest. A clinical feasibility trial. Hypothermia After Cardiac Arrest (HACA) Study Group. *Stroke.* 2000;31(1):86–94.

73. Hypothermia after Cardiac Arrest Study Group. Mild therapeutic hypothermia to improve the neurologic outcome after cardiac arrest. *N Engl J Med.* 2002;346(8):549–56.

74. Bernard SA, Gray TW, Buist MD, et al. Treatment of comatose survivors of out-of-hospital cardiac arrest with induced hypothermia. *N Engl J Med.* 2002;346(8):557–63.

75. Nielsen N, Wetterslev J, Cronberg T, et al. Targeted temperature management at 33 degrees C versus 36 degrees C after cardiac arrest. *N Engl J Med.* 2013;369(23):2197–206.

76. Dumas F, Grimaldi D, Zuber B, et al. Is hypothermia after cardiac arrest effective in both shockable and nonshockable patients?: insights from a large registry. *Circulation.* 2011;123(8):877–86.

77. Perman SM, Grossestreuer AV, Wiebe DJ, Carr BG, Abella BS, Gaieski DF. The utility of therapeutic hypothermia for post-cardiac arrest syndrome patients with an initial non-shockable rhythm. *Circulation.* 2015;132(22):2146–51.

78. Batista LM, Lima FO, Januzzi JL, Jr, Donahue V, Snydeman C, Greer DM. Feasibility and safety of combined percutaneous coronary intervention and therapeutic hypothermia following cardiac arrest. *Resuscitation.* 2010;81(4):398–403.

79. Garot P, Lefevre T, Eltchaninoff H, et al. Six-month outcome of emergency percutaneous coronary intervention in resuscitated patients after cardiac arrest complicating ST-elevation myocardial infarction. *Circulation.* 2007;115(11):1354–62.

80. Dumas F, Cariou A, Manzo-Silberman S, et al. Immediate percutaneous coronary intervention is associated with better survival after out-of-hospital cardiac arrest: insights from the PROCAT (Parisian Region Out of hospital Cardiac ArresT) registry. *Circulation Cardiovasc Interv.* 2010;3(3):200–7.

81. Meloni BP, Zhu H, Knuckey NW. Is magnesium neuroprotective following global and focal cerebral ischaemia? A review of published studies. *Magnesium Res.* 2006;19(2):123–37.

82. Zhu H, Meloni BP, Bojarski C, Knuckey MW, Knuckey NW. Post-ischemic modest hypothermia (35 degrees C) combined with intravenous magnesium is more effective at reducing CA1 neuronal death than either treatment used alone following global cerebral ischemia in rats. *Exper Neurol.* 2005;193(2):361–8.

83. Longstreth WT Jr, Fahrenbruch CE, Olsufka M, Walsh TR, Copass MK, Cobb LA. Randomized clinical trial of magnesium, diazepam, or both after out-of-hospital cardiac arrest. *Neurology.* 2002;59(4):506–14.

84. Zweifler RM, Voorhees ME, Mahmood MA, Parnell M. Magnesium sulfate increases the rate of hypothermia via surface cooling and improves comfort. *Stroke.* 2004;35(10):2331–4.

85. Gisvold SE, Safar P, Hendrickx HH, Rao G, Moossy J, Alexander H. Thiopental treatment after global brain ischemia in pigtailed monkeys. *Anesthesiology.* 1984;60(2):88–96.

86. Ebmeyer U, Safar P, Radovsky A, et al. Thiopental combination treatments for cerebral resuscitation after prolonged cardiac arrest in dogs. Exploratory outcome study. *Resuscitation.* 2000;45(2):119–31.

87. Breivik H, Safar P, Sands P, et al. Clinical feasibility trials of barbiturate therapy after cardiac arrest. *Crit Care Med.* 1978;6(4):228–44.

88. Monsalve F, Rucabado L, Ruano M, Cunat J, Lacueva V, Vinuales A. The neurologic effects of thiopental therapy after cardiac arrest. *Intensive Care Med.* 1987;13(4):244–8.

89. Randomized clinical study of thiopental loading in comatose survivors of cardiac arrest. Brain Resuscitation Clinical Trial I Study Group. *N Engl J Med.* 1986;314(7):397–403.

90. Hashemzadeh E, Movassaghi S, Shafaroodi H, Barmchi AA, Sharifi ZN. Effect of coenzyme q10 (ubiquinone) on hippocampal CA1 pyramidal cells following transient global ischemia/reperfusion in male wistar rat. *J Pharmaceut Health Sci.* 2014;3(1):21–8.

91. Cocchi MN, Giberson B, Berg K, et al. Coenzyme Q10 levels are low and associated with increased mortality in post-cardiac arrest patients. *Resuscitation.* 2012;83(8):991–5.

92. Damian MS, Ellenberg D, Gildemeister R, et al. Coenzyme Q10 combined with mild hypothermia after cardiac arrest: a preliminary study. *Circulation.* 2004;110(19):3011–6.

93. Koliantzaki I, Zakynthinos SG, Mentzelopoulos SD. The potential contribution of corticosteroids to positive cardiac arrest outcomes. In: Gullo A, Ristagno G, eds. *Resuscitation: translational research, clinical evidence, education, guidelines.* Milan, Italy: Springer-Verlag Italia; 2014:143–55.

94. Grafton ST, Longstreth WT Jr. Steroids after cardiac arrest: a retrospective study with concurrent, nonrandomized controls. *Neurology.* 1988;38(8):1315–6.

95. Jastremski M, Sutton-Tyrrell K, Vaagenes P, Abramson N, Heiselman D, Safar P. Glucocorticoid treatment does not improve neurological recovery following cardiac arrest. Brain Resuscitation Clinical Trial I Study Group. *JAMA.* 1989;262(24):3427–30.

96. Annborn M, Bro-Jeppesen J, Nielsen N, et al. The association of targeted temperature management at 33 and 36 degrees C with outcome in patients with moderate shock on admission after out-of-hospital cardiac arrest: a post hoc analysis of the Target Temperature Management trial. *Intensive Care Med.* 2014;40(9):1210–9.

97. Testori C, Sterz F, Holzer M, et al. The beneficial effect of mild therapeutic hypothermia depends on the time of complete circulatory standstill in patients with cardiac arrest. *Resuscitation.* 2012;83(5):596–601.

98. Deng R, Xiong W, Jia X. Electrophysiological monitoring of brain injury and recovery after cardiac arrest. *Int J Mol Sci.* 2015;16(11):25999–26018.

99. Hofmeijer J, Tjepkema-Cloostermans MC, Blans MJ, Beishuizen A, van Putten MJ. Unstandardized treatment of electroencephalographic status epilepticus does not improve outcome of comatose patients after cardiac arrest. *Front Neurol.* 2014;5:39.

100. Lee JH, Kim K, Jo YH, Lee MJ, Hwang JE, Kim MA. Effect of valproic acid combined with therapeutic hypothermia on neurologic outcome in asphyxial cardiac arrest model of rats. *Am J Emerg Med.* 2015;33(12):1773–9.

101. Adrie C, Cariou A, Mourvillier B, et al. Predicting survival with good neurological recovery at hospital admission after successful resuscitation of out-of-hospital cardiac arrest: the OHCA score. *Eur Heart J.* 2006;27(23):2840–5.

102. Oddo M, Schaller MD, Feihl F, Ribordy V, Liaudet L. From evidence to clinical practice: effective implementation of therapeutic hypothermia to improve patient outcome after cardiac arrest. *Crit Care Med.* 2006;34(7):1865–73.

103. Natsukawa T, Sawano H, Natsukawa M, et al. At what level of unconsciousness is mild therapeutic hypothermia indicated for out-of-hospital cardiac arrest: a retrospective, historical cohort study. *J Intensive Care.* 2015;3(1):38.

104. Kim SH, Choi SP, Park KN, Youn CS, Oh SH, Choi SM. Early brain computed tomography findings are associated with outcome in patients treated with therapeutic hypothermia after out-of-hospital cardiac arrest. *Scand J Trauma, Resusc Emerg Med.* 2013;21:57.

105. Rossetti AO, Urbano LA, Delodder F, Kaplan PW, Oddo M. Prognostic value of continuous EEG monitoring during therapeutic hypothermia after cardiac arrest. *Crit Care.* 2010;14(5):R173.

106. Cloostermans MC, van Meulen FB, Eertman CJ, Hom HW, van Putten MJ. Continuous electroencephalography monitoring for early prediction of neurological outcome

in postanoxic patients after cardiac arrest: a prospective cohort study. *Crit Care Med.* 2012;40(10):2867–75.

107. Seder DB, Fraser GL, Robbins T, Libby L, Riker RR. The bispectral index and suppression ratio are very early predictors of neurological outcome during therapeutic hypothermia after cardiac arrest. *Intensive Care Med.* 2010;36(2):281–8.

108. Bouwes A, Binnekade JM, Kuiper MA, et al. Prognosis of coma after therapeutic hypothermia: a prospective cohort study. *Ann Neurol.* 2012;71(2):206–12.

109. Fugate JE, Wijdicks EF, Mandrekar J, et al. Predictors of neurologic outcome in hypothermia after cardiac arrest. *Ann Neurol.* 2010;68(6):907–14.

110. Seder DB, Sunde K, Rubertsson S, et al. Neurologic outcomes and postresuscitation care of patients with myoclonus following cardiac arrest. *Crit Care Med.* 2015;43(5):965–72.

111. Kawai M, Thapalia U, Verma A. Outcome from therapeutic hypothermia and EEG. *J Clin Neurophysiol.* 2011;28(5):483–8.

112. Hirsch KG, Mlynash M, Jansen S, et al. Prognostic value of a qualitative brain MRI scoring system after cardiac arrest. *J Neuroimag.* 2015;25(3):430–7.

113. Hirsch KG, Mlynash M, Eyngorn I, et al. Multi-center study of diffusion-weighted imaging in coma after cardiac arrest. *Neurocrit Care.* 2015;24(1):82–9.

114. Nair SU, Lundbye JB. The occurrence of shivering in cardiac arrest survivors undergoing therapeutic hypothermia is associated with a good neurologic outcome. *Resuscitation.* 2013;84(5):626–9.

115. Ko SB, Ortega-Gutierrez S, Choi HA, et al. Status epilepticus-induced hyperemia and brain tissue hypoxia after cardiac arrest. *Arch Neurol.* 2011;68(10):1323–6.

# 10 Neuroprotection for Acute Ischemic Stroke

Diana Mayor and Michael Tymianski

## GENERAL CONSIDERATIONS

Stroke is the leading cause of acquired neurological disability and the second leading cause of death worldwide, according to the World Health Organization.[1] An estimated 795,000 strokes occur each year in the United States, at a direct and indirect cost exceeding $70 billion.[1] In 2010, the absolute numbers of Western World people affected by stroke had significantly increased since 1990, with 16.9 million people with first stroke, 33 million stroke survivors, 5.9 million stroke-related deaths, and 102 million people with disability-adjusted to life years loss.[2] The most common stroke type, accounting for 85% of cases, is acute ischemic stroke (AIS).[3-5]

## CAUSES OF AND RISKS FOR NEUROLOGICAL INJURY

AIS results from a heterogeneous group of disorders whose final pathway leads to reduction or absence of blood flow due to arterial vascular occlusion.[5-6] Four major mechanisms are responsible for ischemia in acute stroke: cardioembolism, arterio-embolism, small vessel disease, and hemodynamic failure due to other causes.[5,7]

The first three mechanisms result from embolism or in situ thrombosis leading to an abrupt reduction in regional cerebral blood flow (CBF).[5,8] Stroke due to hemodynamic failure usually occurs in patients with moderate arterial stenosis or partial occlusion who have a good collateral blood supply to maintain CBF levels under normal conditions.[9] Under certain conditions, however, such as decreased perfusion (hypotension or low cardiac output) or increased metabolic demand (acidosis), cerebral ischemia may be triggered.[10]

The core area of a stroke is the zone where the blood flow is so drastically reduced that cells cannot recover and subsequently undergo cell death.[11] The tissue that borders the ischemic core is known as the *ischemic penumbra*. This region is dysfunctional due to reduced blood flow, contributing to the clinical deficit, but it has not yet been irreversibly damaged and remains metabolically active.[12-13] If blood flow and oxygen delivery are restored in a timely manner, penumbral tissue is potentially salvageable and the associated clinical deficit is potentially recoverable.[9] Otherwise, this tissue may undergo necrosis or apoptosis within hours or days.

At a molecular level, the decreased blood flow deprives neurons of metabolic substrates. The ischemic cascade begins with adenosine triphosphate (ATP) depletion, which results in failure of the $Na^+/K^+$ pump.[14] Consequently, voltage-sensitive calcium channels are activated, resulting in calcium influx to the cell.[15] The calcium influx results in glutamate release into synapses. Glutamate stimulates α-amino-3-hydroxy-5-methyl-4-isoxazolepropionic acid (AMPA) and N-methyl-D-aspartate (NMDA) receptors, which leads to more calcium influx.[16] The perpetuation of this ischemic cascade leads to excitotoxicity.[17] Intracellular enzymes (proteases, lipases) and the formation of free radicals lead to destruction of cell membranes and mitochondrial breakdown.[18] Multiple other mechanisms have also been proposed, including non-excitotoxic mechanisms involving a range of ion channels, transporters, and intracellular proteins.[18]

The target of neuroprotective therapy for AIS is the ischemic penumbra; the ischemic core is already irreversibly damaged and therefore cannot be salvaged by reperfusion.[19-20] Ischemic penumbra models predict that earlier reperfusion leads to better outcomes in patients with AIS.[11] Over the first few minutes to hours after an acute arterial occlusion, ischemic penumbral tissue progresses to become infarct core, and the potential benefit of restoring blood flow decreases over time.[21] For every minute that an artery is occluded during an ischemic stroke, 2 million neurons die.[22]

## Nonmodifiable Risk Factors for Acute Ischemic Stroke

Risk of AIS is related to age, gender, heredity, and race, and these factors can help identify patients at higher risk.[23] Age is the strongest risk factor; after age 55, the stroke rate doubles for each successive 10 years in both men and women.[24-25] Regarding heredity, the Framingham Study found that parental history of coronary artery disease was strongly associated with acute cerebral ischemia among offspring study members (relative risk = 3.33; 95% confidence interval [CI], 1.27 to 8.72).[26] Stroke incidence and mortality rates vary widely between racial groups; black Americans are more than twice as likely to die of stroke, compared with white Americans.[27] Women using oral contraceptives and those having non-valvular atrial fibrillation have a higher stroke risk than men.[24-25]

## Modifiable Risk Factors for Acute Ischemic Stroke

The single most important modifiable risk factor for ischemic stroke is hypertension. When defined as systolic blood pressure of 160 mm Hg or greater and/or diastolic blood pressure 95 mm Hg or greater, hypertension increases the relative risk by approximately 4.[28] Population surveys show that the prevalence of hypertension steadily increases with age, with a prevalence of approximately 20% at age 50, 30% at age 60, 40% at age 70, 55% at age 80, and 60% at age 90.[29]

Various cardiac diseases are associated with increased risk of stroke. The strongest cardiac precursor of stroke is atrial fibrillation (AF). The Framingham Study showed that the incidence of AF doubles with each successive decade above age 55 and that non-valvular AF was independently associated with a three- to fivefold increased risk for stroke.[30]

Myocardial disease also is a well-established risk factor for stroke.[31–32] The risk of stroke has been shown to increase twofold with coronary artery disease, threefold with electrocardiographic (ECG) left ventricular hypertrophy, and three- to four-fold with cardiac failure.[33] Left ventricular mass assessed by echocardiography also is associated with increased risk for stroke.[33]

Patients with diabetes or insulin resistance have an increased prevalence of ather-ogenic risk factors, atherosclerosis, and stroke.[34] Prospective epidemiological stud-ies and case-control studies of stroke patients have confirmed that diabetes is an independent risk factor, with a relative risk of ischemic stroke from 1.8 to 3.0.[34] In the Framingham study, the risk of brain infarction was double in persons with glu-cose intolerance relative to non-diabetic persons.[35]

Lifestyle factors that are associated with increased stroke risk include obesity, physical inactivity, diet, and cigarette smoking. The relative risk of ischemic stroke increases nearly two times with cigarette smoking, with a dose–response relation-ship.[36] Smoking cessation is associated with a reduction of major risk within 2 to 4 years.[37–38] Obesity (defined as a Metropolitan Life chart relative weight greater than 30% above average) also is a significant independent contributor to ischemic stroke in men aged 35 to 64, and women aged 65 to 94.[35]

## MONITORING FOR INJURY

Although much attention has focused on the first hours after stroke onset, there likely are multiple factors that ultimately affect the stroke outcome in the post-acute phase. One such major factor is whether the patient is admitted to a stroke unit providing careful monitoring.[39] A prospective study that compared out-comes in 268 AIS patients who had continuous monitoring (blood pressure, ECG, oxygen saturation, temperature) for 72 hours in a stroke unit versus routine care (less intense monitoring), showed that more intensive care led to a 2.5-fold increase in the probability of a good outcome at discharge.[40] This may be due to earlier detection and treatment of complications.[41] A small randomized controlled trial in which 54 patients with acute ischemic hemiparetic stroke were randomly assigned to a stroke care monitoring unit (SCMU) versus a conventional stroke unit showed that monitoring for 48 hours was associated with a lower propor-tion of patient deaths and poor outcome at 3 months.[42] The average length of hospital stay also was shorter for the SCMU patients compared to conventional care ($16 \pm 5$ days versus $25 \pm 7$ days).

A Cochrane review of organized inpatient care in a stroke unit concluded that care in a stroke unit was consistently associated with improved outcomes, reducing significantly the odds of death or institutionalized care (odds ratio [OR] 0.82; 95% CI 0.73 to 0.92; $P = 0.0006$), independent of patient age, sex, or stroke severity.[39] Hospitals with organized stroke care would also be more likely to have organized stroke triage mechanisms and uniform approaches to the initial care of patients within the first hours after stroke.

## NEUROPROTECTION STRATEGIES
### Physiologic Interventions

Many clinical factors that require acute intervention may affect stroke outcome. These include blood pressure, fever, blood glucose, oxygenation, concomitant medications, and medical comorbidities. There are significant variations in clinical practices related to these factors among practitioners and institutions. Such variations might be minimized and outcomes improved if stroke patients are channeled to centers with stroke units.

## Blood Pressure Management

Elevated blood pressure is common in the acute stage of ischemic stroke, occurring in two-thirds to three-quarters of patients.[43] Severe hypertension is a contraindication for thrombolytic therapy; however, there are no data defining the level of arterial hypertension that mandates emergent management.[44]

The early hypertension that follows ischemic stroke often reflects undiagnosed or undertreated hypertension, as well as neuroendocrine response to physiological stress.[44] An observational study of AIS patients found that, on arrival to the emergency department, the systolic blood pressure was greater than 139 mm Hg in 77% of patients, and greater than 184 mm Hg in 15%.[43] Furthermore, acute stroke patients with a prior history of hypertension often have higher blood pressure than those without premorbid hypertension on arrival.

Blood pressure control to a normal range after a completed infarct may reduce cerebral edema, reduce hemorrhagic transformation of the cerebral infarction, and accelerate the transition to long-term antihypertensive therapy. In the early phase of care, however, decreasing blood pressure may reduce collateral flow through arteries that have lost autoregulatory function because of ischemia, and increase the size of the cerebral infarction.[44] Blood pressure reduction as late as 48 hours after onset (well after most infarcts are completed) may also be harmful. A placebo-controlled randomized trial that tested oral nimodipine starting within 48 hours after ischemic stroke onset found that functional outcome at 3 months was similar between the two treatment groups, but mortality was significantly higher in the nimodipine group.[45] By contrast, the Acute Candesartan Cilexetil Therapy in Stroke Survivors (ACCESS) trial found that modest blood pressure reduction in the early treatment of stroke (starting an average of 30 hours after stroke onset) in patients with elevated blood pressure showed a strong benefit.[46] Although blood pressure and the Barthel Index of Activities of Daily Living score at 3 months were similar in the two study groups, patients who received the active drug had significantly lower mortality and fewer vascular events at 12 months.[46] The larger Scandinavian Candesartan Acute Stroke Trial (SCAST) also evaluated the benefit of candesartan antihypertensive therapy in AIS patients; however, it failed to show benefit in functional outcome at 6 months despite mean blood pressure reduction of 5–7 mm Hg 1 week after stroke.[47]

## Blood Glucose Management

Both hypoglycemia and hyperglycemia are important modulators of tissue injury and outcomes in AIS. Hypoglycemia can cause focal neurologic signs that mimic stroke and, if severe, can itself result in permanent brain injury.[23] Of patients admitted with AIS, hyperglycemia occurs in 30–63% of those with no prior history of diabetes and even more frequently in patients with a prior history of diabetes.[48-49]

The United Kingdom Glucose Insulin in Stroke Trial (GIST-UK) tested the efficacy of hyperglycemia treatment in AIS.[50] A total of 933 AIS patients were randomly assigned to receive either glucose-insulin-potassium (GIK) infusions to maintain euglycemia or saline. There was no difference in clinical outcomes (mortality at 90 days poststroke) between the two treatment groups.[50] The Stroke Hyperglycemia Insulin Network Effort (SHINE) trial (NCT01369069) is evaluating whether stricter glucose management (by intravenous insulin) to glucose concentrations of 80–130 mg/dL improves clinical outcomes after AIS.[51]

A Cochrane systematic review of 11 randomized control trials involving 1,583 patients evaluated whether intensively monitored insulin therapy (continuous insulin infusion vs. regular subcutaneous insulin depending on glucose level) in the first 24 hours of AIS influences outcome.[52] There were no differences between the treatment and control groups in the outcomes of death or dependency (OR 0.99, 95% CI 0.79 to 1.23) or final neurological deficit (standardized mean difference −0.09, 95% CI −0.19 to 0.01).[52]

## Oxygenation and Airway Management

During periods of acute cerebral ischemia it is important to maintain adequate tissue oxygenation to prevent hypoxia and potential worsening of the neurologic injury. If there is evidence of hypoxia, by blood gas determination or desaturation detected by pulse oximetry, supplemental oxygen should be administered.[23] If the patient has a decreased level of consciousness, tracheal intubation should be considered to reduce aspiration risk.[44,53] It remains to be determined whether supplemental oxygenation by normobaric and hyperbaric means in the setting of adequate oxygenation by pulse oximetry confers any outcome benefit.[54]

## Body Temperature

In the setting of AIS, hyperthermia is associated with poor neurological outcome. This may be due to increased metabolic demands, enhanced release of neurotransmitters, and increased free radical production.[55-57] A meta-analysis demonstrated a twofold increase in short-term mortality in acute stroke patients who were hyperthermic within the first 24 hours of hospitalization.[57]

Three trials evaluated the effect of paracetamol (75 patients) or ibuprofen (24 patients) in achieving normothermia in patients with AIS.[58-59] These studies showed the limitations of antipyretic medications at low doses in achieving normothermia. Treatment with a daily dose of 6,000 mg of paracetamol resulted in a small reduction in body temperature.[58]

A number of small phase II pilot clinical trials have investigated the safety and feasibility of induced hypothermia for AIS. These include the Cooling for Acute Ischemic Brain Damage (COOL-AID) trial and the Intravenous Thrombolysis Plus Hypothermia for Acute Treatment of Ischemic Stroke (ICTUS-L) trial.[60-61] These studies were underpowered for detecting clinical benefit. They also raised questions about the feasibility of inducing hypothermia in relatively awake, spontaneously breathing stroke patients who tend to shiver vigorously and are prone to experience discomfort with hypothermia (unlike intubated trauma and cardiac arrest patients).

## Thrombolysis

In addition to the basic medical interventions just noted, only therapies that may affect vessel recanalization have achieved regulatory approval in the acute phase of AIS. Overall, appropriately selected patients receiving thrombolytic therapy have improved outcomes.[62–65] In patients with failed recanalization, diffusion weighted imaging (DWI) lesion volumes increase, whereas in patients with successful recanalization, especially with middle cerebral artery (MCA) occlusion, DWI lesion increases are significantly attenuated.[66–67] Recanalization, therefore, is a major focus of acute stroke intervention.

Intravenous administration of alteplase is the only widely approved therapy for AIS. In the United States, it is approved for use within 3 hours of stroke onset. It is used off label within 4.5 hours of onset based on the results of the European Cooperative Acute Stroke Study (ECASS) III randomized clinical trial and the large-scale registry study Safe Implementation of Treatment in Stroke-International Stroke Thrombolysis Register (SITS-ISTR), both of which demonstrated the safety and efficacy of alteplase administered 3–4.5 hours after the onset of ischemic stroke symptoms.[62,64–65] More than half of AIS patients who present to the emergency department within the 3-hour window are eligible for rtPA. Ineligibility during the 3-hour window is usually due to mild stroke severity, medical and surgical history, or blood test results indicating a propensity for bleeding (such as a low platelet count).[68–69] Although alteplase has been available since 1996, it is used in only 3–5% of all AIS victims in North America because most patients arrive to a hospital beyond the 3-hour window.[70–71] It can only be administered in hospital after brain imaging excludes a hemorrhagic stroke. The need to initiate rtPA after brain imaging creates significant delays, such that barely 25% of rtPA candidates begin treatment within 140 minutes of stroke onset.[72]

Several clinical trials have implemented imaging selection strategies to evaluate AIS recanalization therapies. Although the Desmoteplase in Acute Ischemic Stroke (DIAS) and Dose Escalation of Desmoteplase for Acute Ischemic Stroke (DEDAS) trials showed that the thrombolytic desmoteplase had a favorable effect, this was not supported by the larger phase III study Desmoteplase in Acute Ischemic Stroke 2 (DIAS-2).[73–75] The Echoplanar Imaging Thrombolysis Evaluation Trial (EPITHET) trial evaluating rtPA administered beyond 3 hours of symptom onset, in which 86% of patients had a mismatch of perfusion weighted imaging (PWI) and DWI suggestive of an ischemic penumbra, similarly failed to show a treatment effect.[76] Data from 502 PWI-DWI mismatch patients who were thrombolyzed beyond 3 hours were examined in a meta-analysis of six trials.[77] The study concluded that "delayed thrombolysis in mismatch patients was not confirmed to improve clinical outcome." It has been proposed, however, that the negative result in the phase III DIAS-2 trial may have been due to a combination of mild stroke severity in the study cohort and small sample size.[78]

The Randomized Trial of Tenecteplase versus Alteplase for Acute Ischemic Stroke studied 75 stroke patients having a perfusion lesion at least 20% greater than the infarct core on computed tomography (CT) perfusion imaging and an associated vessel occlusion on CT angiography.[79] Tenecteplase was associated with significantly better reperfusion and clinical outcomes than Alteplase. It is unclear, however, whether the relevant selection criterion was the CT perfusion mismatch (indicative of a penumbra) or the documented vessel occlusion. A reanalysis of the EPITHET trial data suggests that the site of arterial occlusion strongly predicted clinical outcomes, thus supporting selection based on vessel occlusion imaging.[67] Indeed, the penumbra selection approach was abandoned by the desmoteplase investigators in favor of vessel occlusion criteria in the DIAS-3 Trial. Desmoteplase administration 3–9 hours after onset of stroke symptoms was not associated with increased mortality or severe adverse effects compared to placebo, but it also failed to showed a treatment effect.[80]

## Mechanical Thrombectomy

Endovascular therapy achieves high recanalization rates but benefits a small minority of patients having the combination of a large vessel occlusion (LVO), an evolving penumbra, and timely arrival to a stroke center offering this high-tech intervention.[78,81–83] Seven randomized trials that tested the effectiveness of endovascular therapy and medical therapy (intravenous alteplase when eligible) over medical treatment alone are listed in Table 10.1.[81–85] In all of these trials, endovascular therapy was associated with significantly better neurological outcomes and functional independence compared to intravenous thrombolysis alone. In the MR CLEAN trial, the absolute difference in the rate of functional independence was 13.5% favoring endovascular therapy. Patient randomization was performed after proximal artery occlusion confirmation by CT angiography or CT perfusion imaging.[81]

## Pharmacologic Neuroprotection

Another strategy to reduce progression of stroke is the administration of various neuroprotectants. In the past decade, several randomized controlled trials of neuroprotectant agents for AIS have been performed (see Table 10.2).[86–89] No clinical studies to date, however, have conclusively demonstrated a clinical benefit with any of these pharmacological agents. A significant body of preclinical data may provide clues to the potential utility and the limitations of pharmacological neuroprotection, but preclinical data have their own limitations in extrapolating results to humans. Despite the negative results of pharmacological neuroprotection trials for AIS, there is still optimism for an agent that can reduce the brain's vulnerability to ischemia if administered within a reasonable time frame (≤4 hours).

Because all stroke therapy is highly time-sensitive, the fastest way to administer a neuroprotectant therapy is to administer it before patients arrive to the hospital, typically by paramedics in the field. In the Field Administration of Stroke Therapy – Magnesium (FAST-MAG) trial, 1,700 patients with suspected stroke were randomized to receive either intravenous magnesium sulfate or placebo within a window of 2 hours of symptom onset.[90] A loading dose was initiated by paramedics before the patient arrived at the hospital. Magnesium sulfate did not result in improved 90-day disability outcomes on the modified Rankin scale (mRS).

Perhaps the most promising approach to clinical trials of neuroprotectants is to evaluate these agents as adjuncts to revascularization therapies. The strong evidence that endovascular therapy is effective in improving neurological outcome in patients with large vessel arterial occlusions now provides a human paradigm that simulates the animal models of ischemia-reperfusion that are widely used in preclinical stroke research. The hypothesis is that neuroprotectants may slow the progression of ischemic injury and permit more time for recanalization therapies to exert a benefit or may modulate and minimize reperfusion injury.

## IMPLICATIONS FOR CLINICAL PRACTICE
### Patient Selection

There is a potential benefit to using imaging strategies to pre-select patients for stroke intervention trials in order to selectively treat those who may benefit while protecting those who may not benefit from unnecessary risk. From the perspective of trial conduct, this approach could enrich trial patient samples with "responders,"

Table 10.1 Randomized Trials Testing Effectiveness of Endovascular and Medical Therapy (Intravenous Alteplase when Eligible) over Medical Treatment Alone

| Trial | N | Imaging Selection | NIHSS | Time Window for IAT | TICI 2B-3 for IAT group | mRS 0–2 (%) | | |
|---|---|---|---|---|---|---|---|---|
| | | | | | | IAT | Control | OR [95% CI] |
| **MR CLEAN** | 500 | LVO | ≥2 | ≤6 h | 59% | 33% | 19% | 2.1 [1.4 to 3.4] |
| **EXTEND-IA** | 70 | LVO AND favorable CT perfusion | None | ≤6 h | 86% | 71% | 40% | 4.2 [1.4 to 12] |
| **ESCAPE** | 315 | LVO AND favorable collaterals on multiphase CTA | ≥6 | ≤12 h | 72% | 53% | 29% | 1.7 [1.3 to 2.2] |
| **REVASCAT** | 206 | LVO | ≥6 | ≤8 h | 66% | 44% | 28% | 2.0 [1.1 to 3.5] |
| **SWIFT PRIME** | 196 | LVO AND favorable CT perfusion | 10–30 | ≤6 h | 83% | 60% | 35% | 1.7 [1.2 to 2.3] |
| **THRACE** | 395 | LVO (including basilar) | 10–25 | ≤5 h | NA | 54% | 42% | NA |
| **THERAPY** | 108 | LVO with clot length >8 mm on NCHCT | ≥8 | ≤4.5 h | NA | 38% | 34% | NS |

*MR CLEAN*, Multicenter Randomized Clinical Trial of Endovascular Treatment for Acute Ischemic Stroke in the Netherlands; *EXTEND IA*, Extending the Time for Thrombolysis in Emergency Neurological Deficits—Intra-Arterial; *ESCAPE*, Endovascular Treatment for Small Core and Anterior Circulation Proximal Occlusion with Emphasis on Minimizing CT to Recanalization Times; *REVASCAT*, Randomized Trial of Revascularization with Solitaire FR Device versus Best Medical Therapy in the Treatment of Acute Stroke Due to Anterior Circulation Large Vessel Occlusion Presenting within Eight Hours of Symptom Onset; *SWIFT PRIME*, Solitaire with the Intention for Thrombectomy as Primary Endovascular Treatment; *THRACE*, Thrombectomy in Acute Ischemic Stroke; *THERAPY*, Assess the Penumbra System in the Treatment of Acute Stroke.

Table 10.2 Stroke Neuroprotection Trials Completed Since 2000

| Study Name | Clinicaltrial.org Identifier | Sponsor | Phase | Treatment | Completed | Early Termination | Number of subjects | Enrollment Window |
|---|---|---|---|---|---|---|---|---|
| CLASS-I* | N/A | ArstraZeneca | 2 | Clomethiazole | 2001 | No | 1198 | 12h |
| ASTIN | N/A | | 2 | UK-279,276 | 2002 | Yes (Futility) | 966 | 6h |
| IMAGE S* | N/A | | 3 | MgSO4 vs Placebo | 2003 | No | 2589 | 12h |
| ARTIST-MRI | NCT00044070 | Astellas Phama | 2 | YM872 vs Placebo | 2003 | Yes (Futility) | ? | 6h |
| ARTIST+ | NCT00044057 | Astellas Phama | 2/3 | YM872+tpa vs tPA alone | 2003 | Yes (Futility) | 400 | 6h |
| IL-1-rain AIS* | N/A | University of Manchester | 2 | Interleukin-l receptor antagonist | 2004 | No | 34 | 6h |
| Repinotan | NCT00044915 | Bayer | 3 | Repinotan vs Placebo | 2004 | No | 681 | 4.5h |
| Traxoprodil* | NCT00073476 | Pfizer | 2 | Traxoprodil | 2005 | Yes | 300 | 6h |
| SAINT-I | NCT00119626 | AstraZeneca | 3 | NXY-059 vs Placebo | 2005 | No | 1700 | 6h |
| SAINT-II | NCT00061022 | AstraZeneca | 3 | NXY-059 vs Placebo | 2006 | No | 3306 | 6h |
| SUN N4057 | NCT00272909 | Asubio Pharma | 2 | SUN N4057 vs Placebo | 2007 | Yes | 43 | 9h |
| ESS | NCT00604630 | J&J/Parexel | 3 | EPO vs Placebo | 2008 | No | 522 | 6h |
| ONO-2506 | NCT00229177 | Ono Pharma | 3 | ONO-2506 vs Placebo | 2008 | Yes | 757 | 72h |
| Ginsenoside-Rd* | NCT00591084 | Xiijing Hospital | 2 | Ginsenoside vs Placebo | 2008 | No | 199 | 72h |
| Ginsenoside-Rd* | NCT00815763 | Xiijing Hospital | 3 | Ginsenoside vs Placebo | 2008 | No | 390 | 72h |
| EAST* | NCT00153946 | Japan Cardiovascular Research | 2 | Argatroban+edaravone vs Argatroban | 2008 | No | 808 | 72h |
| ICT uS-L | NCT00283088 | UCSD/NINDS | 1 | Hypothermia vs Placebo | 2009 | No | 59 | 6h |
| Normobaric Oxygen Therapy | NCT00414726 | Mass General/ NINDS | 2 | Normobaric oxygen vs room air | 2009 | No | 85 | 9h |

(continued)

Table 10.2 Continued

| Study Name | Clinicaltrial.org Identifier | Sponsor | Treatment | Phase | Completed | Early Termination | Number of subjects | Enrollment Window |
|---|---|---|---|---|---|---|---|---|
| **TEST** | NCT00331721 | PAION Deustschland | Enecadin | 2 | 2009 | Yes (Invalid Study) | ? | 9h |
| **APCAST** | NCT00533546 | NHLBI | APC | 2(open label) | 2010 | Yes (Recruitment) | ? | 9h |
| **MINOS** | NCT00630396 | NINDS | Minocycline | 1/2 | 2010 | No | 60 | 6h |
| **TANDEM-1** | NCT00777140 | German Trials I Pujol Hospital | Desferal + tPA vs tPA | 2 | 2011 | No | 62 | 3h |
| **AXIS-2** | NCT00132470 | Cygnis Pharma Ag | GCSF vs Placebo | 2 | 2011 | No | 328 | 9h |
| **CASTA\*** | NCT00868283 | Ever Neuro Pharma GmbH | Cerebrolysin vs Placebo | 4 | 2011 | No | 1070 | 12h |
| **ENACT** | NCT00728182 | NoNO Inc. | NA-1 vs Placebo | 2 | 2011 | No | 185 | |
| **ALIAS** | NCT00235495 | U of Miami/NINDS | Albumin vs Placebo | 3 | 2012 | Yes (Recruitment) | 843 | 6h |
| **MACSI\*** | NCT00893867 | D-Pharma Ltd | Dp-99 vs Placebo | 3 | 2012 | Yes | 770 | 9h |
| **ICTUS** | NCT00331890 | Ferrer InterATIONAL | Citicholine vs Placebo | 3 | 2012 | Yes (Futility) | 2078 | 24h |
| **ICTuS 2/3** | NCT01123161 | UCSD/NINDS | Hypothermia vs Placebo | 2/3 | 2015 | Yes | 120 | 6h |
| **FAST-MAG** | NCT00059332 | UCLA/NINDS | MgSO4 vs Placebo (Prehospital) | 3 | 2015 | No | 1700 | 2h |
| **URICO-ICTUS** | NCT00860366 | Carlos III Health Institute | Uric Acid+tPA vs tPA | 3 | 205 | No | 421 | 4.5h |
| **FRONTIER** | NCT02315443 | NoNO Inc. | NA-1 vs Placebo (Prehospital) | 3 | Ongoing | No | 558 | 3h |

\* Studies that excluded patients if rtPA was used

resulting in less variability in response to treatment and necessitating smaller sample sizes. Imaging selection strategies beyond the plain, non–contrast-enhanced CT scan might be useful in selecting patients into studies evaluating AIS treatments, including recanalization therapies.

Four main approaches have been considered for selecting patients who would be amenable to brain salvage by a therapeutic intervention: (1) imaging the penumbra using magnetic resonance imaging (MRI DWI/PWI) mismatch or CT perfusion techniques, (2) imaging stroke volumes, (3) imaging the site of arterial occlusion, and (4) using an imaging-based scoring system as a surrogate for these approaches.

All penumbra imaging trials to date have focused on the relationship between the region of hypoperfused viable tissue, operationally defined by MR or CT, and response to reperfusion therapy. The intuitive rationale for penumbra imaging as a selection criterion for reperfusion studies is supported by the DEFUSE-2 trial, which provided evidence that patients exhibiting a larger perfusion defect than suggested by imaging of the ischemic core (mismatch) can benefit from intravenous thrombolysis, whereas those without mismatch do not.[91] This rationale has been further tested, albeit less successfully, in a number of reperfusion trials that selected patients based on penumbra imaging.[67,73–75,79]

The recent endovascular trials provide an important clue to a potentially useful approach to imaging selection of responders to intervention, including pharmacological neuroprotection. These trials all used imaging criteria for inclusion/exclusion and showed a clinical benefit of the intervention. These criteria therefore must identify patients who are most likely to exhibit an ischemic penumbra (the desired target of therapy) at the time of subject enrollment. Although the precise details of imaging differed between the trials, they all had a common approach for selecting subjects with a treatable LVO and, using direct or indirect means, the presence of sufficient collateral circulation to support a viable penumbra with reversible injury.[81–85] The simplest way of achieving this, in both clinical trials and clinical practice, is to image an LVO (typically of the MCA) on a CT angiogram while simultaneously demonstrating little or no early ischemic injury on a noncontrast CT using the Alberta Stroke Program Early CT Score (ASPECTS) score. More complex perfusion or collateral imaging adds significant technical challenges and delays due to image reconstruction, making trials using these methods more challenging compared to studies that employ only clinical criteria of CT angiogram alone. There continues to be controversy about the best approach for perfusion and collateral imaging, which makes the agreement among institutions that is required for large-scale multicenter trials difficult.

To date, all imaging strategies used in trials have been designed to select patients who would have the best response to reperfusion therapies (see Table 10.3) as opposed to neuroprotection. Nonetheless, the use of revascularization may enhance the therapeutic effect of neuroprotectants, and therefore imaging selection of responders to revascularization may also apply to neuroprotection studies.

## Current Guidelines

Current American Heart Association and American Stroke Association (AHA/ASA) 2013 guidelines recommend performing non–contrast-enhanced CT or MRI before intravenous rtPA administration to exclude intracerebral hemmorhage (ICH), which is an absolute contraindication (class I; level of evidence A).[23] The 2015 update of AHA/ASA Guidelines recommend a noninvasive intracranial

Table 10.3 Stroke Trials Using Imaging Strategies for Patient Selection

| Study Type | Study Name | Clinicaltrial.org Identifier | Sponsor | Treatment | Phase | Completed | Early Termination | Number of subjects | Enrollment Window |
|---|---|---|---|---|---|---|---|---|---|
| **Studies using stroke lesion size criteria for enrollment** | | | | | | | | | |
| Neuroprotection | AXIS-2 | NCT00132470 | Cygnis Pharma AG | GCSF vs Placebo | 2 | 2011 | No | 328 | 12h |
| Neuroprotection | Reponitan | NCT00044915 | Bayer | Repinotan vs Placebo | 3 | 2004 | No | 240 | 4.5h |
| Device | IMS-II | NCT00359424 | NINDS | tPA vs tPA-IA therapy | 3 | 2012 | Yes (Futility) | 587 | 3h |
| **Studies that measured infarct volume on enrollment** | | | | | | | | | |
| Neuroprotection | ESS | NCT00604630 | J&J/Parexel | EPO vs Placebo | 3 | 2008 | No | 522 | 6h |
| Neuroprotection | ARTIST-MRI | NCT00044070 | Astellas Pharma | YM872 vs Placebo | 2 | 2003 | Yes (Futility) | ? | 6h |
| Thrombolytic | EPITHET | NCT00238537 | Melbourne Health | tPA vs Placebo | 2 | 2007 | No | 101 | >3h |
| **Studies that confirmed symptomatic intracranial occlusion on enrollment by CTA or MRA** | | | | | | | | | |
| Thrombolytic/ Device | ESCAPE | NCT01778335 | University of Calgary | Endovascular Thrombectomy/ Thrombolysis vs tPA alone | 3 | 2014 | Yes (Efficacy) | 316 | 12h |
| Thrombolytic/ Device | EXTEND-IA | NCT01492725 | Neuroscience Trials Australia | Solitaire device/tPA vs tPA alone | 2 | 2014 | Yes (Efficacy) | 70 | 4.5h |
| Thrombolytic/ Device | SWIFT PRIME | NCT01657461 | Medtronic - MITG | Solitaire FR device/ tPA vs tPA alone | 3 | 2015 | Yes (Efficacy) | 196 | 6h |
| Thrombolytic/ Device | REVASCAT | NCT01692379 | Fundacio Ictus Malaltia Vascular | Solitaire FR device/ tPA vs tPA alone | 3 | 2015 | Yes (Efficacy) | 206 | 8h |

vascular study (CT angiography, CT perfusion imaging) during the initial imaging evaluation if either intra-arterial fibrinolysis or mechanical thrombectomy is contemplated, provided that this imaging does not delay intravenous rtPA if indicated (class I, level of evidence A).[92]

With respect to physiological interventions for patients with AIS, the 2013 AHA/ASA Guidelines recommend that, in patients who are eligible for treatment with intravenous rtPA and have elevated blood pressure, blood pressure should be carefully lowered to a systolic blood pressure of less than 185 mm Hg and a diastolic blood pressure of less than 110 mm Hg before fibrinolytic therapy is initiated (class I; level of evidence B).[23] Oxygen saturation should be maintained at greater than 94% by providing supplemental oxygen (class I; level of evidence C).[23] Patients presenting with hyperthermia (temperature >38°C) should undergo an examination to identify and treat the source(s) of hyperthermia and should be treated with antipyretic medications (class I; level of evidence C).[23]

Recommendations on intravenous rtPA administration are unchanged from the 2013 Guidelines. Intravenous rtPA must be administered to all eligible patients as quickly as possible (door-to-needle time should be less than 60 minutes) within the 0- to 3-hour window (class I, level of evidence A), or within the 3- to 4.5-hour window (class I, level of evidence B), even if considering other adjunctive therapies (class I, level of evidence A).[23] With regard to oral administration of antiplatelet agents, the 2013 guidelines recommend oral administration of aspirin (initial dose is 325 mg) within 24–48 hours after stroke onset for most patients to reduce the risk of stroke recurrence (class I; level of evidence A).[23]

In the 2015 update of AHA/ASA Guidelines for the early management of AIS, a new class I, level of evidence A recommendation is that patients should receive endovascular therapy with a stent retriever if they meet all the following criteria: (a) pre-stroke mRS score of 0–1, (b) acute ischemic stroke receiving intravenous rtPA within 4.5 hours of onset according to guidelines from professional medical societies, (c) causative occlusion of the internal carotid artery or proximal MCA (M1), (d) age 18 years or older, (e) National Institutes of Health Stroke Scale (NIHSS) score of 6 or higher, (f) ASPECTS of 6 or more, and (g) treatment can be initiated (groin puncture) within 6 hours of symptom onset.[92]

The 2013 AHA/ASA guideline recommended the use of specialized stroke care (i.e., stroke units) that incorporates rehabilitation and intense monitoring of AIS patients (class I; level of evidence A).[23]

## FUTURE DIRECTIONS

The main objective of stroke care is a rapid intervention after the onset of the stroke. Greater importance should therefore be placed on public health programs that improve prehospital care and optimize delivery of reperfusion therapies to patients.

Clinical trials to evaluate the best approach to stroke care and neuroprotection are ongoing. Previous clinical trial designs have focused on methodologies for implementing various recanalization therapies, including the development of sophisticated imaging technologies for patient selection. To date, however, it is unclear whether trial strategies developed to evaluate various recanalization strategies also apply to neuroprotectant agents. Nonetheless, the ability of reperfusion studies to select patients with salvageable brain tissue teaches that intervention, either through reperfusion or neuroprotection, is possible. Rigorous trial design, implementation, and outcome assessment will be needed to evaluate new therapeutic options in the future.

Neuroprotectants should be evaluated as early as possible after stroke onset, ideally in the first "golden hour," when every stroke victim still has brain tissue to salvage. Pharmacological neuroprotectants may be best suited for use as adjuvants to reperfusion therapies, extending the window during which repefusion may be of benefit and improving clinical outcomes.

## REFERENCES

1. Mozaffarian D, Benjamin EJ, Go AS, et al; American Heart Association Statistics Committee; Stroke Statistics Subcommittee. Heart disease and stroke statistics—2016 update: a report from the American Heart Association. *Circulation.* 2016; 133(4):e38–e360.

2. Feigin VL, Forouzanfar MH, Krishnamurthi R, et al. Global and regional burden of stroke during 1990–2010: findings from the Global Burden of Disease Study 2010. *Lancet (London, England).* 2014;383(9913):245–54.

3. van der Worp HB, van Gijn J. Clinical practice. Acute ischemic stroke. *N Engl J Med.* 2007;357(6):572–9.

4. Khaja AM. Acute ischemic stroke management: administration of thrombolytics, neuroprotectants, and general principles of medical management. *Neurol Clin.* 2008;26(4):943–61, viii.

5. Jovin TG, Demchuk AM, Gupta R. Pathophysiology of acute ischemic stroke. *Continuum.* 2008;14:28–45.

6. A classification and outline of cerebrovascular diseases. II. *Stroke.* 1975;6(5):564–616.

7. Musuka T, Wilton S, Traboulsi M, Hill M. Diagnosis and management of acute ischemic stroke: speed is critical. *CMAJ.* 2015;187(12):887–93.

8. Arboix A. Cardiovascular risk factors for acute stroke: risk profiles in the different subtypes of ischemic stroke. *W J Clin Cases.* 2015;3(5):418–29.

9. Doyle KP, Simon RP, Stenzel-Poore MP. Mechanisms of ischemic brain damage. *Neuropharmacology.* 2008;55(3):310–8.

10. Dirnagl U, Iadecola C, Moskowitz MA. Pathobiology of ischaemic stroke: an integrated view. *Trends Neurosci.* 1999;22(9):391–7.

11. Liu S, Levine SR, Winn HR. Targeting ischemic penumbra: part I—from pathophysiology to therapeutic strategy. *J Exper Stroke Translational Med.* 2010;3(1):47–55.

12. Donnan GA, Davis SM. Neuroimaging, the ischaemic penumbra, and selection of patients for acute stroke therapy. *Lancet Neurol.* 2002;1(7):417–25.

13. Woodruff TM, Thundyil J, Tang S-C, Sobey CG, Taylor SM, Arumugam TV. Pathophysiology, treatment, and animal and cellular models of human ischemic stroke. *Mol Neurodegeneration.* 2011;6(1):11.

14. Budd SL. Mechanisms of neuronal damage in brain hypoxia/ischemia: focus on the role of mitochondrial calcium accumulation. *Pharmacol Therapeutics.* 1998;80(2):203–29.

15. Arundine M, Tymianski M. Molecular mechanisms of glutamate-dependent neurodegeneration in ischemia and traumatic brain injury. *Cell Mol Life Sci.* 2004;61(6):657–68.

16. Barber PA, Demchuk AM, Hirt L, Buchan AM. Biochemistry of ischemic stroke. *Adv Neurol.* 2003;92:151–64.

17. Clark RK, Lee EV, Fish CJ, et al. Development of tissue damage, inflammation and resolution following stroke: an immunohistochemical and quantitative planimetric study. *Brain Res Bull.* 1993;31(5):565–72.

18. Dugan LL, Choi DW. Excitotoxicity, free radicals, and cell membrane changes. *Ann Neurol.* 1994;35 Suppl:S17–21.

19. Saver JL. Time is brain--quantified. *Stroke*. 2006;37(1):263–6.

20. Prabhakaran S, Ruff I, Bernstein R. Acute stroke intervention- A systematic review. *JAMA*. 2015;313(14):1451.

21. Astrup J, Siesjö BK, Symon L. Thresholds in cerebral ischemia—the ischemic penumbra. *Stroke*. 12(6):723–5.

22. Balami JS, Hadley G, Sutherland B, Karbalai H, Buchan AM. The exact science of stroke thrombolysis and the quiet art of patient selection. *Brain*. 2013;136(Pt 12):3528–53.

23. Jauch EC, Saver JL, Adams HP, et al.; American Heart Association Stroke Council; Council on Cardiovascular Nursing; Council on Peripheral Vascular Disease; Council on Clinical Cardiology. Guidelines for the early management of patients with acute ischemic stroke: a guideline for healthcare professionals from the American Heart Association/American Stroke Association. *Stroke*. 2013;44(3):870–947.

24. Brown RD, Whisnant JP, Sicks JD, O'Fallon WM, Wiebers DO. Stroke incidence, prevalence, and survival: secular trends in Rochester, Minnesota, through 1989. *Stroke*. 1996;27(3):373–80.

25. Wolf PA, D'Agostino RB, O'Neal MA, et al. Secular trends in stroke incidence and mortality. The Framingham Study. *Stroke*. 1992;23(11):1551–5.

26. Kiely DK, Wolf PA, Cupples LA, Beiser AS, Myers RH. Familial aggregation of stroke. The Framingham Study. *Stroke*. 1993;24(9):1366–71.

27. Howard G, Anderson R, Sorlie P, Andrews V, Backlund E, Burke GL. Ethnic differences in stroke mortality between non-Hispanic whites, Hispanic whites, and blacks. The National Longitudinal Mortality Study. *Stroke*. 1994;25(11):2120–5.

28. Whisnant JP. Effectiveness versus efficacy of treatment of hypertension for stroke prevention. *Neurology*. 1996;46(2):301–7.

29. Prevention of stroke by antihypertensive drug treatment in older persons with isolated systolic hypertension. Final results of the Systolic Hypertension in the Elderly Program (SHEP). SHEP Cooperative Research Group. *JAMA*. 1991;265(24):3255–64.

30. Benjamin EJ, Levy D, Vaziri SM, D'Agostino RB, Belanger AJ, Wolf PA. Independent risk factors for atrial fibrillation in a population-based cohort. The Framingham Heart Study. *JAMA*. 1994;271(11):840–4.

31. Feinberg WM, Blackshear JL, Laupacis A, Kronmal R, Hart RG. Prevalence, age distribution, and gender of patients with atrial fibrillation. Analysis and implications. *Arch Intern Med*. 1995;155(5):469–73.

32. Wolf PA, Abbott RD, Kannel WB. Atrial fibrillation as an independent risk factor for stroke: the Framingham Study. *Stroke*. 1991;22(8):983–8.

33. Bikkina M, Levy D, Evans JC, et al. Left ventricular mass and risk of stroke in an elderly cohort. The Framingham Heart Study. *JAMA*. 1994;272(1):33–6.

34. Burchfiel CM, Curb JD, Rodriguez BL, Abbott RD, Chiu D, Yano K. Glucose intolerance and 22-year stroke incidence. The Honolulu Heart Program. *Stroke*. 1994;25(5):951–7.

35. Shinozaki K, Naritomi H, Shimizu T, et al. Role of insulin resistance associated with compensatory hyperinsulinemia in ischemic stroke. *Stroke*. 1996;27(1):37–43.

36. Shinton R, Beevers G. Meta-analysis of relation between cigarette smoking and stroke. *BMJ*. 1989;298(6676):789–94.

37. Wolf PA, D'Agostino RB, Kannel WB, Bonita R, Belanger AJ. Cigarette smoking as a risk factor for stroke. The Framingham Study. *JAMA*. 1988;259(7):1025–9.

38. Kawachi I, Colditz GA, Stampfer MJ, et al. Smoking cessation and decreased risk of stroke in women. *JAMA*. 1993;269(2):232–6.

39. Stroke Unit Trialists' Collaboration. Organised inpatient (stroke unit) care for stroke. *Cochrane Database Syst Rev*. 2013;(9):CD000197.

40. Cavallini A, Micieli G, Marcheselli S, Quaglini S. Role of monitoring in management of acute ischemic stroke patients. *Stroke.* 2003;34(11):2599–603.

41. Menon BK, Campbell BC V, Levi C, Goyal M. Role of imaging in current acute ischemic stroke workflow for endovascular therapy. *Stroke.* 2015;46(6):1453–61.

42. Sulter G, Elting JW, Langedijk M, Maurits NM, De Keyser J. Admitting acute ischemic stroke patients to a stroke care monitoring unit versus a conventional stroke unit: a randomized pilot study. *Stroke.* 2003;34(1):101–4.

43. Qureshi AI, Ezzeddine MA, Nasar A, et al. Prevalence of elevated blood pressure in 563,704 adult patients with stroke presenting to the ED in the United States. *Am J Emerg Med.* 2007;25(1):32–8.

44. Adams HP. Management of patients with acute ischaemic stroke. *Drugs.* 1997;54 Suppl 3:60–9; discussion 69–70.

45. Kaste M, Fogelholm R, Erilä T, et al. A randomized, double-blind, placebo-controlled trial of nimodipine in acute ischemic hemispheric stroke. *Stroke.* 1994;25(7):1348–53.

46. Schrader J, Lüders S, Kulschewski A, et al.; Acute Candesartan Cilexetil Therapy in Stroke Survivors Study Group. The ACCESS Study: evaluation of Acute Candesartan Cilexetil Therapy in Stroke Survivors. *Stroke.* 2003;34(7):1699–703.

47. Sandset EC, Bath PMW, Boysen G, et al.; SCAST Study Group. The angiotensin-receptor blocker candesartan for treatment of acute stroke (SCAST): a randomised, placebo-controlled, double-blind trial. *Lancet.* 2011;377(9767):741–50.

48. Gentile NT, Seftchick MW, Huynh T, Kruus LK, Gaughan J. Decreased mortality by normalizing blood glucose after acute ischemic stroke. *Acad Emerg Med.* 2006;13(2):174–80.

49. Williams LS, Rotich J, Qi R, et al. Effects of admission hyperglycemia on mortality and costs in acute ischemic stroke. *Neurology.* 2002;59(1):67–71.

50. Gray CS, Hildreth AJ, Sandercock PA, et al.; GIST Trialists Collaboration. Glucose-potassium-insulin infusions in the management of post-stroke hyperglycaemia: the UK Glucose Insulin in Stroke Trial (GIST-UK). *Lancet Neurol.* 2007;6(5):397–406.

51. Connor JT, Broglio KR, Durkalski V, Meurer WJ, Johnston KC. The Stroke Hyperglycemia Insulin Network Effort (SHINE) trial: an adaptive trial design case study. *Trials.* 2015;16:72.

52. Bellolio MF, Gilmore RM, Ganti L. Insulin for glycaemic control in acute ischaemic stroke. *Cochrane Database Syst Rev.* 2014;(1):CD005346.

53. Grotta J, Pasteur W, Khwaja G, Hamel T, Fisher M, Ramirez A. Elective intubation for neurologic deterioration after stroke. *Neurology.* 1995;45(4):640–4.

54. Bansal S, Sangha KS, Khatri P. Drug treatment of acute ischemic stroke. *Am J Cardiovasc Drugs.* 2013;13(1):57–69.

55. Azzimondi G, Bassein L, Nonino F, et al. Fever in acute stroke worsens prognosis. A prospective study. *Stroke.* 1995;26(11):2040–3.

56. Castillo J, Dávalos A, Marrugat J, Noya M. Timing for fever-related brain damage in acute ischemic stroke. *Stroke.* 1998;29(12):2455–60.

57. Prasad K, Krishnan PR. Fever is associated with doubling of odds of short-term mortality in ischemic stroke: an updated meta-analysis. *Acta Neurologica Scand.* 2010;122(6):404–8.

58. Dippel DW, van Breda EJ, van Gemert HM, et al. Effect of paracetamol (acetaminophen) on body temperature in acute ischemic stroke: a double-blind, randomized phase II clinical trial. *Stroke.* 2001;32(7):1607–12.

59. Dippel DWJ, van Breda EJ, van der Worp HB, et al.; PISA-Investigators. Effect of paracetamol (acetaminophen) and ibuprofen on body temperature in acute ischemic stroke PISA,

a phase II double-blind, randomized, placebo-controlled trial [ISRCTN98608690]. *BMC Cardiovascr Dis.* 2003;3:2.

60. De Georgia, MA, Krieger DW, Abou-Chebl A, et al. Cooling for Acute Ischemic Brain Damage (COOL AID): a feasibility trial of endovascular cooling. *Neurology,* 2004;63(2):312–7.

61. Hemmen TM, Raman R, Guluma KZ, et al. Intravenous thrombolysis plus hypothermia for acute treatment of ischemic stroke (ICTuS-L): final results. *Stroke,* 2010;41(10):2265–70.

62. Group TNI of ND and S rt-PSS. Tissue plasminogen activator for acute ischemic stroke. The National Institute of Neurological Disorders and Stroke rt-PA Stroke Study Group. *N Engl J Med.* 1995;333(24):1581–7.

63. Rha J-H, Saver JL. The impact of recanalization on ischemic stroke outcome: A meta-analysis. *Stroke.* 2007;38(3):967–73.

64. Hacke W, Kaste M, Bluhmki E, et al. Thrombolysis with alteplase 3 to 4.5 hours after acute ischemic stroke. *N Engl J Med.* 2008;359(13):1317–29.

65. Hacke W, Donnan G, Fieschi C, et al.; ATLANTIS Trials Investigators; ECASS Trials Investigators; NINDS rt-PA Study Group Investigators. Association of outcome with early stroke treatment: pooled analysis of ATLANTIS, ECASS, and NINDS rt-PA stroke trials. *Lancet.* 2004;363(9411):768–74.

66. Seitz RJ, Oberstrass H, Ringelstein A, Wittsack H-J, Siebler M. Failed recovery from thrombolysis is predicted by the initial diffusion weighted imaging lesion. *Cerebrovasc Dis.* 2011;31(6):580–7.

67. De Silva DA, Brekenfeld C, Ebinger M, et al.; Echoplanar Imaging Thrombolytic Evaluation Trial (EPITHET) Investigators. The benefits of intravenous thrombolysis relate to the site of baseline arterial occlusion in the Echoplanar Imaging Thrombolytic Evaluation Trial (EPITHET). *Stroke.* 2010;41(2):295–9.

68. Barber PA, Zhang J, Demchuk AM, Hill MD, Buchan AM. Why are stroke patients excluded from TPA therapy? An analysis of patient eligibility. *Neurology.* 2001;56(8):1015–20.

69. Kleindorfer D, Kissela B, Schneider A, et al. Eligibility for recombinant tissue plasminogen activator in acute ischemic stroke: a population-based study. *Stroke.* 2004;35(2):e27–9.

70. Adeoye O, Hornung R, Khatri P, Kleindorfer D. Recombinant tissue-type plasminogen activator use for ischemic stroke in the United States: a doubling of treatment rates over the course of 5 years. *Stroke.* 2011;42(7):1952–5.

71. George MG, Tong X, McGruder H, et al. Paul Coverdell National Acute Stroke Registry Surveillance—four states, 2005–2007. *MMWR Surveill Summ.* 2009;58(7):1–23.

72. Fonarow GC, Smith EE, Saver JL, et al. Timeliness of tissue-type plasminogen activator therapy in acute ischemic stroke: patient characteristics, hospital factors, and outcomes associated with door-to-needle times within 60 minutes. *Circulation.* 2011;123(7):750–8.

73. Hacke W, Albers G, Al-Rawi Y, et al.; DIAS Study Group. The Desmoteplase in Acute Ischemic Stroke Trial (DIAS): a phase II MRI-based 9-hour window acute stroke thrombolysis trial with intravenous desmoteplase. *Stroke.* 2005;36(1):66–73.

74. Furlan AJ, Eyding D, Albers GW, et al.; DEDAS Investigators. Dose Escalation of Desmoteplase for Acute Ischemic Stroke (DEDAS): evidence of safety and efficacy 3 to 9 hours after stroke onset. *Stroke.* 2006;37(5):1227–31.

75. Hacke W, Furlan AJ, Al-Rawi Y, et al. Intravenous desmoteplase in patients with acute ischaemic stroke selected by MRI perfusion-diffusion weighted imaging or perfusion

CT (DIAS-2): a prospective, randomised, double-blind, placebo-controlled study. *Lancet Neurol.* 2009;8(2):141–50.

76. Davis SM, Donnan GA, Parsons MW, et al. Effects of alteplase beyond 3 h after stroke in the Echoplanar Imaging Thrombolytic Evaluation Trial (EPITHET): a placebo-controlled randomised trial. *Lancet Neurol.* 2008;7(4):299–309.

77. Mishra NK, Albers GW, Davis SM, et al. Mismatch-based delayed thrombolysis: a meta-analysis. *Stroke.* 2010;41(1):e25–33.

78. Davis SM, Donnan GA. MR mismatch and thrombolysis: appealing but validation required. *Stroke.* 2009;40(8):2910.

79. Parsons M, Spratt N, Bivard A, et al. A randomized trial of tenecteplase versus alteplase for acute ischemic stroke. *N Engl J Med.* 2012;366(12):1099–107.

80. Albers GW, von Kummer R, Truelsen T, et al.; DIAS-3 Investigators. Safety and efficacy of desmoteplase given 3–9 h after ischaemic stroke in patients with occlusion or high-grade stenosis in major cerebral arteries (DIAS-3): a double-blind, randomised, placebo-controlled phase 3 trial. *Lancet Neurol.* 2015;14(6):575–84.

81. Campbell BCV, Mitchell PJ, Kleinig TJ, et al. Endovascular therapy for ischemic stroke with perfusion-imaging selection. *N Engl J Med.* 2015;372(11):1009–18.

82. Berkhemer OA., Fransen PSS, Beumer D, et al. A randomized trial of intraarterial treatment for acute ischemic stroke. *N Engl J Med.* 2015;372(1):11–20.

83. Saver JL, Goyal M, Bonafe A, et al.; SWIFT PRIME Investigators. Stent-retriever thrombectomy after intravenous t-PA vs. t-PA alone in stroke. *N Engl J Med.* 2015;372(24):2285–96.

84. Goyal M, Demchuk AM, Menon BK, et al.; ESCAPE Trial Investigators. Randomized assessment of rapid endovascular treatment of ischemic stroke. *N Engl J Med.* 2015;372(11):1019–30.

85. Molina CA, Chamorro A, Rovira À, et al. REVASCAT: a randomized trial of revascularization with SOLITAIRE FR device vs. best medical therapy in the treatment of acute stroke due to anterior circulation large vessel occlusion presenting within eight-hours of symptom onset. *Int J Stroke.* 2015;10(4):619–26.

86. Dávalos A, Alvarez-Sabín J, Castillo J, et al.; International Citicoline Trial on acUte Stroke (ICTUS) trial investigators. Citicoline in the treatment of acute ischaemic stroke: an international, randomised, multicentre, placebo-controlled study (ICTUS trial). *Lancet.* 2012;380(9839):349–57.

87. Ringelstein EB, Thijs V, Norrving B, et al.; AXIS 2 Investigators. Granulocyte colony-stimulating factor in patients with acute ischemic stroke: results of the AX200 for Ischemic Stroke trial. *Stroke.* 2013;44(10):2681–7.

88. Shuaib A, Lees KR, Lyden P, et al.; SAINT II Trial Investigators. NXY-059 for the treatment of acute ischemic stroke. *N Engl J Med.* 2007;357(6):562–71.

89. Ehrenreich H, Weissenborn K, Prange H, et al. Recombinant human erythropoietin in the treatment of acute ischemic stroke. *Stroke.* 2009;40(12):e647–56.

90. Saver JL, Starkman S, Eckstein M, et al. Prehospital use of magnesium sulfate as neuroprotection in acute stroke. *N Engl J Med.* 2015;372(6):528–36.

91. Albers GW, Thijs VN, Wechsler L, et al. Magnetic resonance imaging profiles predict clinical response to early reperfusion: the diffusion and perfusion imaging evaluation for understanding stroke evolution (DEFUSE) study. *Ann Neurol.* 2006;60(5):508–17.

92. Powers WJ, Derdeyn CP, Biller J, et al.; American Heart Association Stroke Council. 2015 AHA/ASA Focused Update of the 2013 guidelines for the early management of patients with acute ischemic stroke regarding endovascular treatment. *Stroke.* 2015;46(10):3020–35.

# 11 Neuroprotection for Intracerebral Hemorrhage

Julius Griauzde, Neeraj Chaudhary,

Joseph J. Gemmete, Aditya S. Pandey,

and Guohua Xi

## GENERAL CONSIDERATIONS

Intracerebral hemorrhage (ICH) is a devastating condition which accounts for 10–15% of acute strokes.[1] Forty percent of patients with ICH die within 30 days, and only 38% survive at 1 year after ictus.[1] The pathophysiology of neurological injury in ICH is complex and heterogeneous. The mechanisms involved remain incompletely understood, and neuroprotective strategies are largely unproved. Our understanding of the most effective neuroprotective management strategy is expanding and many novel approaches are currently under investigation.

## MECHANISMS OF AND RISKS FOR NEUROLOGICAL INJURY
### Primary Mechanisms of Injury

ICH is the result of rupture of chronically damaged or weakened blood vessels. Following vessel rupture, extravasated blood products spread into the adjacent brain parenchyma. Early neurological injury in the setting of ICH begins as a result of the mass effect of the hematoma. This results in increased surrounding tissue pressure and distorts both macroscopic and cellular architecture.[2] Surrounding cerebral vessels are often distorted as well, resulting in hypoperfusion of the tissue immediately surrounding the hematoma.[3] Furthermore, mass effect on the ventricular outflow as well as intraventricular extension of blood products significantly alters cerebrospinal fluid (CSF) flow dynamics resulting in hydrocephalus, which further elevates intracranial pressure (ICP) and worsens the neurological injury.[4]

## Secondary Mechanisms of Injury

### Inflammation

Following the initial phase of injury, presence of an intracerebral hematoma results in a profound inflammatory response that begins a cascade of multiple pathologic pathways. One of the initial inciting events in secondary neurological injury is the release of thrombin for hemostasis. Thrombin promotes blood–brain barrier (BBB) disruption, edema formation, and inflammatory cell activation.[5] Thrombin also triggers apoptotic cascades in neuronal cells, leading to cell death.[6]

The inflammatory milieu of the ICH activates leucocytes and matrix metalloproteinases, which disrupt the BBB and further potentiate inflammatory cell infiltration and edema formation.[7] Several types of inflammatory cells have been identified as pathologic actors in the response to ICH including neutrophils, lymphocytes, and mast cells, as well as the complement system.[8–9] Central nervous system (CNS) support cells such as microglia and astrocytes also have been shown to potentiate the inflammatory response to ICH.[10–11] The inflammatory cells, CNS support cells, and complement system break down the hemorrhagic components of the ICH, resulting in release of hemoglobin, iron, and oxidized free radicals that cause further compound neuronal damage and trigger apoptotic cascades.[12–13]

### Excitotoxicity and Neuronal Death

Excitotoxicity has been extensively studied in ischemic stroke. Although its role in ICH is not fully defined, it is believed to have several congruent mechanisms to ischemic neurological injury. In ischemic stroke models, excitotoxicity occurs as a result of rapid release of glutamate in ischemic brain parenchyma.[14] Glutamate neurotoxicity has also been implicated in neuronal cell death following ICH as a result of elevated glutamate concentration.[15] Additionally, thrombin that is released soon after ICH has been shown to upregulate excitatory N-methyl-D-aspartate (NMDA) receptors, increasing their functionality and response to excitatory neurotransmitters.[15] Increased glutamate release and response alters neuronal calcium homeostasis, which can trigger apoptotic cascades and act as a contributor to direct neuronal death.[16] In several models of ICH, elevated levels of pro-apoptotic factors, including nuclear factor κ-light-chain-enhancer of activated B cells (NF-κB), Fas and, caspases have been demonstrated.[17–18]

### Red Blood Cell Lysis, Hemoglobin, and Brain Iron Overload

Extravasated blood in ICH undergoes degradation, which leads to red blood cell (RBC) lysis and release of free hemoglobin and other breakdown products. RBCs increase cerebral edema, and the products of their lysis cause oxidative stress and brain injury. Further catabolism leads to the release of hemoglobin and its breakdown products, including iron. The presence of these compounds in ICH has been shown to increase cerebral edema, worsen hydrocephalus, and promote brain tissue loss.[19] Brain iron overload is a significant contributor to neuronal injury because iron potentiates oxidative stress, causes DNA damage, and worsens hydrocephalus.[20]

## Risks for Neurological Injury

The most commonly cited risk factors for ICH include hypertension, advanced age, cerebral amyloid angiopathy, alcohol abuse, and male sex.[1] Hypertension and cerebral amyloid angiopathy together account for about 90% of primary intracranial hemorrhage.[1] Less common risk factors for ICH include primary or metastatic intracranial neoplasms, arterial venous malformations, and cerebrovascular aneurysms.[1] Pharmacologic agents associated with increased risk of ICH include anticoagulants, antiplatelet agents, and substances of abuse (typically cocaine and amphetamines).[21]

# MONITORING FOR NEUROLOGICAL INJURY
## Monitoring for Acute Injury

Both clinical and imaging factors can be used to measure the extent of acute neurological injury and to prognosticate outcomes in patients with ICH. The Glasgow Coma Scale (GCS) score is the strongest outcome predictor in patients with ICH.[22] Additional clinical factors associated with worse outcome include prior anticoagulant or antiplatelet use, prior ischemic stroke, increased age, elevated admission blood glucose, limb paresis, and communication disorders.[22]

Noncontrast computed tomography (NCCT) of the head is the primary modality for evaluating the extent of acute injury in ICH. The volume of ICH is a powerful predictor of 30-day morbidity and mortality in ICH patients.[23] ICH hematoma volume is typically measured using the ABC/2 method.[24] Volumes greater than 30 cubic centimeters (cc) are associated with significantly worse outcomes.[22] Hematoma expansion within the first 24 hours is seen in up to 38% of ICH patients and is associated with a significantly higher risk of poor outcomes and mortality.[25–26] Intraventricular extension of ICH, infratentorial location, and hydrocephalus are also associated with poor outcomes.[22,27] The "ICH score" is a validated and widely accepted method for stratifying ICH patients. It is composed of both clinical and imaging factors including GCS, ICH volume (greater or less than 30 cc), intraventricular extension, infratentorial location, and patient age (greater or less than 80 years).[22]

CT angiography (CTA) is an important adjunct to NCCT in risk stratification of patients with ICH. The CTA "spot sign," a high attenuation focus within an ICH that represents active extravasation, is an imaging predictor of worse outcome, mortality, and hematoma progression.[28–30] CTA also is helpful in the identification of underlying vascular lesions in ICH patients.[21]

## Monitoring for Secondary Injury

Secondary neurological injury following ICH is a preventable cause of significant morbidity and mortality. Secondary injury following ICH can result from hematoma expansion, hydrocephalus, elevated intracranial pressure, electrolyte and metabolic disturbances, and seizure activity. Monitoring for possible causes of secondary injury is therefore of great clinical importance. First and foremost, clinical neurological exams should be performed at frequent, regular intervals. Any change in the neurological exam results warrants emergent investigation. Imaging, laboratory investigations, ICP monitoring, and electroencephalograms (EEGs) should be performed rapidly to identify and correct any abnormalities and avert any significant secondary neurological injury.

## Imaging

NCCT, CTA, and magnetic resonance imaging (MRI) of the head are vital to the workup of ICH patients with neurological changes. Concerning NCCT findings include intraventricular extension of hemorrhage, development or worsening of hydrocephalus, worsening mass effect on normal parenchyma, and finally, parenchymal herniation. In the case of a suspected underlying lesions or secondary ischemic changes, CTA and MRI can be employed following NCCT.

## Laboratory Investigations

Following an acute change in neurological status, blood gas analysis, coagulation assay, and metabolic panel can be evaluated. Blood gas analysis can be used to identify the need for intubation or a change in ventilator settings. A coagulation panel is helpful in evaluating progress of anticoagulant reversal, which is of particular importance in patients with an expanding hematoma. Metabolic and electrolyte panels help identify correctable abnormalities, such as hyponatremia and hyperglycemia. Hyponatremia occurs in up to 50% of neurosurgical patients and can lead to cerebral edema, mental status changes, seizures, and even death.[31] Hyperglycemia also is very prevalent in neurological injury patients and has been correlated with an increased risk of cerebral and infectious complications.[32]

## ICP Monitoring

ICH patients are often sedated or have depressed mental status. Therefore, clinical monitoring for changes in neurological exam due to worsening ICP elevation can be quite challenging. Direct ICP monitoring allows for rapid identification of acute changes in patient status and helps warn caretakers of worsening neurological injury in a timely fashion.

## Electroencephalography

Continuous EEG monitoring should be considered in ICH patients with decreased mental status because seizures, which are often a sign of new insult or worsening neurological injury, can be clinically occult in these cases. Additionally, patients with a history of a seizure disorder or presenting symptoms of seizure should be monitored.

## NEUROPROTECTION STRATEGIES
### Physiologic Interventions

Several physiologic interventions have been suggested for neuroprotection in acute neurological injury. These include airway management, ICP monitoring, management of electrolyte and metabolic abnormalities, infection prophylaxis and control, incentive spirometry, sequential compression devices, early ambulation, and nutritional support. None of these is unique to ICH patients and all are centered on providing high-quality intensive care. Admission to a neurological intensive care unit (NICU) or stroke unit allows for continuous monitoring of ICH patients by highly trained observers. In large cohort studies, ICH patients admitted to a NICU or stroke unit have significantly lower rates of mortality and institutional living at 90 days, when compared to patients who were admitted to general intensive care units.[33–34]

## Pharmacologic Interventions

### Coagulation

**Cohort Studies** Anticoagulant therapy is associated with a significantly increased risk of ICH (up to 10 times higher than in patients not on anticoagulation).[35] Warfarin-related ICH is associated with larger hemorrhage volume at onset and double the mortality rate of non–warfarin associated ICH.[36] An international normalized ratio (INR) greater than 2.0 within 24 hours of ICH predisposes to hematoma enlargement, and higher levels of INR are strongly correlated with increased risk of mortality in ICH patients.[37–38] Patients taking heparin and patients with poor platelet function or thrombocytopenia also are at increased risk of major bleeding.[39–40] Reversal of anticoagulation within 4 hours of ICH is associated with lower rates of hematoma enlargement.[41]

Reversal of warfarin and other vitamin K antagonists can be achieved with oral or intravenous vitamin K, fresh frozen plasma, or prothrombin complex concentrates (PCC).[42–43] Reversal with PCC is much faster than both vitamin K and fresh frozen plasma.[43–44] Early platelet transfusion in patients with poor platelet function or on antiplatelet therapy is associated with smaller final hemorrhage size and improved independence at 3 months.[45] Platelet transfusions have also been suggested as a remedy for antiplatelet agents, although efficacy has been disputed by some authors.[40] Unfractionated heparin can be rapidly reversed with protamine, and low-molecular-weight heparin compounds can be reversed by recombinant activated factor VII (rFVIIa).[46–47] Newer anticoagulant agents such as dabigatran (a direct thrombin inhibitor) present a more complex dilemma because there are currently no effective reversal agents, although dialysis has been presented as a potential therapy.[48]

**Pilot Studies** Intravenous desmopressin acetate improves platelet activity after acute ICH and it is well-tolerated.[49] Further studies are needed to evaluate the actual effect on ICH.

**Randomized Control Trials** A randomized control trial (RCT) comparing the safety and preliminary efficacy of fresh frozen plasma and PCC in normalizing INR in Coumadin-associated ICH was terminated and is under official review, but no results have been reported.[50] The investigators of the Platelet Transfusion in Cerebral Hemorrhage (PATCH) trial recently found that ICH patients on antiplatelet therapy who received platelet transfusions had greater odds of death or dependence than those patients who received the standard of care.[51] The Recombinant Activated Factor VII (rFVIIA) for Acute Intracerebral Hemorrhage trial evaluated the effect of hemostatic therapy with rFVIIa on ICH patients. This trial showed that treatment within 4 hours of ICH onset limits the growth of the hematoma, reduces mortality, and improves functional outcomes.[52] Unfortunately, the follow-up Efficacy and Safety of Recombinant Activated Factor VII for Acute Intracerebral Hemorrhage (FAST) trial showed no significant improvement in survival or functional outcomes despite reduced hematoma growth.[53]

## Blood Pressure Control

**Cohort Studies** Retrospective studies have identified inadequate blood pressure control as a poor prognostic indicator in ICH patients.[54] Other studies have correlated increased mean blood pressure with greater risk of mortality in putaminal and thalamic hemorrhages.[55] In a large cohort study, Kuramatsu et al. demonstrated that a systolic blood pressure (SBP) of less than 160 mm Hg was associated with a lower rate of hematoma enlargement.[41] This finding, however, was not borne out in an exploratory analysis of the FAST trial.[56]

**Randomized Control Trials** The Antihypertensive Treatment in Acute Cerebral Hemorrhage (ATACH) trial showed no adverse events and no significant effect on neurological outcome with aggressive blood pressure management using an SBP goal of less than 140 mm Hg.[57] The Intracerebral Hemorrhage Acutely Decreasing Arterial Pressure Trial (ICH ADAPT) further confirmed the safety of intensive blood pressure management in ICH by demonstrating that rapid blood pressure lowering does not reduce peri-hematomal cerebral blood flow and therefore does not cause cerebral ischemia.[58] In the Intensive Blood Pressure Reduction in Acute Cerebral Hemorrhage Trial (INTERACT I), patients presenting within 6 hours of ictus were randomized into two subgroups: (1) aggressive blood pressure management with an SBP goal of less than 140 mm Hg, or (2) standard management with a SBP goal of less than 180 mm Hg. This study showed no excess adverse events and no increase in worsened neurological outcomes in the aggressive treatment group.[59] The follow-up INTERACT II trial showed no significant reduction in the rate of death or severe disability in the aggressive SBP management group; however, patients in the aggressive management group did have a significantly lower modified Rankin score (mRs) at 90 days.[60] The Antihypertensive Treatment in Acute Cerebral Hemorrhage II (ATACH II) trial found that treating ICH patients to target systolic blood pressures of 110–139 mm Hg did not reduce rates of death or disability when compared to standard target systolic blood pressures of 140–179 mm Hg.[61]

## Temperature Regulation

**Cohort Studies** Fever has been identified as a poor prognostic indicator in ICH patients and has been correlated with hematoma growth.[62] A post hoc analysis of an RCT demonstrated that the use of acetaminophen to control temperature is beneficial in patients with a body temperature of 37–39°C.[63]

**Pilot Studies** A pilot study has shown that hypothermia reduces peri-hemorrhagic edema in patients with large ICH.[64] No RCTs have been completed to evaluate temperature regulation in ICH, although the Cooling in Intracerebral Hemorrhage (CINCH) trial is ongoing.[65]

## Glycemic Control

**Cohort Studies**  Cohort studies have found correlations between hyperglycemia on admission in ICH patients and increased infectious and neurological complications, as well as worse overall outcomes.[66] Other studies support these findings, showing that tight glucose control is associated with lower infection rates and improved neurological outcomes.[67] Hyperglycemia has also been independently associated with risk of early death in ICH.[68]

**Randomized Control Trials**  The Normoglycemia in Intensive Care Evaluation–Survival Using Glucose Algorithm Regulation (NICE-SUGAR) study, conducted on a population of ICU patients (not just NICU or ICH patients), found that a blood glucose goal of 81–108 mg/dL was associated with increased mortality compared to a blood glucose target of less than 180 mg/dL.[69] A subgroup analysis in traumatic brain injury patients from this trial demonstrated no significant difference in clinical outcome between intensive and standard glycemic control groups.[70] Additional RCTs have shown conflicting outcomes of intensive blood glucose control, with some suggesting improved survival with lower morbidity, while others show increased hypoglycemic events and potentially worsened outcomes.[71]

## Seizure Prophylaxis

**Cohort Studies**  Seizures occur in up to 21% of patients following ICH, with occurrence most likely in patients with lobar ICH.[32,72] Cohort studies addressing antiepileptic prophylaxis (AEP) in this patient population have yielded mixed results. In one study, AEP was shown to significantly reduce the risk of seizure in patients with lobar ICH.[32] In another study, there was no significant association with AEP use and risk of early seizures, long-term epilepsy, disability, or death.[73] A post hoc analysis of an RCT and a prospective cohort study have demonstrated that AEP is associated with increased risk of poor outcomes.[74]

**Randomized Control Trials**  A recent RCT showed that early to late post-ICH AEP with valproic acid (VPA) did not prevent the occurrence of seizures. The treatment group did, however, demonstrate a lower National Institute of Health Stroke Scale (NIHSS) score at 12-month follow-up, raising the possibility of a neuroprotective role of VPA prophylaxis.[72]

## Miscellaneous Agents

**Cohort and Pilot Studies**  Citicoline is an anti-inflammatory neuroprotectant that acts by preventing cell membrane breakdown and decreasing levels of free fatty acids.[75] In a pilot RCT, citicoline was shown to be safe (primary trial goal), but it did not show any significant improvement in NIHSS score or volume of residual lesion.[76]

Rosuvastatin, an HMG CoA-reductase inhibitor, is typically used in the management of hyperlipidemia. In animal models it has neuroprotective properties by an anti-inflammatory mechanism.[77] In a retrospective cohort study, prior statin use has also been correlated with reduced mortality and decreased peri-hematomal edema in ICH.[78] A large retrospective analysis demonstrated that inpatient statin use improved outcomes after ICH and that cessation substantially worsened outcomes.[79] A nonrandomized prospective pilot study demonstrated nonsignificant trends toward lower in-hospital mortality as well as other promising outcomes; however, because none of these differences was statistically significant, the study was not definitive.[80] An RCT evaluating the effect of simvastatin on peri-hematomal edema in ICH was terminated because of poor recruitment and no results were reported (www.clinicaltrials.gov; study identifier NCT00718328).

Celecoxib is a nonsteroidal anti-inflammatory agent that selectively inhibits the prostaglandin COX-2 and has been shown to reduce brain edema and cell death in preclinical studies.[81] The Administration of Celecoxib for Treatment of Intracerebral Hemorrhage (ACE-ICH) trial is a randomized pilot study evaluating the effects of celecoxib on peri-hematomal edema in ICH. Although the study has been completed, no results have been reported yet (www.clinicaltrials.gov; study identifier NCT00526214).

Hemoglobin breakdown products, especially iron, promote free radical formation and edema in ICH.[82] Deferoxamine is an iron chelator that attenuates the detrimental effects of free iron and reduces neurological injury following ICH in animal models.[83-84] Deferoxamine has also been found to display anti-inflammatory effects.[85] A pilot phase I trial of deferoxamine in ICH demonstrated that intravenous infusion is safe and well-tolerated up to a dose of 62 mg/kg.[86]

**Randomized Control Trials** Both mannitol and glycerol are believed to exhibit neuroprotective effects by reducing cerebral edema and improving cerebrovascular hemodynamics.[87-88] RCTs evaluating the neuroprotective benefits of both agents in hemorrhagic stroke did not demonstrate significant difference in mortality and functional outcomes between the experimental and control groups.[88-89]

NXY-059 is a nitrone that exhibits neuroprotective effects by acting as an antioxidant, scavenging and combining with reactive oxygen species.[90] In a large RCT, NXY-059 was shown to be associated with significantly reduced disability

Table 11.1 Randomized Controlled Trials Showing Neuroprotective Benefit in Intracerebral Hemorrhage (ICH)

| Trial | Intervention Group | Outcome |
|---|---|---|
| Phase IIB rFVIIa | 40, 80, or 160 μg/kg of rFVIIa within 4 hours of ICH | ↓Hematoma growth ↓Mortality ↑Functional outcomes |
| FAST (Phase III rFVIIa) | 80 μg/kg of rFVIIa within 4 hours of ICH | ↓Hematoma growth ↔Mortality ↔Functional outcomes |
| INTERACT II | Intensive SBP control <140 within 6 hours of ICH | ↓ mRs ↔Mortality ↔Functional outcomes |
| Valproic acid prophylaxis | Therapeutic VPA at 2 hours after ICH for 1 month | ↔ seizure in first year post-ICH ↓NIHSS at 12 months |

**Table 11.2** Ongoing Trials for Neuroprotection in Intracerebral Hemorrhage (ICH)

| Trial | Intervention |
| --- | --- |
| CINCH | Therapeutic hypothermia (35°C) for 8 days |
| iDEF | Deferoxamine 32 mg/kg/day intravenous for 3 days |
| SHRINC | Escalating doses of pioglitazone for 3 days, then 30 mg orally for duration of study |
| MISTIE III | Minimally invasive surgery plus rt-PA |

at 90 days after ischemic stroke when compared to the control condition.[91] The Cerebral Hematoma and NXY Treatment trial (CHANT) showed that NXY-059 is safe and well-tolerated in ICH patients, but no significant therapeutic benefit was observed when comparing intervention and control groups.[92]

The NMDA receptor is an excitatory neurotransmitter receptor that is activated when it binds with glutamate and glycine.[93] Overactivity of excitatory pathways has been identified as a contributor to neurotoxicity in acute stroke models.[94] One RCT has evaluated the neuroprotective effects of NMDA receptor blockers in acute stroke. The Glycine Antagonist in Neuroprotection (GAIN) ICH trial showed no significant difference in functional outcomes between ICH patients given gavestinel (NMDA receptor blocker) and placebo.[95]

Pioglitazone is a peroxisome proliferator–activated receptor γ agonist used for the treatment of diabetes mellitus. In preclinical studies, it has displayed neuroprotective properties by acting as an anti-inflammatory and inhibiting matrix metalloproteinase and microglial activation.[96–97] The Safety of Pioglitazone for Hematoma Resolution in Intracerebral Hemorrhage (SHRINC) trial is under way, with a primary safety outcome of mortality at discharge.[97]

The High-Dose Deferoxamine in Intracerebral Hemorrhage (HI-DEF) trial was suspended early because of an increased incidence of acute respiratory distress syndrome (www.clinicaltrials.gov; study identifier NCT01662895).[98] Modifications to dosing have been made. The Intracerebral Hemorrhage Deferoxamine (iDEF) trial is scheduled for completion in 2018 (www.clinicaltrials.gov; study identifier NCT02175225).

The Minimally Invasive Surgery Plus Rt-PA for ICH Evacuation Phase III (MISTIE III) trial is scheduled for completion in 2019 (www.clinicaltrials.gov; study identifier NCT01827046).

A summary of RCTs showing a neuroprotective benefit in ICH is provided in Table 11.1, and a summary of ongoing RCTs is provided in Table 11.2.

## IMPLICATIONS FOR CLINICAL PRACTICE
### Coagulation

Despite the lack of RCTs confirming benefit, rapid reversal of anticoagulation is indicated in ICH patients based on strong observational data and widespread consensus. Cohort studies have suggested that early platelet transfusion is beneficial in patients with poor platelet function or on antiplatelet therapy. The PATCH trial contradicts these findings and therefore platelet transfusion is not recommended in these patients.[51] Despite some positive data, there is insufficient evidence for routine use of rFVIIa for hemostasis in ICH.

## Blood Pressure Control

Aggressive blood pressure management with an SBP goal of 140 mm Hg is safe, but does not result in a lower rate of death or disability when compared to standard reduction of SBP to a goal of 140–179 mm Hg.[59-61]

## Temperature Regulation

Cooling with a goal of normothermia is reasonable in patients with ICH and fever. Further recommendations will depend on the result of the ongoing CINCH trial.[65]

## Glycemic Control

Benefits of tight glucose control in ICU were not confirmed in a meta-analysis of critically ill neurological patients.[70,99] Meta-analyses have shown worsened risks of hypoglycemia with no mortality benefit in tight glucose control and worse neurological outcomes in nonstringent glucose control.[100] Moderate rather than strict glucose control is reasonable, with a therapeutic goal of normoglycemia and avoidance of hypoglycemia.[100]

## Seizure Prophylaxis

Currently there is insufficient evidence that AEP is neuroprotective in ICH patients, and, in fact, it may be associated with worse outcomes.[74] Special consideration for AEP should be given to patients who have a lobar location of ICH or who have a history of seizures.[32]

## Miscellaneous Agents

Mannitol, glycerol, gavestinel, and NXY-059 have shown no significant neuroprotective benefit in RCTs and are therefore not recommended. Although some small and preliminary studies have shown mild benefits with statin therapy in ICH, there is insufficient evidence to recommend the use of statins as a neuroprotectant in ICH. RCTs to evaluate the neuroprotective benefits of pioglitazone and deferoxamine in ICH are currently ongoing, and there is insufficient evidence to recommend their routine use.

## FUTURE DIRECTIONS

Several compounds have been shown to have neuroprotective properties in animal models of ICH and other types of neurological injury. These therapies act by improving coagulation, enhancing clot removal, and chelating iron. There is, however, no convincing scientific evidence that any of these agents benefit ICH patients. Future studies should evaluate the role of combination therapies that may disrupt secondary injury cascades at several different points.

## REFERENCES

1. Qureshi AI, Tuhrim S, Broderick JP, Batjer HH, Hondo H, Hanley DF. Spontaneous intracerebral hemorrhage. *N Engl J Med.* 2001;344(19):1450–60.

2. Zazulia AR, Diringer MN, Derdeyn CP, Powers WJ. Progression of mass effect after intracerebral hemorrhage. *Stroke.* 1999;30(6):1167–73.

3. Zazulia AR, Diringer MN, Videen TO, et al. Hypoperfusion without ischemia surrounding acute intracerebral hemorrhage. *J Cereb Blood Flow Metab.* 2001;21(7):804–10.

4. Diringer MN, Edwards DF, Zazulia AR. Hydrocephalus: a previously unrecognized predictor of poor outcome from supratentorial intracerebral hemorrhage. *Stroke.* 1998;29(7):1352–7.

5. Xi G, Keep RF, Hua Y, Xiang J, Hoff JT. Attenuation of thrombin-induced brain edema by cerebral thrombin preconditioning. *Stroke.* 1999;30(6):1247–55.

6. Donovan FM, Pike CJ, Cotman CW, Cunningham DD. Thrombin induces apoptosis in cultured neurons and astrocytes via a pathway requiring tyrosine kinase and RhoA activities. *J Neurosci.* 1997;17(14):5316–26.

7. Keep RF, Xiang J, Ennis SR, et al. Blood-brain barrier function in intracerebral hemorrhage. *Acta Neurochir Suppl.* 2008;105:73–7.

8. Hua Y, Xi G, Keep RF, Hoff JT. Complement activation in the brain after experimental intracerebral hemorrhage. *J Neurosurg.* 2000;92(6):1016–22.

9. Xi G, Hua Y, Keep RF, Younger JG, Hoff JT. Systemic complement depletion diminishes perihematomal brain edema in rats. *Stroke.* 2001;32(1):162–7.

10. Wang J. Preclinical and clinical research on inflammation after intracerebral hemorrhage. *Prog Neurobiol.* 2010;92(4):463–77.

11. Zhao X, Sun G, Ting SM, et al. Cleaning up after ICH: the role of Nrf2 in modulating microglia function and hematoma clearance. *J Neurochem.* 2015;133(1):144–52.

12. Nakamura T, Keep RF, Hua Y, Hoff JT, Xi G. Oxidative DNA injury after experimental intracerebral hemorrhage. *Brain Res.* 2005;1039(1–2):30–6.

13. Han N, Ding SJ, Wu T, Zhu YL. Correlation of free radical level and apoptosis after intracerebral hemorrhage in rats. *Neurosci Bull.* 2008;24(6):351–8.

14. Drejer J, Benveniste H, Diemer NH, Schousboe A. Cellular origin of ischemia-induced glutamate release from brain tissue in vivo and in vitro. *J Neurochem.* 1985;45(1):145–51.

15. Sharp F, Liu DZ, Zhan X, Ander BP. Intracerebral hemorrhage injury mechanisms: glutamate neurotoxicity, thrombin, and Src. *Acta Neurochir Suppl.* 2008;105:43–6.

16. Bano D, Young KW, Guerin CJ, et al. Cleavage of the plasma membrane Na+/Ca2+ exchanger in excitotoxicity. *Cell.* 2005;120(2):275–85.

17. Zhu X, Tao L, Tejima-Mandeville E, et al. Plasmalemma permeability and necrotic cell death phenotypes after intracerebral hemorrhage in mice. *Stroke.* 2012;43(2):524–31.

18. Qureshi AI, Suri MF, Ostrow PT, et al. Apoptosis as a form of cell death in intracerebral hemorrhage. *Neurosurgery.* 2003;52(5):1041–7; discussion 1047–8.

19. Chen YC, Chen CM, Liu JL, Chen ST, Cheng ML, Chiu DT. Oxidative markers in spontaneous intracerebral hemorrhage: leukocyte 8-hydroxy-2'-deoxyguanosine as an independent predictor of the 30-day outcome. *J Neurosurg.* 2011;115(6):1184–90.

20. Chaudhary N, Gemmete JJ, Thompson BG, Xi G, Pandey AS. Iron: potential therapeutic target in hemorrhagic stroke. *World Neurosurgery.* 2013;79(1):7–9.

21. Griauzde J, Dickerson E, Gemmete J. Hemorrhagic stroke. In: Saba L, Raz E, editors. *Neurovascular imaging.* New York: Springer; 2014:1–34.

22. Hemphill JC 3rd, Bonovich DC, Besmertis L, Manley GT, Johnston SC. The ICH score: a simple, reliable grading scale for intracerebral hemorrhage. *Stroke.* 2001;32(4):891–7.

23. Broderick JP, Brott TG, Duldner JE, Tomsick T, Huster G. Volume of intracerebral hemorrhage. A powerful and easy-to-use predictor of 30-day mortality. *Stroke.* 1993;24(7):987–93.

24. Kothari RU, Brott T, Broderick JP, et al. The ABCs of measuring intracerebral hemorrhage volumes. *Stroke.* 1996;27(8):1304–5.

25. Davis SM, Broderick J, Hennerici M, et al. Hematoma growth is a determinant of mortality and poor outcome after intracerebral hemorrhage. *Neurology.* 2006;66(8): 1175–81.

26. Fujii Y, Takeuchi S, Sasaki O, Minakawa T, Tanaka R. Multivariate analysis of predictors of hematoma enlargement in spontaneous intracerebral hemorrhage. *Stroke.* 1998;29(6):1160–6.

27. Godoy DA, Pinero G, Di Napoli M. Predicting mortality in spontaneous intracerebral hemorrhage: can modification to original score improve the prediction? *Stroke.* 2006;37(4):1038–44.

28. Dowlatshahi D, Wasserman JK, Momoli F, et al. Evolution of computed tomography angiography spot sign is consistent with a site of active hemorrhage in acute intracerebral hemorrhage. *Stroke.* 2014;45(1):277–80.

29. Wada R, Aviv RI, Fox AJ, et al. CT angiography "spot sign" predicts hematoma expansion in acute intracerebral hemorrhage. *Stroke.* 2007;38(4):1257–62.

30. Delgado Almandoz JE, Yoo AJ, Stone MJ, et al. The spot sign score in primary intracerebral hemorrhage identifies patients at highest risk of in-hospital mortality and poor outcome among survivors. *Stroke.* 2010;41(1):54–60.

31. Rahman M, Friedman WA. Hyponatremia in neurosurgical patients: clinical guidelines development. *Neurosurgery.* 2009;65(5):925–35; discussion 935–6.

32. Passero S, Rocchi R, Rossi S, Ulivelli M, Vatti G. Seizures after spontaneous supratentorial intracerebral hemorrhage. *Epilepsia.* 2002;43(10):1175–80.

33. Diringer MN, Edwards DF. Admission to a neurologic/neurosurgical intensive care unit is associated with reduced mortality rate after intracerebral hemorrhage. *Crit Care Med.* 2001;29(3):635–40.

34. Terent A, Asplund K, Farahmand B, et al. Stroke unit care revisited: who benefits the most? A cohort study of 105,043 patients in Riks-Stroke, the Swedish Stroke Register. *J Neurol Neurosurg Psychiatry.* 2009;80(8):881–7.

35. Wintzen AR, de Jonge H, Loeliger EA, Bots GT. The risk of intracerebral hemorrhage during oral anticoagulant treatment: a population study. *Ann Neurol.* 1984;16(5):553–8.

36. Flaherty ML, Tao H, Haverbusch M, et al. Warfarin use leads to larger intracerebral hematomas. *Neurology.* 2008;71(14):1084–9.

37. Yasaka M, Minematsu K, Naritomi H, Sakata T, Yamaguchi T. Predisposing factors for enlargement of intracerebral hemorrhage in patients treated with warfarin. *Thromb Haemost.* 2003;89(2):278–83.

38. Rosand J, Eckman MH, Knudsen KA, Singer DE, Greenberg SM. The effect of warfarin and intensity of anticoagulation on outcome of intracerebral hemorrhage. *Arch Intern Med.* 2004;164(8):880–4.

39. Levine MN, Raskob G, Beyth RJ, Kearon C, Schulman S. Hemorrhagic complications of anticoagulant treatment: the Seventh ACCP Conference on Antithrombotic and Thrombolytic Therapy. *Chest.* 2004;126(3 Suppl):287S–310S.

40. Taylor G, Osinski D, Thevenin A, Devys JM. Is platelet transfusion efficient to restore platelet reactivity in patients who are responders to aspirin and/or clopidogrel before emergency surgery? *J Trauma Acute Care Surg.* 2013;74(5):1367–9.

41. Kuramatsu JB, Gerner ST, Schellinger PD, et al. Anticoagulant reversal, blood pressure levels, and anticoagulant resumption in patients with anticoagulation-related intracerebral hemorrhage. *JAMA.* 2015;313(8):824–36.

42. Dezee KJ, Shimeall WT, Douglas KM, Shumway NM, O'Malley PG. Treatment of excessive anticoagulation with phytonadione (vitamin K): a meta-analysis. *Arch Intern Med.* 2006;166(4):391–7.

43. Fredriksson K, Norrving B, Stromblad LG. Emergency reversal of anticoagulation after intracerebral hemorrhage. *Stroke.* 1992;23(7):972–7.

44. van Aart L, Eijkhout HW, Kamphuis JS, et al. Individualized dosing regimen for prothrombin complex concentrate more effective than standard treatment in the reversal of oral anticoagulant therapy: an open, prospective randomized controlled trial. *Thromb Res.* 2006;118(3):313–20.

45. Naidech AM, Liebling SM, Rosenberg NF, et al. Early platelet transfusion improves platelet activity and may improve outcomes after intracerebral hemorrhage. *Neurocrit Care.* 2012;16(1):82–7.

46. van Veen JJ, Maclean RM, Hampton KK, et al. Protamine reversal of low molecular weight heparin: clinically effective? *Blood Coagul Fibrinolysis.* 2011;22(7):565–70.

47. Firozvi K, Deveras RA, Kessler CM. Reversal of low-molecular-weight heparin-induced bleeding in patients with pre-existing hypercoagulable states with human recombinant activated factor VII concentrate. *Am J Hematol.* 2006;81(8):582–9.

48. Chang DN, Dager WE, Chin AI. Removal of dabigatran by hemodialysis. *Am J Kidney Dis.* 2013;61(3):487–9.

49. Naidech AM, Maas MB, Levasseur-Franklin KE, et al. Desmopressin improves platelet activity in acute intracerebral hemorrhage. *Stroke.* 2014;45(8):2451–3.

50. Steiner T, Freiberger A, Griebe M, et al. International normalised ratio normalisation in patients with coumarin-related intracranial haemorrhages—the INCH trial: a randomised controlled multicentre trial to compare safety and preliminary efficacy of fresh frozen plasma and prothrombin complex—study design and protocol. *Int J Stroke.* 2011;6(3):271–7.

51. Baharoglu MI, Cordonnier C, Al-Shahi Salman R, et al. Platelet transfusion versus standard care after acute stroke due to spontaneous cerebral haemorrhage associated with antiplatelet therapy (PATCH): a randomised, open-label, phase 3 trial. *Lancet.* 2016;387(10038):2605-13.

52. Mayer SA, Brun NC, Begtrup K, et al. Recombinant activated factor VII for acute intracerebral hemorrhage. *N Engl J Med.* 2005;352(8):777–85.

53. Mayer SA, Brun NC, Begtrup K, et al. Efficacy and safety of recombinant activated factor VII for acute intracerebral hemorrhage. *N Engl J Med.* 2008;358(20):2127–37.

54. Dandapani BK, Suzuki S, Kelley RE, Reyes-Iglesias Y, Duncan RC. Relation between blood pressure and outcome in intracerebral hemorrhage. *Stroke.* 1995;26(1):21–4.

55. Terayama Y, Tanahashi N, Fukuuchi Y, Gotoh F. Prognostic value of admission blood pressure in patients with intracerebral hemorrhage. Keio Cooperative Stroke Study. *Stroke.* 1997;28(6):1185–8.

56. Broderick JP, Diringer MN, Hill MD, et al. Determinants of intracerebral hemorrhage growth: an exploratory analysis. *Stroke.* 2007;38(3):1072–5.

57. Qureshi AI, Palesch YY, Martin R, et al. Effect of systolic blood pressure reduction on hematoma expansion, perihematomal edema, and 3-month outcome among patients with intracerebral hemorrhage: results from the antihypertensive treatment of acute cerebral hemorrhage study. *Arch Neurol.* 2010;67(5):570–6.

58. Butcher KS, Jeerakathil T, Hill M, et al. The Intracerebral Hemorrhage Acutely Decreasing Arterial Pressure Trial. *Stroke.* 2013;44(3):620–6.

59. Arima H, Huang Y, Wang JG, et al. Earlier blood pressure-lowering and greater attenuation of hematoma growth in acute intracerebral hemorrhage: INTERACT pilot phase. *Stroke.* 2012;43(8):2236–8.

60. Anderson CS, Heeley E, Huang Y, et al. Rapid blood-pressure lowering in patients with acute intracerebral hemorrhage. *N Engl J Med.* 2013;368(25):2355–65.

61. Qureshi AI, Palesch YY, Barsan WG, et al. Intensive Blood-Pressure Lowering in Patients with Acute Cerebral Hemorrhage. *N Engl J Med.* 2016;375(11):1033–43.

62. Schwarz S, Hafner K, Aschoff A, Schwab S. Incidence and prognostic significance of fever following intracerebral hemorrhage. *Neurology.* 2000;54(2):354–61.

63. den Hertog HM, van der Worp HB, van Gemert HM, et al. The Paracetamol (Acetaminophen) In Stroke (PAIS) trial: a multicentre, randomised, placebo-controlled, phase III trial. *Lancet Neurol.* 2009;8(5):434–40.

64. Kollmar R, Staykov D, Dorfler A, Schellinger PD, Schwab S, Bardutzky J. Hypothermia reduces perihemorrhagic edema after intracerebral hemorrhage. *Stroke.* 2010;41(8):1684–9.

65. Kollmar R, Juettler E, Huttner HB, et al. Cooling in intracerebral hemorrhage (CINCH) trial: protocol of a randomized German-Austrian clinical trial. *Int J Stroke.* 2012;7(2):168–72.

66. Passero S, Ciacci G, Ulivelli M. The influence of diabetes and hyperglycemia on clinical course after intracerebral hemorrhage. *Neurology.* 2003;61(10):1351–6.

67. Ooi YC, Dagi TF, Maltenfort M, et al. Tight glycemic control reduces infection and improves neurological outcome in critically ill neurosurgical and neurological patients. *Neurosurgery.* 2012;71(3):692–702; discussion 702.

68. Kimura K, Iguchi Y, Inoue T, et al. Hyperglycemia independently increases the risk of early death in acute spontaneous intracerebral hemorrhage. *J Neurol Sci.* 2007;255(1–2):90–4.

69. Griesdale DE, de Souza RJ, van Dam RM, et al. Intensive insulin therapy and mortality among critically ill patients: a meta-analysis including NICE-SUGAR study data. *CMAJ.* 2009;180(8):821–7.

70. NICE-SUGAR Study Investigators for the Australian and New Zealand Intensive Care Society Clinical Trials Group and the Canadian Critical Care Trials Group, Finfer S, Chittock D, Li Y, et al. Intensive versus conventional glucose control in critically ill patients with traumatic brain injury: long-term follow-up of a subgroup of patients from the NICE-SUGAR study. *Intensive Care Med.* 2015;41(6):1037–47.

71. van den Berghe G, Wouters P, Weekers F, et al. Intensive insulin therapy in critically ill patients. *N Engl J Med.* 2001;345(19):1359–67.

72. Gilad R, Boaz M, Dabby R, Sadeh M, Lampl Y. Are post intracerebral hemorrhage seizures prevented by anti-epileptic treatment? *Epilepsy Res.* 2011;95(3):227–31.

73. Reddig RT, Nixdorf KE, Jensen MB. The prophylactic use of an antiepileptic drug in intracerebral hemorrhage. *Clin Neurol Neurosurg.* 2011;113(10):895–7.

74. Messe SR, Sansing LH, Cucchiara BL, et al. Prophylactic antiepileptic drug use is associated with poor outcome following ICH. *Neurocrit Care.* 2009;11(1):38–44.

75. Clark W, Gunion-Rinker L, Lessov N, Hazel K. Citicoline treatment for experimental intracerebral hemorrhage in mice. *Stroke.* 1998;29(10):2136–40.

76. Secades JJ, Alvarez-Sabin J, Rubio F, et al. Citicoline in intracerebral haemorrhage: a double-blind, randomized, placebo-controlled, multi-centre pilot study. *Cerebrovasc Dis.* 2006;21(5–6):380–5.

77. Seyfried D, Han Y, Lu D, Chen J, Bydon A, Chopp M. Improvement in neurological outcome after administration of atorvastatin following experimental intracerebral hemorrhage in rats. *J Neurosurg.* 2004;101(1):104–7.

78. Naval NS, Abdelhak TA, Zeballos P, Urrunaga N, Mirski MA, Carhuapoma JR. Prior statin use reduces mortality in intracerebral hemorrhage. *Neurocrit Care.* 2008;8(1):6–12.

79. Flint AC, Conell C, Rao VA, et al. Effect of statin use during hospitalization for intracerebral hemorrhage on mortality and discharge disposition. *JAMA Neurol.* 2014;71(11):1364–71.

80. Tapia-Perez H, Sanchez-Aguilar M, Torres-Corzo JG, et al. Use of statins for the treatment of spontaneous intracerebral hemorrhage: results of a pilot study. *Cent Eur Neurosurg.* 2009;70(1):15–20.

81. Chu K, Jeong SW, Jung KH, et al. Celecoxib induces functional recovery after intracerebral hemorrhage with reduction of brain edema and perihematomal cell death. *J Cereb Blood Flow Metab.* 2004;24(8):926–33.

82. Goldstein L, Teng ZP, Zeserson E, Patel M, Regan RF. Hemin induces an iron-dependent, oxidative injury to human neuron-like cells. *J Neurosci Res.* 2003;73(1):113–21.

83. Nakamura T, Keep RF, Hua Y, Schallert T, Hoff JT, Xi G. Deferoxamine-induced attenuation of brain edema and neurological deficits in a rat model of intracerebral hemorrhage. *J Neurosurg.* 2004;100(4):672–8.

84. Gu Y, Hua Y, Keep RF, Morgenstern LB, Xi G. Deferoxamine reduces intracerebral hematoma-induced iron accumulation and neuronal death in piglets. *Stroke.* 2009;40(6):2241–3.

85. Tanji K, Imaizumi T, Matsumiya T, et al. Desferrioxamine, an iron chelator, upregulates cyclooxygenase-2 expression and prostaglandin production in a human macrophage cell line. *Biochim Biophys Acta.* 2001;1530(2–3):227–35.

86. Selim M, Yeatts S, Goldstein JN, et al. Safety and tolerability of deferoxamine mesylate in patients with acute intracerebral hemorrhage. *Stroke.* 2011;42(11):3067–74.

87. Plotnikov MB. [Antiedemic action of glycerin in intracerebral hemorrhage]. *Farmakol Toksikol.* 1981;44(5):568–71.

88. Misra UK, Kalita J, Ranjan P, Mandal SK. Mannitol in intracerebral hemorrhage: a randomized controlled study. *J Neurol Sci.* 2005;234(1–2):41–5.

89. Yu YL, Kumana CR, Lauder IJ, et al. Treatment of acute cerebral hemorrhage with intravenous glycerol. A double-blind, placebo-controlled, randomized trial. *Stroke.* 1992;23(7):967–71.

90. Marshall JW, Cummings RM, Bowes LJ, Ridley RM, Green AR. Functional and histological evidence for the protective effect of NXY-059 in a primate model of stroke when given 4 hours after occlusion. *Stroke.* 2003;34(9):2228–33.

91. Lees KR, Zivin JA, Ashwood T, et al. NXY-059 for acute ischemic stroke. *N Engl J Med.* 2006;354(6):588–600.

92. Lyden PD, Shuaib A, Lees KR, et al. Safety and tolerability of NXY-059 for acute intracerebral hemorrhage: the CHANT Trial. *Stroke.* 2007;38(8):2262–9.

93. Choi DW. Methods for antagonizing glutamate neurotoxicity. *Cerebrovasc Brain Metab Rev.* 1990;2(2):105–47.

94. Lee ST, Chu K, Jung KH, et al. Memantine reduces hematoma expansion in experimental intracerebral hemorrhage, resulting in functional improvement. *J Cereb Blood Flow Metab.* 2006;26(4):536–44.

95. Haley EC Jr, Thompson JL, Levin B, et al. Gavestinel does not improve outcome after acute intracerebral hemorrhage: an analysis from the GAIN International and GAIN Americas studies. *Stroke.* 2005;36(5):1006–10.

96. Zhao X, Sun G, Zhang J, et al. Hematoma resolution as a target for intracerebral hemorrhage treatment: role for peroxisome proliferator-activated receptor gamma in microglia/macrophages. *Ann Neurol.* 2007;61(4):352–62.

97. Gonzales NR, Shah J, Sangha N, et al. Design of a prospective, dose-escalation study evaluating the Safety of Pioglitazone for Hematoma Resolution in Intracerebral Hemorrhage (SHRINC). *Int J Stroke.* 2013;8(5):388–96.

98. Yeatts SD, Palesch YY, Moy CS, Selim M. High dose deferoxamine in intracerebral hemorrhage (HI-DEF) trial: rationale, design, and methods. *Neurocrit Care.* 2013;19(2):257–66.

99. Wiener RS, Wiener DC, Larson RJ. Benefits and risks of tight glucose control in critically ill adults: a meta-analysis. *JAMA.* 2008;300(8):933–44.

100. Kramer AH, Roberts DJ, Zygun DA. Optimal glycemic control in neurocritical care patients: a systematic review and meta-analysis. *Crit Care.* 2012;16(5):R203.

# 12 Neuroprotection for Mechanical Circulatory Support

Lauren E. Dunn, Joshua Z. Willey,

and Ronald M. Lazar

## GENERAL CONSIDERATIONS

Since the introduction of mechanical circulatory support (MCS) as a viable option for heart failure patients, physicians have been faced with new clinical challenges arising from this technology. The neurologic events associated with these devices are of significant concern, representing some of the most frequently encountered complications after device placement.[1] Due to their relatively recent introduction, however, there exist few clinical trials that examine the incidence and outcomes of neurologic complications in the setting of MCS. Most of the literature available focuses on observational studies and institutional experience. This chapter will explore the most frequently encountered neurologic complications of MCS, as well as describe current management strategies.

### History and Background

Although the pneumatically powered ventricular assist device (VAD) was first successfully implanted in a human patient by Michael DeBakey in 1966, it wasn't until the 1990s that long-term MCS as a bridge to cardiac transplant became a clinical reality. Following the REMATCH trial in 2001, the US Food and Drug Administration (FDA) approved the HeartMate Vented Electric VAD as destination therapy, or permanent circulatory support for those heart failure patients ineligible for cardiac transplant.[2] Today, patients receive VADs for one of three heart-failure indications: (1) bridge to transplantation, (2) bridge to recovery, and (3) destination therapy.

VAD technology has evolved considerably over the years, and the internal mechanics of the various devices dictate a patient's need for antiplatelet agents, anticoagulation, or both—a topic highly germane to the neurologist. Today, most implanted VADs are "second-generation" or continuous flow devices, and include the HeartMateII and Jarvik 2000.[3] So called "third-generation" pumps are currently being used in small numbers as bridge to transplant devices and have been designed for durability, compact size, and optimization of blood flow to reduce thrombus formation and hemolysis.

Despite their tenuous clinical status at the time of implantation, VAD patients often do quite well, with 6-month survival statistics approaching 90% in some studies.[2,4] Data indicate that these devices also improve quality of life in heart failure patients and that these benefits begin soon after implantation and persist for the duration of mechanical support.[5] Current American Heart Association Guidelines recommend consideration of a VAD for patients with refractory end-stage heart failure whose 1-year mortality approaches 50% with maximal medical therapy.[6] In 2011, more than 1,500 patients received VADs in the United States. While this number is small, there are millions of American patients with heart failure, and VAD use is only expected to increase.[7]

In addition to the VAD for chronic support, advanced cardiac care also makes use of percutaneous assist devices in acute decompensated heart failure. These devices include the intra-aortic balloon pump (IABP), the TandemHeart, and the Impella. Generally, these devices are used in patients who have suffered devastating myocardial infarctions or are undergoing high-risk percutaneous coronary intervention. Unlike the VADs, which take over for a failing heart, the percutaneous assist devices provide support by reducing myocardial oxygen demand via direct unloading of the left ventricle and increasing coronary perfusion due to diastolic augmentation. Along with VADs, they require anticoagulation; however, their duration of use is much shorter, usually less than 2 weeks. Their short-term use reduces myocardial infarct size and allows the patient to proceed more safely to coronary intervention.[8]

Lastly, some patients with refractory cardiac or respiratory failure are now being treated with extracorporeal membrane oxygenation (ECMO). This technology was pioneered in the 1950s by surgeon John Gibbon as a means of blood oxygenation during prolonged cardiac surgeries.[9] In the 1970s, ECMO was applied with success to neonates with congenital cardiac defects or severe respiratory failure.[10–11] The use of ECMO in adults outside of the operating room expanded following the CESAR trial in 2006, which showed reduced rates of death and severe disability in patients with refractory, acute respiratory distress syndrome (ARDS) who were treated with ECMO, when compared to conventional ventilation strategies.[12] Further interest was generated following promising reports of improved outcomes in ARDS patients during the 2009 H1N1 epidemic. ECMO used for respiratory support, referred to as veno-venous, or VV-ECMO, provides no hemodynamic support. Blood is extracted from the vena cava or femoral vein and returned to the right atrium. In the ECMO circuit, blood is passed through an oxygenator, where gas exchange occurs across a semi-permeable membrane.[13]

In addition to treating patients with hypoxemic respiratory failure, ECMO is being used for hemodynamic support in the setting of severe cardiac failure (due to cardiac arrest, refractory septic shock, or cardiogenic shock). The mode of ECMO used for hemodynamic support is known as VA-ECMO, or veno-arterial ECMO. In this setting, venous blood is removed from the right atrium and returned to the arterial systemic circulation, bypassing the heart and lungs. Locations of arterial cannulation include right femoral artery (preferred), right subclavian artery, and right common carotid. VA-ECMO can also be installed "centrally," which is usually the approach when a patient cannot be weaned off cardiopulmonary bypass during cardiac surgery. In central VA-ECMO, blood is returned to the ascending aorta directly.[14]

As with other forms of MCS, ECMO requires anticoagulation, usually with unfractionated heparin, to prevent thrombus formation in the circuit. This, in conjunction with unique clinical situations arising from venous and arterial cannulation, puts ECMO patients at risk for neurologic complications, which will be described later.[15]

Observational studies have shown that patients with respiratory indications for ECMO tend to have better outcomes than those who receive ECMO for cardiac complications, which may reflect the severity and irreversibility of the underlying cardiac conditions.[16-17] These cardiac patients are also more likely to experience neurologic problems while cannulated.[16] Overall survival for adult ECMO patients is around 50%, which reflects the severe medical illness of this population.[15]

## CAUSES OF AND RISKS FOR NEUROLOGICAL INJURY

Second-generation VADs support the circulation by providing continuous flow of blood (up to 10 L/min in the case of the HeartMateII) from the apex of the left ventricle to the ascending aorta. Blood flows from the left ventricle into a pump containing a rotor, which converts the radial velocity of blood flow into an axial direction and directs it into the ascending aorta. A percutaneous lead exits the body where it connects to an externally worn computer and battery pack (Figure 12.1).

All VADs approved for use today require concomitant anticoagulation to reduce the risk of thrombosis associated with the rotor pump and valves.[18] As a result, thrombosis and hemorrhage are the two most common complications associated with MCS.[3] Unfortunately, these complications frequently manifest with neurologic events, notably ischemic and hemorrhagic stroke. Observational studies suggest that the incidence of stroke among VAD patients is approximately 15% per year.[19-20] Not only does stroke offset the primary benefits of MCS, namely improved quality of life and survival, but, at some centers, it is also a leading disqualification for patients who would otherwise receive a cardiac transplant.[21-22]

Stroke risk in the VAD patient is amplified by pre-existing comorbidities, such as atrial fibrillation. Interestingly, hypertension is the strongest risk factor for stroke in the general population, but its contribution to stroke risk in the VAD population has not been well established.[23] Even if not the primary cause of stroke, traditional stroke risk factors likely contribute to the infarct volume by affecting the viability of cerebral arterioles and the presence of collateral circulation. Several studies have identified female gender as a significant risk factor for ischemic and hemorrhagic stroke, though the physiology underlying this association has not been clarified.[24-25]

The device itself probably increases the likelihood of stroke due to fibrin deposition throughout the assembly. Device thrombosis, defined as in situ clot formation, occurs with higher incidence in the newer VADs due to their smaller size and smaller device components.[26] Device thrombosis, however, does not always lead to stroke, nor is it necessarily the source of embolism when stroke does occur.[21] Chronic low blood flow due to device malfunction or inadequate settings can also predispose to ischemic events. Strokes of this etiology manifest as infarcts in arterial border-zone areas, with patients clinically demonstrating proximal quadriparesis in the case of anterior cerebral artery (ACA)-middle cerebral artery (MCA)

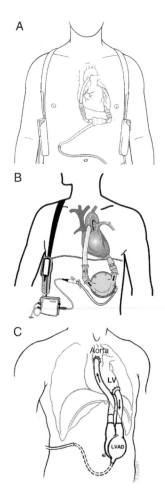

FIGURE 12.1  Ventricular Assist Devices. Figure (A) shows the HeartMate II LVAD, in which blood is pumped continuously from the left ventricle to the ascending aorta. Figure (B) shows the HeartMate XVE LVAD, a pulsatile device, and Figure (C) the Implantable Ventricular Assist Device (IVAD), a versatile device that can function as an LVAD, RVAD, or BiVAD.

Reproduced with permission from Starling RC, Naka Y, Boyle AJ, et al. Results of the Post-US Food and Drug Administration-approval study with a continuous flow left ventricular assist device as a bridge to heart transplantation: a prospective study using the INTERMACS (Interagency Registry for Mechanically Assisted Circulatory Support). *J Am Coll Cardiol.* 2011;57(19):1890–8.

watershed stroke and cortically based visual abnormalities if the MCA-posterior cerebral artery (PCA) zone is affected. Watershed infarcts may also be seen in VA-ECMO patients in whom the common carotid is used for arterial cannulation.

In contrast to the hypoperfusion mechanism of watershed infarcts, VAD patients are also at risk for cerebral hyperperfusion. An identical syndrome is seen in patients who undergo carotid endarterectomy. In a patient with severe carotid stenosis or poor forward flow due to end-stage heart failure, cerebral arterioles are maximally dilated to maintain cerebral blood flow. Following restoration of normal cardiac output via VAD, cerebral edema results when damaged arterioles are unable to constrict in response to the sudden increase in cerebral blood flow. Clinically, cerebral hyperperfusion is manifested by altered mental status, headache, seizure, or focal deficits.[27] Diagnosis can be made with transcranial Doppler, which demonstrates increased flow velocities (up to 300%) through the MCA, or computed tomography (CT) perfusion studies. Noncontrast CT scan is often normal in the acute period, although white matter edema may be seen. Intracerebral hemorrhage (ICH) is the most serious adverse outcome.[28–29]

Due to the anticoagulation/antiplatelet requirements of VADs, patients who experience ischemic stroke are already taking a combination of agents; current guidelines recommend aspirin 81 mg/day and warfarin with an international normalized ratio (INR) goal of 2–2.5 for the HeartMate II. Suboptimal regimens have been found to contribute to thrombus formation; however, patients who stop anticoagulation due to gastrointestinal bleeding do not frequently have strokes.[8,30] Systemic infection has been found to be the most consistent and significant risk factor for ischemic stroke, increasing the risk of stroke by nearly twofold in one institution's experience.[31] The presence of infection in the setting of stroke suggests septic emboli as an etiology. However, even in the absence of documented septic emboli, systemic infection has the potential to alter the coagulation cascade and inflammatory profile.

Patients with left ventricular assist devices (LVAD) are also at risk for hemorrhagic stroke due to their need for long-term anticoagulation, as well as due to an acquired form of von Willebrand factor (vWF) deficiency. After 30 days, nearly all patients on continuous flow VAD support develop loss of large-molecular-weight vWF multimers. These multimers play a key role in primary hemostasis through interactions with platelets. This acquired coagulopathy, however, may be unrelated to ICH.

Endocarditis, due to bacteremia and other systemic infection, also increases the risk for hemorrhage. Lobar hemorrhage, in particular, may suggest an underlying infectious etiology, such as mycotic aneurysm or septic arteritis. A patchy hemorrhage with surrounding hypodensity that corresponds to an arterial territory is suggestive of hemorrhagic infarction. With regard to hemorrhagic transformation (HT) of ischemic stroke, little is known about risk factors leading to this event in LVAD patients. Institutional experience suggests that large stroke volume (>50% of the MCA territory) and cardioembolic etiology are likely risk factors for HT, as they are in the general stroke population.[21]

Air embolism has also been reported as a rare but devastating neurologic consequence of MCS. This complication occurs as a result of intracardiac or intradevice air, most likely introduced at the time of device placement, repair, or exchange. A case of fatal air embolism has also been reported as a consequence of small defects in the diaphragm separating the pump from the blood chambers.[32]

In addition to the vascular consequences just mentioned, LVAD patients are at risk for the same acute neurologic illnesses that plague all critical care patients. These include but are not limited to seizures and status epilepticus, central nervous system infection, critical illness myopathy, compressive neuropathy due to prolonged positioning, and toxic-metabolic encephalopathy.

Patients supported temporarily with percutaneous devices, such the Impella and IABP, are similarly affected by ischemic and hemorrhagic stroke. In the Europella registry of Impella patients, the reported stroke rate was 0.7% among a cohort of 144 patients.[33] IABPs are perhaps a higher risk for ischemic stroke due to their placement directly in the aorta and retrograde blood flow from the descending aorta into the brachiocephalic vessels during the diastolic counter-pulsation phase. A meta-analysis found an absolute increase in stroke risk of 2% in IABP patients compared to similar patients without the device.[34]

Rates of neurologic complications in ECMO patients range from 7% to 50%, varying across institutions and observational databases.[15,35-36] Neurologic sequelae of ECMO are poorly characterized, likely due to low numbers and poor overall survival. Severe neurologic injury is also a frequent reason for ECMO withdrawal, which influences data on the intrinsic mortality of neurologic complications.[35] Reassuringly, however, many of those patients who survive to 30 days after hospital discharge demonstrate no lasting neurologic deficits.[37]

ECMO patients are exposed to the same risk factors that predispose VAD patients to ischemic stroke. Rates of ischemic stroke in ECMO patients range from 3.6% to 8%, and rates of ICH range from 2.5% to 10%. Rates of seizure are much lower (0.2% to 2.5%) and have not been found to affect mortality.[15,35-36] ECMO and IABP patients are at high risk for limb ischemia, which is a consequence of femoral arterial cannulation and subsequent occlusion of that vessel. Limb ischemia may present as loss of distal pulses, pallor, or poor distal arterial flow as detected by duplex ultrasonography.[38] Alternatively, patients may develop ischemic neuropathy in the affected limb that may manifest as foot drop or leg weakness. Management of these neurologic complications is similar to those strategies used for LVAD patients.

## MANAGEMENT OF ACUTE NEUROLOGICAL COMPLICATIONS

The management of acute neurologic events in the VAD patient is not significantly different from that in any other patient. In fact, recommendations regarding management of this population come from the application of existing evidence in the general population. One of the challenges of managing neurologic events in the VAD population, however, stems from their location on cardiac and surgical services, where frequent neurologic checks and exam documentation are not as standardized as on neuro units. Failure to recognize or delays in recognizing acute neurologic changes limits the available treatment options and likely leads to worse outcomes. Some institutions have designated a dedicated vascular neurologist who assists in management of neurologic issues in VAD patients. Columbia University, for example, has implemented a standardized approach to neurologic deficits in this unique population.[21]

### Acute Ischemic Stroke

Given the acuity of stroke and its high incidence in the VAD population, any neurologic deficits should be treated as an acute ischemic stroke until proven otherwise. As outlined in the Columbia University algorithm (Box 12.1), this approach includes documenting "last known normal," performing a focused neurologic exam, and obtaining a noncontrast CT of the head as soon as possible. While the inpatient VAD apparatus can be large and cumbersome, this should not impede prompt neuroimaging. It should be noted, however, that VADs are not compatible with magnetic resonance imaging (MRI).

Clinical trials regarding the efficacy of intravenous recombinant tissue plasminogen activator (rTPA) have not included patients on mechanical circulatory support, and some experts believe that the drug may have limited clinical efficacy in strokes in VAD patients. Thrombi formed within VADs may have a composition (specifically fibrin and denatured protein) that is not amenable to thrombolysis.[39]

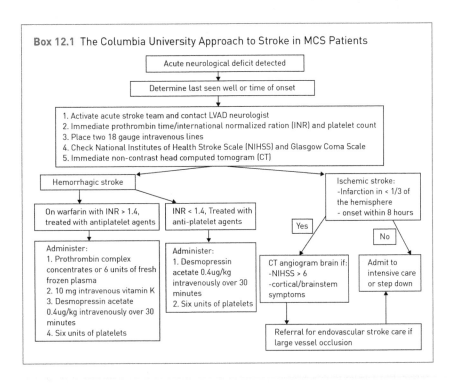

Box 12.1 The Columbia University Approach to Stroke in MCS Patients

Additionally, these patients are at high risk for hemorrhagic complications of rTPA due to the embolic nature of their strokes, the higher potential for systemic infection (which increases the likelihood of septic emboli), and concomitant anticoagulant usage. For these reasons, the use of rTPA in VAD patients should be undertaken with extreme caution.

Recent studies demonstrating the efficacy of endovascular stroke treatment have greatly expanded the options available to acute stroke patients. While these trials did not include patients ineligible for systemic thrombolysis, it is reasonable to consider endovascular therapy for VAD patients.[40] Current American Heart Association/American Stroke Association (AHA/ASA) guidelines recommend endovascular therapy in stroke patients who demonstrate a National Institute of Health Stroke Scale (NIHSS) score of 6 or greater, causative internal carotid or proximal MCA (M1) occlusion, small infarct core as determined by Alberta Stroke Program Early CT Score (ASPECTS) or perfusion imaging, and are ready to undergo groin puncture within 6 hours after symptom onset.[41] In the general stroke population, the incidence of symptomatic ICH (sICH) was not found to be increased in patients who underwent endovascular therapy provided the preceding guidelines were followed.[42-43] There are clinical challenges in managing sedation and anesthesia for endovascular treatment of unstable VAD patients, who may be prone to hemodynamic compromise when anesthetic agents are used. Involving experienced anesthesia leaders in creating protocols and teams to manage these challenging clinical situations is an important aspect of clinical care for these patients. Vessel imaging, as obtained via CT angiography, may be less feasible for the advanced cardiac patient who is likely to have impaired renal function. The applicability of endovascular treatment in the VAD population depends on an individual assessment of risk, predicted disability, and a multidisciplinary discussion of goals of care.

## Intracerebral Hemorrhage

Management of ICH also poses a complex clinical dilemma in the VAD patient. Initial treatment should focus on securing the airway, as indicated, and blood pressure control. Guidelines for primary stroke prevention in VAD patients recommend mean arterial pressures of less than 90 mm Hg, which would also be a reasonable goal in the patient experiencing ICH.[21] A CT scan should be repeated within 24 hours to ensure the hemorrhage has not expanded.

The decision whether to reverse anticoagulation in the setting of ICH is a difficult one. Rapid reversal may lead to device thrombosis, although the likelihood of that event has been shown to be small in one cases series (1 thrombus in 38 episodes of reversal).[44] Given the high mortality associated with hematoma expansion in ICH associated with warfarin use, reversal of anticoagulation is a reasonable option for VAD patients.[45] Current AHA guidelines recommend reversing warfarin with prothrombin complex concentrates (PCC) or fresh frozen plasma. PCC is preferred due to the small volume of infusion and high concentration of vitamin K–dependent clotting factors. An INR within the normal range (usually ≤1.4, though this is laboratory dependent) should be targeted and maintained for 72 hours. VAD patients with ICH are also eligible for platelet transfusion since they are often receiving dual antiplatelet therapy and develop an acquired vWF deficiency. In the setting of larger hematomas (>30 mL), transfusion of platelets and administration of desmopressin (0.3 µg/kg), which enhances platelet adhesion, are recommended. ICH in the setting of therapeutic heparin infusions should be treated with intravenous protamine and cessation of the anticoagulant.

Given the risk of intradevice thrombosis associated with anticoagulation reversal, markers for hemolysis should be monitored daily. These include lactate dehydrogenase, haptoglobin, indirect bilirubin, creatinine, hemoglobin/hematocrit, and plasma free hemoglobin. Increased pump power, changes in pulsatility index, and overt left ventricular failure may also indicate device-related thrombosis.[26]

In the case of suspected hemorrhagic conversion of ischemic stroke (vs. primary ICH), reversal of anticoagulation should be pursued more cautiously. If a primary thrombotic or embolic event has taken place, aggressive reversal could precipitate further strokes.[21]

As with any ICH or stroke patient, normal sodium concentrations and normothermia should be maintained. If cerebral edema occurs, measures to reduce intracranial pressure should be implemented, including elevating the head of the bed to 30 degrees, analgesia and sedation, and avoidance of hypotonic fluids. There is no evidence to support the use of glucocorticoids in this setting. Prophylactic use of antiepileptic drugs in the setting of ICH or stroke has not been shown to be beneficial.[46] There may, however, be a role for their use if a large, lobar hemorrhage is present, or if a convulsion could cause dangerous hemodynamic derangements or dislodgement of the VAD in certain patients.

## Emergency Neurosurgical Intervention

Decompressive hemicraniectomy may be indicated in patients with impaired level of consciousness due to a malignant MCA stroke or a large ICH. Significant mortality benefit is conferred when hemicraniectomy is performed in patients younger than 60 who experience large hemispheric stroke, although studies did not include VAD patients.[47] Data suggest, however, that patients with baseline disability experience less benefit from surgery. Additionally, the decision to proceed to surgery is complicated by the VAD patient's need for antiplatelet and/or anticoagulation and should be pursued only after a detailed risk assessment and consideration of the patient's goals of care. Emergency craniotomy for evacuation of large ICH causing brainstem herniation is also a vexing clinical challenge, with meager documentation of good outcomes to support this practice.

## Resumption of Anticoagulation

Resumption of aspirin following ischemic stroke can occur on the day after imaging confirms a hemorrhagic stroke has not taken place. If there has been hemorrhagic transformation, aspirin can be restarted when the bleed is stable on serial imaging for at least 24 hours. Evidence of device thrombosis may prompt earlier resumption of antiplatelet therapy even if the hemorrhagic zone has expanded. Like many management decisions in the VAD population, a balance needs to be struck between neurologic risk and cardiac risk.

Anticoagulation is generally safe to resume 24 hours after ischemic stroke if no hemorrhagic transformation is present and the total infarct size is less than 50% of the MCA territory, since larger infarcts are more susceptible to hemorrhagic transformation. With large territory infarcts, anticoagulation can usually be restarted 5 days after the event, assuming stability on imaging at that time. Resumption of anticoagulation when a primary ICH has occurred is based on clinical judgment and experience, with some experts waiting until 5 days after the resumption of aspirin to ensure that the bleed is stable with platelet inhibition. Known cerebral amyloid angiopathy in a VAD patient who has experienced an ICH may preclude further anticoagulation. The extent to which amyloid angiopathy may affect the VAD population will likely be an important future issue as device use is expanded to older patients.

## Hyperperfusion Syndrome

In the case of cerebral hyperperfusion syndrome, management centers around prompt recognition of symptoms and rapid reduction in systemic blood pressure, which in turn reduces cerebral perfusion pressure. Labetalol and intravenous nicardipine have been recommended specifically for this purpose. Blood pressure should be strictly controlled until cerebral autoregulation is restored.

## Air Embolism

Air embolism is treated with hyperbaric therapy to reduce the size of the emboli, or 100% oxygen to promote resorption of poorly soluble nitrogen within the emboli. The source of emboli should be located and corrected. If systemic venous air emboli are suspected, patients should be placed in the left lateral decubitus or Trendelenburg position to restrict bubbles to the right ventricle of the heart. This maneuver prevents entry into the pulmonary arteries or passage into the left atrium via a patent foramen ovale.

# Limb Ischemia

Younger ECMO patients tend to be at increased risk for lower limb ischemia due to the larger arterial cannulae used in this population.[38] Many centers insert a down-flow cannula into the superficial femoral artery to maintain perfusion of the leg, though this practice is not being used prophylactically at all centers as it requires additional surgical dissection of the groin.[13,38] This complication highlights the importance of involvement of neurologists in the care of patients on mechanical circulatory support. Leg weakness may be the result of a central or peripheral neurologic insult, and localization of the injury is necessary for effective treatment, especially in critically ill patients in whom prompt CNS imaging is not always an option.

## FUTURE DIRECTIONS

MCS is certain to become more commonplace and safer in the future. The prevalence of heart failure in the United States is only expected to increase with our aging population.[48] It is already evident that the number of hearts available for transplantation will not keep up with this increase in demand. In one observational study, the rate of ECMO in adult patients was found to increase by an astounding 650% over 10 years.[36] Mechanical circulatory support provides temporary and long-term cardiac benefit to this critically ill population. As with any medical intervention, the neurological risks of these devices must be integrated into the treatment model for these patients. Moreover, MCS is an extremely expensive therapy and diverts significant amounts of resources to small numbers of patients. Concurrent neurologic complications have been found to increase the hospitalization costs of ECMO patients by more than US$100,000.[36] MCS providers are thus mandated to minimize neurologic complications both to improve patient outcomes and to ensure the economic sustainability of these therapies. Education of the cardiac care team regarding neurologic complications and early involvement of a neurologist are paramount to ensuring neuroprotection in this population.

## REFERENCES

1. Lazar RM, Shapiro PA, Jaski BE, et al. Neurological events during long-term mechanical circulatory support for heart failure: the Randomized Evaluation of Mechanical Assistance for the Treatment of Congestive Heart Failure (REMATCH) experience. *Circulation.* 2004;109(20):2423–7.

2. Kirklin JK, Naftel DC. Mechanical circulatory support: registering a therapy in evolution. *Circ Heart Fail.* 2008;1(3):200–5.

3. Kirklin JK, Naftel DC, Pagani FD, et al. Sixth INTERMACS annual report: a 10,000-patient database. *J Heart Lung Transplant.* 2014;33(6):555–64.

4. Starling RC, Naka Y, Boyle AJ, et al. Results of the post-U.S. Food and Drug Administration-approval study with a continuous flow left ventricular assist device as a bridge to heart transplantation: a prospective study using the INTERMACS (Interagency Registry for Mechanically Assisted Circulatory Support). *J Am Coll Cardiol.* 2011;57(19):1890–8.

5. Maciver J, Ross HJ. Quality of life and left ventricular assist device support. *Circulation.* 2012;126(7):866–74.

6. Jessup M, Abraham WT, Casey DE, et al. 2009 focused update: ACCF/AHA Guidelines for the Diagnosis and Management of Heart Failure in Adults: a report of the American College of Cardiology Foundation/American Heart Association Task Force on Practice Guidelines: developed in collaboration with the International Society for Heart and Lung Transplantation. *Circulation.* 2009;119(14):1977–2016.

7. Go AS, Mozaffarian D, Roger VL, et al.; American Heart Association Statistics Committee and Stroke Statistics Subcommittee. Heart disease and stroke statistics—2013 update: a report from the American Heart Association. *Circulation.* 2013;127(1):e6–e245.

8. Naidu SS. Novel percutaneous cardiac assist devices: the science of and indications for hemodynamic support. *Circulation.* 2011;123(5):533–43.

9. Mosier JM, Kelsey M, Raz Y, et al. Extracorporeal membrane oxygenation (ECMO) for critically ill adults in the emergency department: history, current applications, and future directions. *Crit Care.* 2015;19:431.

10. Bartlett RHG, Jefferies MR, Huxtable RF, Haiduc NJ, Fong SW. Extracorporeal membrane oxygenation (ECMO) cardiopulmonary support in infancy. *Trans Am Soc Artific Intern Organs.* 1976;22:80–93.

11. Baffes TGF, Bicoff JP, Whitehill JL. Extracorporeal circulation for support of palliative cardiac surgery in infants. *Arch Thoracic Surg.* 1970;10(4):354–63.

12. Peek GJ, Mugford MT, Wilson A, et al.; CESAR trial collaboration. Efficacy and economic assessment of conventional ventilatory support versus extracorporeal membrane oxygenation for severe adult respiratory failure (CESAR): a multicentre randomised controlled trial. *Lancet.* 2009;374(9698):1351–63.

13. Marasco SF, Lukas G, McDonald M, McMillan J, Ihle B. Review of ECMO (extra corporeal membrane oxygenation) support in critically ill adult patients. *Heart Lung Circ.* 2008;17 Suppl 4:S41–7.

14. Abrams D, Combes A, Brodie D. Extracorporeal membrane oxygenation in cardiopulmonary disease in adults. *J Am Coll Cardiol.* 2014;63(25 Pt A):2769–78.

15. Mateen FJ, Muralidharan R, Shinohara RT, Parisi JE, Schears GJ, Wijdicks EF. Neurological injury in adults treated with extracorporeal membrane oxygenation. *Arch Neurol.* 2011;68(12):1543–9.

16. Guttendorf J, Boujoukos AJ, Ren D, Rosenzweig MQ, Hravnak M. Discharge outcome in adults treated with extracorporeal membrane oxygenation. *Am J Crit Care.* 2014;23(5):365–77.

17. Conrad SA, Rycus PT, Dalton H. Extracorporeal Life Support Registry Report 2004. *ASAIO J.* 2005;51(1):4–10.

18. Stehlik J, Johnson SA, Selzman CH. Gold standard in anticoagulation assessment of left ventricular assist device patients?: how about bronze. *JACC Heart Failure.* 2015;3(4):323–6.

19. Tsukui H, Abla A, Teuteberg JJ, et al. Cerebrovascular accidents in patients with a ventricular assist device. *J Thoracic Cardiovasc Surg.* 2007;134(1):114–23.

20. Yuan N, Arnaoutakis GJ, George TJ, et al. The spectrum of complications following left ventricular assist device placement. *J Card Surg.* 2012;27(5):630–8.

21. Willey JZ, Demmer RT, Takayama H, Colombo PC, Lazar RM. Cerebrovascular disease in the era of left ventricular assist devices with continuous flow: risk factors, diagnosis, and treatment. *J Heart Lung Transplant.* 2014;33(9):878–87.

22. Patlolla V, Mogulla V, DeNofrio D, Konstam MA, Krishnamani R. Outcomes in patients with symptomatic cerebrovascular disease undergoing heart transplantation. *J Am Coll Cardiol.* 2011;58(10):1036–41.

23. Willey JZ. Blood pressure and stroke risk in left ventricular assist devices. *J Heart Lung Transplant.* 2015;34(4):497–8.

24. Morris AA, Pekarek A, Wittersheim K, et al. Gender differences in the risk of stroke during support with continuous-flow left ventricular assist device. *J Heart Lung Transplant.* 2015;34(12):1570–7.

25. Bogaev RC, Pamboukian SV, Moore SA, et al.; HeartMate II Clinical Investigators. Comparison of outcomes in women versus men using a continuous-flow left ventricular assist device as a bridge to transplantation. *J Heart Lung Transplant.* 2011;30(5):515–22.

26. Tchantchaleishvili V, Sagebin F, Ross RE, Hallinan W, Schwarz KQ, Massey HT. Evaluation and treatment of pump thrombosis and hemolysis. *Ann Cardiothoracic Surg.* 2014;3(5):490–5.

27. Lietz K, Brown K, Ali SS, et al. The role of cerebral hyperperfusion in postoperative neurologic dysfunction after left ventricular assist device implantation for end-stage heart failure. *J Thoracic Cardiovasc Surg.* 2009;137(4):1012–9.

28. Mussivand T. Neurological dysfunction associated with mechanical circulatory support: complications that still need attention. *Artific Organs.* 2008;32(11):831-4.

29. Lieb M, Shah U, Hines GL. Cerebral hyperperfusion syndrome after carotid intervention: a review. *Cardiol Rev.* 2012;20(2):84–9.

30. Najjar SS, Slaughter MS, Pagani FD, et al.; HVAD Bridge to Transplant ADVANCE Trial Investigators. An analysis of pump thrombus events in patients in the HeartWare ADVANCE bridge to transplant and continued access protocol trial. *J Heart Lung Transplant.* 2014;33(1):23–34.

31. Kato TS, Schulze PC, Yang J, et al. Pre-operative and post-operative risk factors associated with neurologic complications in patients with advanced heart failure supported by a left ventricular assist device. *J Heart Lung Transplant.* 2012;31(1):1–8.

32. Elkind MSV, Chin SS, Rose EA. Massive air embolism with left ventricular assist device. *Neurology.* 2002;58(11):1694.

33. Sjauw KD, Konorza T, Erbel R, et al. Supported high-risk percutaneous coronary intervention with the Impella 2.5 device the Europella registry. *J Am Coll Cardiol.* 2009;54(25):2430–4.

34. Sjauw KD, Engstrom AE, Vis MM, et al. A systematic review and meta-analysis of intra-aortic balloon pump therapy in ST-elevation myocardial infarction: should we change the guidelines? *Eur Heart J.* 2009;30(4):459–68.

35. Lan C, Tsai PR, Chen YS, Ko WJ. Prognostic factors for adult patients receiving extracorporeal membrane oxygenation as mechanical circulatory support--a 14-year experience at a medical center. *Artif Organs.* 2010;34(2):E59–64.

36. Nasr DM, Rabinstein AA. Neurologic complications of extracorporeal membrane oxygenation. *J Clin Neurol.* 2015;11(4):383–9.

37. Risnes I, Wagner K, Nome T, et al. Cerebral outcome in adult patients treated with extracorporeal membrane oxygenation. *Ann Thoracic Surg.* 2006;81(4):1401–6.

38. Foley PJ, Morris RJ, Woo EY, et al. Limb ischemia during femoral cannulation for cardiopulmonary support. *J Vasc Surg.* 2010;52(4):850–3.

39. Starling RC, Moazami N, Silvestry SC, et al. Unexpected abrupt increase in left ventricular assist device thrombosis. *N Engl J Med.* 2014;370(1):33–40.

40. Al-Mufti F, Bauerschmidt A, Claassen J, Meyers PM, Colombo PC, Willey JZ. Neuroendovascular interventions for acute ischemic strokes in patients supported with left ventricular assist devices: a single-center case series and review of the literature. *World Neurosurg.* 2016;88:199–204.

41. Powers WJ, Derdeyn CP, Biller J, et al.; American Heart Association Stroke Council. 2015 American Heart Association/American Stroke Association Focused Update of the 2013 Guidelines for the Early Management of Patients with Acute Ischemic Stroke Regarding Endovascular Treatment: a guideline for healthcare professionals from the American Heart Association/American Stroke Association. *Stroke*. 2015;46(10):3020–35.

42. Campbell BC, Mitchell PJ, Kleinig TJ, et al.; EXTEND-IA Investigators. Endovascular therapy for ischemic stroke with perfusion-imaging selection. *N Engl J Med*. 2015;372(11):1009–18.

43. Berkhemer OA, Fransen PS, Beumer D, et al.; MR CLEAN Investigators. A randomized trial of intraarterial treatment for acute ischemic stroke. *N Engl J Med*. 2015;372(1):11–20.

44. Jennings DL, Jacob M, Chopra A, Nemerovski CW, Morgan JA, Lanfear DE. Safety of anticoagulation reversal in patients supported with continuous-flow left ventricular assist devices. *ASAIO J*. 2014;60(4):381–4.

45. Brouwers HB, Chang Y, Falcone GJ, et al. Predicting hematoma expansion after primary intracerebral hemorrhage. *JAMA Neurol*. 2014;71(2):158–64.

46. Jauch EC, Cucchiara B, Adeoye O, et al. Part 11: adult stroke: 2010 American Heart Association Guidelines for Cardiopulmonary Resuscitation and Emergency Cardiovascular Care. *Circulation*. 2010;122(18 Suppl 3):S818–28.

47. Huttner HB, Schwab S. Malignant middle cerebral artery infarction: clinical characteristics, treatment strategies, and future perspectives. *Lancet Neurol*. 2009;8(10):949–58.

48. Heidenreich PA, Albert NM, Allen LA, et al.; American Heart Association Advocacy Coordinating Committee; Council on Arteriosclerosis, Thrombosis and Vascular Biology; Council on Cardiovascular Radiology and Intervention; Council on Clinical Cardiology; Council on Epidemiology and Prevention; Stroke Council. Forecasting the impact of heart failure in the United States: a policy statement from the American Heart Association. *Circulation Heart Failure*. 2013;6(3):606–19.

# 13 Neuroprotection in Sepsis and Acute Respiratory Distress Syndrome

Neha S. Dangayach, Charles L. Francoeur,

Stephan A. Mayer, and Tarek Sharshar

## GENERAL CONSIDERATIONS

Sepsis and acute respiratory distress syndrome (ARDS) result from insults that trigger complex immune and inflammatory systemic responses. The acute brain dysfunction that occurs in these patients is one of the most frequent and earliest manifestation of sepsis-related multiple organ dysfunction syndrome (MODS). This syndrome can evolve from simple confusion with inattention and disorganized thinking, to delirium with fluctuating level of consciousness to coma.[1] Sepsis-associated encephalopathy (SAE) is defined as any brain dysfunction that is related to septic illness that is not a direct consequence of central nervous system infection (e.g., meningitis), hypoperfusion, or hypoxia. It is the product of multiple interacting factors, including neurotransmitter derangements, microglial activation, mitochondrial dysfunction, blood–brain barrier (BBB) disruption, and dysregulation of the immune system with an imbalanced inflammatory response.[2–3] Knowledge of the complex pathophysiology of SAE has been hampered by multiple definitions of the syndrome and the fact that it is an evolving concept in search of standardized and highly generalizable diagnostic criteria.

### Epidemiology

The incidence of SAE varies enormously depending on how it is defined and diagnosed and the population studied. In peritonitis patients, it ranges from a mere 9% incidence when defined as coma, to 50% when defined as any kind of alteration of mental status.[4]

SAE undoubtedly represents a significant proportion of ICU delirium. In ARDS patients, the incidence of delirium has been observed to be 70%.[5] The role that SAE may play as a distinct entity is difficult to ascertain, given the large number of coexisting metabolic derangements (i.e., hypoxia, hypoglycemia, acidosis, renal failure) that can alter cerebral function and the effects of medications (especially sedatives, analgesics and antibiotics). Patients with underlying hepatic or renal dysfunction that impairs clearance of drugs and drug metabolites are more prone to developing medication-induced encephalopathy.

## Outcome

SAE has been associated with increased mortality risk.[6] Among ventilated patients, the presence of delirium was associated with up to a threefold increase in mortality.[7] Among septic patients with SAE, a greater severity of encephalopathy was associated with lower survival.[4]

An emerging concept is that SAE is not a simple, reversible syndrome, but rather is an injury with long-lasting consequences.[7] The BRAIN-ICU study enrolled patients who had respiratory failure or shock in a medical or surgical ICU and no pre-existing cognitive impairment.[8] Patients were evaluated for in-hospital delirium and cognitive function at 3 and 12 months after hospital discharge. At 3 months, 40% of this cohort had global cognition scores 1.5 standard deviations (SDs) below the population mean, and 26% had scores 2.0 SDs below the population mean. Cognitive impairment occurred in both younger and older patients and persisted at 12 months, as 34% of the sample had global cognition scores 1.5 SD below the population mean and 24% had scores 2.0 SD below the population mean. In a cohort study of patients with severe sepsis, there was a 10% absolute increase in the prevalence of moderate to severe cognitive impairment within an 8-year follow-up period.[9] Survivors of sepsis had three times the odds of long-term moderate to severe cognitive impairment compared to those who did not develop sepsis. This association was not seen after general hospital admissions that did not involve sepsis. Among ARDS survivors, up to 47% demonstrated neurocognitive sequelae at 2 years.[10] A study that examined the relationship between SAE and long-term cognitive outcome found that attention was particularly impaired (median time since ICU discharge was 6 years).[11] In the ARDS Cognitive Outcomes Study (ACOS), 122 ARDS survivors underwent telephone neuropsychological assessments at 2 and 12 months.[12] Long-term cognitive dysfunction was present in more than half the survivors.

These data speak to the burden upon patients and their caregivers related to long-term deficits, from what was previously thought to be a completely reversible encephalopathy. The deleterious impact of SAE on quality of life is also well-documented, and the societal and financial consequences are enormous due to the inability of many survivors to return to work, higher health care resources utilization, and earlier institutionalization.[13] There is an urgency for the critical care community to better understand the mechanisms underlying neurological injury secondary to sepsis and ARDS in order to prevent long-term disastrous consequences.

## MECHANISMS OF AND RISKS FOR NEUROLOGIC INJURY

The pathophysiology of SAE involves two key processes: (1) neuroinflammation due to BBB dysfunction, microglial activation, and cytokine-mediated neurological injury; and (2) ischemia due to impaired cerebral perfusion, endothelial activation, loss of cerebral autoregulation, and microcirculatory dysfunction.[14–16] These two processes are not mutually exclusive.

BBB disruption causes the brain to come in contact with circulating tumor necrosis factor-α (TNFα) and interleukin 1 (IL-1). This leads to endothelial dysfunction and an increase in mediators of inflammation, such as vascular cell adhesion molecule 1 (VCAM-1) and intercellular adhesion molecule 1 (ICAM-1), that is proportional to the extent of BBB disruption. This in turn causes increased production of reactive oxygen species and inducible nitric oxide synthase (iNOS), which upregulates the production of reactive NOS, glial activation, and mitochondrial dysfunction. This leads to further BBB disruption, endothelial activation, inflammation, and cytotoxic edema. Microvascular dysfunction causes cerebral ischemia, which eventually leads to fibrinoid necrosis. The most important cytokine mediators of SAE appear to be IL-1 and TNFα. Neuroinflammation and dysregulation of cerebral perfusion leads to mitochondrial dysfunction and apoptosis and creates an imbalance between inhibitory and excitotoxic neurotransmitters.[17]

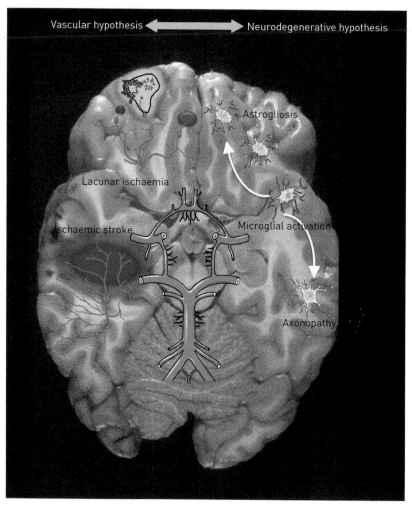

FIGURE 13.1 Mechanisms of sepsis-associated encephalopathy.
From Mazeraud A, Pascal Q, Verdonk F, Heming N, Chrétien F, Sharshar T. Neuroanatomy and physiology of brain dysfunction in sepsis. Clin Chest Med. 2016;37(2):333–45.

In the ischemic process, micro- and macro-circulatory failure, in combination with clotting disorders, results in impaired oxygen and nutrient supply and leads to ischemia and hemorrhage. In the neuroinflammatory process, the key step is endothelial activation that induces microcirculatory dysfunction and BBB alteration, which allows the passage of neurotoxic mediators into the brain, notably inflammatory mediators (see Figure 13.1 and Table 13.1).[18] The main consequence of these two processes is cellular dysfunction, notably via oxidative stress, that affects all brain cells. Activation of microglial cells has also been observed and implicated. Alteration of neurotransmission accounts for the clinical features of encephalopathy. Long-term cognitive decline may be related to Alzheimer's disease–type processes involving microglial activation and vascular-type processes related to diffuse ischemic damage.

## Risks for Acute Neurological Dysfunction

Studies examining risk factors for neurological impairment in septic and ARDS patients have resulted in inconsistent findings due to varying definitions of neurological impairment. In the general ICU population, pre-existing factors consistently recognized as risk factors for delirium include pre-existing dementia, history of hypertension, a history of alcohol abuse, and higher severity of illness at admission. Age and benzodiazepine usage have been found to be predictive in some studies, but not others.[19] In the ARDS population, the most recent studies assessing patients with the Confusion Assessment Method- Intensive Care Unit (CAM-ICU) report similar findings, with ARDS itself being a strong predictor for delirium after adjustment for known confounders.[5] It is more difficult to determine risk factors specific to SAE because there are very few studies and varying definitions of SAE. Overall, greater severity of illness appears to be related to higher incidence of SAE, without any other strong predictors.

Patient-related factors that increase the risk of delirium and SAE include higher Acute Physiology and Chronic Health Evaluation II (APACHE-II) scores; renal dysfunction; elevated blood urea nitrogen, bilirubin, lactate, and sodium levels; lower Glasgow Coma Scale (GCS) scores; and lower pH, serum albumin, platelet, and blood pressure levels.[20–22] SAE-related delirium can be seen in patients with gram-positive/gram-negative bacteremia, with the most common sources being biliary or intestinal infections.[21] Certain organisms and infections that predispose to the development of SAE include biliary tract/intestinal infections, *Staphylococcus aureus*, *Enterococcus faecium*, *Acinetobacter* spp., and *Pseudomonas aeruginosa*.[21]

## Other Metabolic and Inflammatory Changes

Dysregulation of nuclear factor-κB (NF-κB), which plays a key role in the inflammatory response and has diverse functions in the nervous system, interrupts leptin/insulin secretion at the hypothalamic level and leads to hyperglycemia.[23] Hypernatremia is common in SAE due to relative vasopressin deficiency, possibly due to disruption of central sodium-level sensing mechanisms.[23–24] There is an imbalance between pro- and anti-inflammatory mediators that causes pathological changes in vital organs and systems, including metabolic changes such as hyperglycemia, hyponatremia, and hyperlactatemia.[25] The effects of hepatic or renal dysfunction add to worsening encephalopathy in patients with SAE due to

**Table 13.1** Homeostatic Cellular Function in the Brain and Pathophysiology During Sepsis-Induced Encephalopathy[18]

| | Cell Type | Homeostatic Function | Cellular Changes | Mechanisms | Consequences |
|---|---|---|---|---|---|
| Glial cells | Astrocytes | Synaptic plasticity, neurovascular coupling, microenvironment homeostasy, BBB formation | Astrogliosis in mouse model but not in patients | Unknown | ↑BBB permeability Neuroinflammation Mediator of tissue damage |
| | Oligodendrocytes | Myelin sheath formation and maintenance | Unknown | Unknown | Worse myelination development, potential cognitive impairment |
| | Microglial cells | Innate immune system of the central nervous system Inflammatory cell recruitment | Microgliosis, modification of their activation state, M1 or M2 phenotype | Vagal nerve stimulation, 107 IL-1β and TNFα exposure Other activating factors | Excitotoxic compound release iNOS expression Neuroinflammation |
| Blood vessels | Endothelial cells | Blood vessel lining in their lumen Role in coagulation, vasoconstriction and vasodilation, inflammation | Endothelial activation Inflammatory mediator leakage and production Cell recruitment | TNFα and other cytokine exposure | ↑BBB permeability Microthrombi Infarct Ischemic lesions |
| | Pericytes | Blood vessel stabilization, vasoconstriction, vasodilation | Unknown | — | ↑BBB Premeability Microthrombi, ischemic lesion, infarct Supply/demand oxygen inadequation |
| Choroid plexus | Ependymal cell | Cerebrospinal fluid production and resorption | Unknown | — | — |
| | Neurons | Information processing | Dysfunction (long-term potentiation) apoptosis | Glutamate excitotoxicity Metabolic impairment | Cognitive impairment |

↑ represents an increase ; BBB, blood-brain barrier; IL, interleukin; iNOS, inducible nitric oxide synthase; TNF, tumor necrosis factor.

prolonged or inadequate clearance of medications. This may potentiate the sedative effects of benzodiazepines and their active metabolites. Fever also occurs with cytokine effects on the hypothalamus. Cytokines such as TNFα cause direct and indirect endothelial damage.[26] IL-1, IL-2, IL-8 are increased in inflammatory delirium, while IL-10 and amyloid-β are increased in noninflammatory delirium.[27–28] Increased severity of sepsis and multiorgan dysfunction leads to the development of SAE plus neuromyopathy.[29–30]

## Long-Term Neurological Deficits

Approximately one-third of critically ill patients present with long-term neuropsychological impairment, including memory, attention, verbal fluency, and executive function impairment.[8] In the general ICU population, the strongest predictors of long-term global cognition impairment are episodes of acute brain dysfunction and the presence of sepsis.[8] Longer duration of delirium is associated with worse long-term global cognition independently of sedative or analgesic medication use, age, pre-existing cognitive impairment, coexisting conditions, or coexisting organ failure during ICU care. In ARDS patients, duration of hypoxia and of hypotension correlates with poorer cognitive performance at discharge and 1 year after discharge.[10] Contrary to previous paradigms, ICU length of stay, APACHE II score, duration of sedation and analgesia, and duration of intubation do not predict long-term neurocognitive impairment. In septic patients, use of mechanical ventilation was not associated with worse cognitive outcome. In the general ICU population, benzodiazepines, analgesics, and other sedatives were not associated with long-term cognitive impairment. Cognitive decline after an episode of sepsis that is complicated by acute brain dysfunction has a detrimental impact on long-term quality of life.[9] Thus, the available evidence shows that acute brain dysfunction is the mediator by which all other clinical risk factors produce or predict long-term cognitive impairment. Avoidance of acute SAE is probably the best way to prevent long-term consequences.[31]

## MONITORING FOR NEUROLOGICAL INJURY

Patients with sepsis and septic shock require very close multimodal monitoring to diagnose acute brain dysfunction.

### Clinical Examination

Sepsis alerts are commonly triggered when patients meet certain criteria for respiratory rate, temperature, blood pressure, and altered mentation.[32] This risk can be assessed using a bedside clinical score, the quick Sepsis-related Organ Failure Assessment (qSOFA). The new consensus definition of sepsis includes altered mentation, which highlights that acute brain dysfunction occurs early in the course of sepsis.[32]

Monitoring for neurological injury in patients with sepsis or ARDS, as in any other critically ill patient population, usually starts with clinical examination. This can be performed using validated structured assessment tools, such as the CAM-ICU, the Intensive Care Delirium Screening Checklist (ICDSC), or the GCS, along with a focused neurological exam to look for focal neurological signs or neck stiffness.[14] Both the CAM-ICU and ICDSC have been validated for detecting delirium.

Current Society of Critical Care Medicine (SCCM) guidelines recommend routine delirium screening in the ICU.[19]

The accuracy of a focused neurological examination in septic ICU patients may be confounded by the degree of sedation. Variability in the pharmacokinetics of sedative medications related to hepatic or renal dysfunction further complicate clinical assessments. For this reason, neurological assessments should always be performed off sedation whenever possible.

Clinical examination, however, only provides a snapshot of the patient's condition and can potentially miss fluctuations or progressive neurological injury unless there are scheduled sedation breaks to facilitate clinical examination. In patients with primary neurological disorders (e.g., traumatic brain injury) and in neurosurgical patients, hourly examinations (aka "neurochecks") are warranted in the acute setting for detecting worsening from intracranial hemorrhage or cerebral edema. Prolonged use, however, may be harmful due to sleep deprivation.[33] For patients with ARDS or sepsis without primary neurological injury, it is not clear how frequently neurochecks should be performed.

## Continuous Electroencephalography

There are different types of abnormal continuous electroencephalography (cEEG) patterns that may be seen in SAE, including triphasic waves, generalized periodic epileptiform discharges (GPEDs), lateralized epileptiform discharges, and generalized slowing.[21] Young et al. studied 69 septic patients, 49 of whom had some degree of encephalopathy that was categorized as either mild or severe.[34] They identified five classes of EEG patterns that were associated with worsened outcome in ascending order of severity: (1) normal EEG, (2) excessive $\theta$ (theta), (3) predominant $\delta$ (delta), (4) triphasic waves, and (5) suppression or burst suppression. Mortality was also associated with the severity of EEG abnormality, with an incidence of 0% in patients with normal EEG, 19% in patients with excessive $\theta$, 36% in patients with predominant $\delta$, 50% in patients with triphasic waves, and 67% in patients with suppression or burst suppression. It is important to note that a burst suppression EEG pattern in SAE, unlike in anoxic-ischemic encephalopathy, may not always indicate a grave prognosis since recovery is possible with ongoing support.

With the advent of electronic databases and computerized recording, it has become feasible to record large amounts of EEG data from many critically ill patients simultaneously.[35] Critically ill patients with sepsis frequently have coexisting toxic-metabolic insults that may cause both mental status changes and seizures. These include but are not limited to hyponatremia, hypoglycemia and hyperglycemia, hypocalcemia, drug intoxication and withdrawal, uremia, hepatic failure, and hypertensive encephalopathy.[36]

In a study of 201 medical ICU patients without brain injury who underwent cEEG, 22% were found to have had periodic epileptiform discharges (PEDs) or seizures. Sepsis and acute renal failure were significantly associated with electrographic seizures.[37] In a retrospective study of critically ill patients who underwent cEEG monitoring, 21% of the patients with toxic metabolic encephalopathies were found to have had nonconvulsive seizures.[38] Comatose patients were more likely to have their first seizure recorded after more than 24 hours of monitoring, compared to noncomatose patients (20% vs. 5%; odds ratio [OR] 4.5, $P = 0.018$).

Nonictal EEG abnormalities are observed even in septic patients with relatively normal cognition in about 50% of cases.[21] The prevalence of electrographic seizures has been found to be 10–16% among septic patients, with nonconvulsive status epilepticus (NCSE) in about 11%.[39-40] Nonconvulsive seizures have been associated with poor outcome in two cohorts of critically ill septic patients, one from a medical ICU and another from a surgical ICU.[37,41] In the surgical ICU septic patients, nonconvulsive seizures were associated with a 10 times higher odds of a poor outcome.

EEG interpretation for critically ill patients requires expertise. There is excellent inter-rater agreement for generalized periodic discharges ($k = 0.81$), but inter-rater agreement for triphasic waves (a subtype of generalized periodic discharges), which are usually associated with metabolic encephalopathy, is poor ($k = 0.33$).[42] Triphasic waves are usually not associated with seizures, whereas other generalized periodic discharges are associated with seizures. A prospective study of ICU patients with sepsis that examined standard EEG recordings performed for 20 minutes within 3 days of ICU admission observed low voltage in 65%, predominant $\theta$ rhythm in 48%, absence of reactivity in 25%, PEDs in 19%, electrographic seizures in 15%, and triphasic waves in 6%.[43] The presence of an electrographic seizure was associated with delirium, and the presence of a $\delta$-predominant rhythm was associated with subsequent development of delirium.[43] The absence of EEG reactivity has been associated with increased mortality in two studies of septic patients.[40,43] Thus, nonconvulsive seizures and periodic discharges commonly occur in septic patients. Early recognition and treatment may help reduce mortality and morbidity in these patients.

## Evoked Potentials

Sensory evoked potentials (SEPs) are a sensitive means of detecting SAE. The prevalence of SAE is greater when detected by SEPs than when identified by clinical criteria.[44] In a study of 68 medical ICU patients studied within 48 hours of severe sepsis or septic shock, subcortical SEP (N13–N20 peaks) pathways were impaired in 34% of patients, and cortical SEP (N20–N70) pathways were impaired in 84% of patients, indicating diffuse dysfunction. In another study, peak latencies were significantly prolonged in patients with severe sepsis and septic shock.[45]

An advantage of evoked potential studies is that sedation does not affect their reliability, unlike cEEG. A recent systematic review of EEG and SEP concluded that both cEEG and evoked potentials are sensitive for diagnosing SAE (although not specific) because they can be abnormal before clinical symptoms develop.[39]

EEG and evoked potentials provide both diagnostic and prognostic information. They are, however, resource intensive, as well-trained individuals are needed to record and interpret these studies. It is easier to perform cEEG in critically ill patients, in contrast to evoked potentials. Similar to a clinical examination, evoked potentials provide a snapshot of a patient's condition, as compared to cEEG which provides continuous neuromonitoring. Current recommendations for cEEG monitoring in critically ill patients suggest that cEEG should be used to monitor comatose patients with unexplained and persistent altered consciousness.[46] At centers where it is available, cEEG monitoring should be utilized early in patients with sepsis or ARDS who develop encephalopathy.

## Cerebrospinal Fluid

Cerebrospinal fluid (CSF) studies are usually normal in patients with SAE.[47–48] CSF has been reported to be normal in an autopsy study of patients with sepsis and cerebral microabscesses.[48]

## Serological Biomarkers

In a systematic review, Zenaide et al. concluded that neuron-specific enolase (NSE) and S-100 calcium-binding protein B (S-100B) are well-established nonspecific markers of neurological injury, not just in disease processes such as hypoxic ischemic encephalopathy and traumatic brain injury, but also in sepsis.[49] These serological markers, along with clinical examination and neurophysiological studies, may aid in identifying septic or ARDS patients at risk for developing SAE, but further work is needed before biomarkers are integrated into standard clinical practice.

## Brain Imaging

Computed tomography (CT) or magnetic resonance imaging (MRI) may be difficult to obtain in patients with sepsis or ARDS, particularly when they are hemodynamically unstable or have very high oxygenation demands.[50–51] In patients with new-onset encephalopathy and fever, CT of the chest, abdomen, and pelvis may reveal a source of infection, while CT of the head may reveal the presence of an intracranial abscess, stroke, or hemorrhage. The optimal timing for obtaining a brain MRI in septic shock remains unknown. In patients who do not have focal neurological deficits, MRI of the brain may be completely normal or show evidence of multifocal infarcts, microhemorrhages, or leukoencephalopathy. The most consistent MRI finding in SAE is cytotoxic edema.[52] The utility of brain MRI in this patient population may increase when performed in the setting of focal neurological signs or progressive worsening in mental status or coma.[53]

Functional neuroimaging techniques, such as xenon CT, CT-perfusion, positron emission tomography (PET), functional MRI, and MR spectroscopy can be used to measure global and regional blood flow or metabolism.[54] These techniques have been studied in animal models of sepsis, but they have not been investigated in prospective studies of patients with sepsis and ARDS.

## Cerebral Autoregulation Monitoring

Patients with sepsis usually suffer from early microcirculatory impairment.[55] Sepsis is associated with cardiovascular changes that may lead to development of tissue hypoperfusion. Early recognition of sepsis and tissue hypoperfusion is critical to implement appropriate hemodynamic support and in preventing irreversible organ damage.[56] Optimization of cerebral perfusion in SAE patients is challenging, and appropriate monitoring techniques for cerebral perfusion and detection of autoregulatory dysfunction have not been well established. Small cohort studies have utilized noninvasive monitoring techniques, such as transcranial Doppler for monitoring cerebral autoregulation using $CO_2$ reactivity.[57] Similarly, near-infrared spectroscopy (NIRS) has been evaluated in small cohort studies.[58–59] Further data are required before integration of these techniques into clinical practice (see Figure 13.2 for a simplified diagnostic algorithm for patients with suspected SAE).[60]

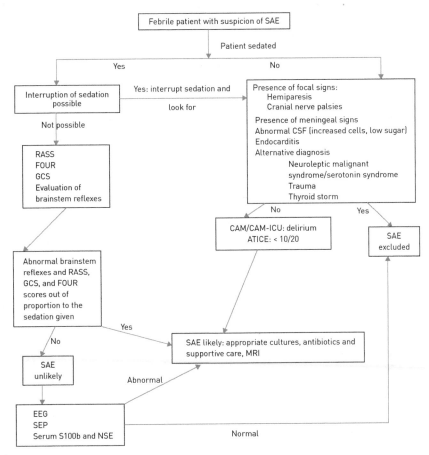

FIGURE 13.2 Algorithm for diagnosis of sepsis associated encephalopathy.
*RASS,* Richmond Agitation-Sedation Scale; *FOUR,* Full Online of Unresponsiveness; *GCS,* Glasgow
Coma Scale; *SEP,* somatosensory evoked potentials; *NSE,* neuron-specific enolase; *CAM/CAM-ICU,* Confusion Assessment Method (Intensive Care Unit); *ATICE,* Adaptation to Intensive Care
Environment.
From Chaudhry N, Duggal A. Sepsis associated encephalopathy. *Adv Med.* 2014;2014:762320.

## NEUROPROTECTION STRATEGIES
### Physiological Interventions

Similar to all ICU patients, sepsis and ARDS patient care should include daily sedation breaks, spontaneous breathing trials, prevention of hyperglycemia, sleep promotion strategies, and early mobilization. These efforts may help reduce the risk of delirium.

### Cerebral Blood Flow and Cerebral Autoregulation

In a retrospective analysis, hypotension was the only predictor of SAE.[22] Mean arterial pressure, however, is not the only determinant of cerebral blood flow (CBF). CBF is also affected by chemical, metabolic, neural, and myogenic factors.[61] CBF is very sensitive to changes in arterial partial pressure of carbon dioxide ($PaCO_2$); hypercapnia increases CBF, whereas hypocapnia decreases it. Cerebral autoregulation may be impaired early during sepsis.[62] Multiple small studies show conflicting data on the effect of $CO_2$ and cerebral autoregulation. Determining an appropriate $CO_2$ goal is therefore limited by inadequate methods for assessing autoregulation at the bedside, use of sedative and vasoactive medication, and variable responses in intubated versus non-intubated patients.[63]

## Glycemic Control

Tight glycemic control (90–108 mg/dL) has been refuted as a method for improving outcome in multiple studies since the original Van den Berghe study in septic patients, although continuous insulin infusions are still commonly used to minimize variability in the range of 120–180 mg/dL.[25,64] Krinsley et al. identified patients at risk for developing severe hypoglycemia in a retrospective study and found that septic shock, diabetes mellitus, and higher APACHE-II scores were associated with an increased risk of severe hypoglycemia and mortality.[65] Both hyperglycemia (a powerful pro-inflammatory mediator) and hypoglycemia are harmful in patients with sepsis and septic shock.[66]

## Therapeutic Temperature Modulation

Targeted temperature management (TTM) has been used as a neuroprotective strategy in animal models of sepsis and septic shock. Schortgen et al. conducted a randomized controlled trial of surface cooling for 48 hours in febrile patients with septic shock to achieve normothermia, compared to no external cooling.[67] Surface cooling resulted in a reduction in vasopressor requirements and early (14-day) mortality (19% vs. 34%, $P = 0.013$). Villar et al. also found that mild hypothermia (32–35°C) reduced mortality in a small pilot study of ARDS patients.[68] Additional studies are needed to conclusively show benefit of such a strategy in this patient population.[69]

## Pharmacologic Interventions

Pharmacologic treatment and prevention of delirium is an active area of research, but few investigators have focused on SAE. The Safety and Efficacy of Dexmedetomidine Compared with Midazolam (SEDCOM) trial was an international multicenter double-blind randomized controlled trial (RCT) comparing sedation with dexmedetomidine (an $\alpha_2$ adrenoreceptor agonist) versus benzodiazepines in 375 mechanically ventilated medical/surgical ICU patients.[70] It demonstrated an impressive reduction in delirium incidence, from 77% in the benzodiazepine group to 54% in the dexmedetomidine group ($P$ <0.001). This corroborated the findings of an earlier double-blind RCT of 106 mechanically ventilated medical/surgical ICU patients, the Maximizing Efficacy of Targeted Sedation and Reducing Neurological Dysfunction (MENDS) trial.[71] In this study, patients in the dexmedetomidine group had more days alive without delirium or coma (7 vs. 3; $P = 0.01$) and a lower prevalence of coma (63% vs. 92%; $P$ <0.001). An a priori subgroup analysis of septic patients found that septic patients who received dexmedetomidine had more delirium-free days, more ventilator-free days, and a 70% reduction in the hazard ratio for death at 28 days compared to septic patients who received lorazepam.[72] The daily risks of delirium were also strongly reduced (OR 0.3 [0.1, 0.9]). The putative neuroprotective mechanisms of dexmedetomidine include anti-inflammatory, antiapoptotic, and sympatholytic effects, as well as sleep architecture preservation.

One small RCT analyzed the effect of the now defunct drotrecogin alfa on S-100B levels in 54 SAE patients with pneumonia-induced septic shock.[73] There was a decrease in S-100B levels in the intervention group, but it was not clinically significant. Another small RCT investigated the effect of a perfusion of n-3 fatty acids for 7 days in septic patients.[74] They did not find any difference in incidence of SAE or levels of S-100B and NSE. To our knowledge, no human trials specific to SAE have evaluated clinical outcomes. Numerous interventions have been studied in animal models, with various degrees of success. These include erythropoietin (EPO), intravenous immunoglobulin (IVIG), valproic acid, and L-ascorbate.[75–78] The main outcomes studied have been neuronal loss/apoptosis or behavioral/cognitive impairment. Currently, none of these has been translated into human clinical trials.

Concerning ARDS-induced delirium and long-term cognitive outcome, two RCTs explored the effect of specific treatments. The EDEN trial, a multicenter, open-label, randomized study comparing initial low-dose trophic feeds (10–30 mL/h) versus full enteral feeding on survival and ventilation duration in 1,000 ARDS patients, found no difference in the incidence of cognitive impairment at 12 months.[79–81] The Statins for Acutely Injured Lungs from Sepsis (SAILS) trial assessed short-term effects of rosuvastatin versus placebo on mortality and ventilation duration in sepsis-associated ARDS.[82] It did not improve outcome and may have contributed to increased hepatic and renal dysfunction. Some observational studies showed a potential benefit of statins on the incidence of delirium in critically ill patients through a putative reduction in systemic inflammation. An ancillary study of the SAILS trial assessed the daily incidence of ICU delirium using the CAM-ICU, as well as long-term cognitive outcome at 6 and 12 months.[83] Seventy-two percent of the patients experienced delirium. The mean proportion of time in delirium was 34% of ICU days; however, rosuvastatin was not associated with a reduction in delirium. At 12 months, 30% of the patients had some cognitive impairment, but again there was no significant difference between the rosuvastatin versus placebo groups.

Thus, the existing literature has not identified specific pharmacologic treatment for ARDS-associated delirium in ICU settings.

## IMPLICATIONS FOR CLINICAL PRACTICE

The available evidence clearly demonstrates an association between acute brain dysfunction and poor outcome in sepsis and ARDS patients. Current clinical practice guidelines, however, do not address detection, prevention, or treatment of the associated encephalopathy.[84] Recent guidelines that define best practices for management of delirium in adult ICU patients should be applied to septic and ARDS patients, although the strength of the recommendations for any specific treatment is weak.[19]

Strategies that incorporate treatment of underlying sepsis, adequate pain management, and minimal sedation as part of an integrated pain, agitation, and delirium protocol are recommended for all ICUs. Early mobilization should be prioritized, and normal sleep patterns should be facilitated. Benzodiazepines should probably be avoided, especially in patients with delirium, and dexmedetomidine should be considered in high-risks patients. Routine neurologic exam should be part of every sepsis and ARDS patient assessment, including monitoring for development of delirium using either the CAM-ICU or the ICDSC.[85-86] Once a diagnosis of SAE or delirium is established, antipsychotics may be used on an as-needed basis.

## FUTURE DIRECTIONS

Targeted neuroprotective strategies for monitoring and early detection of neuro-inflammation, autoregulatory dysfunction, and neurophysiological dysfunction are needed for patients who are at risk of developing SAE. Physiologic, pharmacologic, and nonpharmacologic strategies for neuroprotection need further investigation in patients with severe sepsis and septic shock. Whether these strategies will help in preventing or ameliorating the long-term consequences of sepsis on cognitive function also requires investigation.

## REFERENCES

1. Freund H, Atamian S, Holroyde J, Fischer JE. Plasma amino acids as predictors of the severity and outcome of sepsis. *Ann Surg.* 1979;190(5):571–76.
2. Sonneville R, Verdonk F, Rauturier C, et al. Understanding brain dysfunction in sepsis. *Ann Intensive Care.* 2013;3(1):15.
3. Xu Z, Huang Y, Mao P, Zhang J, Li Y. Sepsis and ARDS: the dark side of histones. *Mediators Inflamm.* 2015;2015:205054.
4. Eidelman LA, Putterman D, Putterman C, Sprung CL. The spectrum of septic encephalopathy: Definitions, etiologies, and mortalities. *JAMA.* 1996;275(6):470–3.
5. Hsieh SJ, Soto GJ, Hope A, Ponea A, Gong MN. The association between acute respiratory distress syndrome, delirium, and in-hospital mortality in intensive care unit patients. *Am J Respir Crit Care Med.* 2015;191(1):71–8.
6. Young GB, Bolton CF, Austin TW, Archibald YM, Gonder J, Wells GA. The encephalopathy associated with septic illness. *Clin Invest Med.* 1990;13(6):297–304.
7. Widmann CN, Heneka MT. Long-term cerebral consequences of sepsis. *Lancet Neurol.* 2014;13(6):630–6.
8. Pandharipande PP, Girard TD, Jackson JC, et al.; BRAIN-ICU Study Investigators. Long-term cognitive impairment after critical illness. *N Engl J Med.* 2013;369(14):1306–16.
9. Iwashyna TJ, Ely EW, Smith DM, Langa KM. Long-term cognitive impairment and functional disability among survivors of severe sepsis. *JAMA.* 2010;304(16):1787–94.
10. Hopkins RO, Weaver LK, Collingridge D, Parkinson RB, Chan KJ, Orme JF Jr. Two-year cognitive, emotional, and quality-of-life outcomes in acute respiratory distress syndrome. *Am J Respir Crit Care Med.* 2005;171(4):340–7.
11. Rothenhäusler HB, Ehrentraut S, Stoll C, Schelling G, Kapfhammer HP. The relationship between cognitive performance and employment and health status in long-term survivors of the acute respiratory distress syndrome: results of an exploratory study. *Gen Hosp Psychiatry.* 2001;23(2):90–6.
12. Carlson CG, Huang DT. The Adult Respiratory Distress Syndrome Cognitive Outcomes Study: long-term neuropsychological function in survivors of acute lung injury. *Crit Care.* 2013;17(3):317.
13. Herridge MS, Tansey CM, Matté A, et al.; Canadian Critical Care Trials Group. Functional disability 5 years after acute respiratory distress syndrome. *N Engl J Med.* 2011;364(14):1293–304.
14. Adam N, Kandelman S, Mantz J, Chrétien F, Sharshar T. Sepsis-induced brain dysfunction. *Expert Rev Anti Infect Ther.* 2013;11(2):211–21.

15. Iacobone E, Bailly-Salin J, Polito A, Friedman D, Stevens RD, Sharshar T. Sepsis-associated encephalopathy and its differential diagnosis. *Crit Care Med.* 2009;37(10 Suppl):S331–6.

16. Siami S, Annane D, Sharshar T. The encephalopathy in sepsis. *Crit Care Clin.* 2008;24(1):67–82.

17. Basler T, Meier-Hellmann A, Bredle D, Reinhart K. Amino acid imbalance early in septic encephalopathy. *Intensive Care Med.* 2002;28(3):293–8.

18. Mazeraud A, Pascal Q, Verdonk F, Heming N, Chrétien F, Sharshar T. Neuroanatomy and physiology of brain dysfunction in sepsis. *Clin Chest Med.* 2016;37(2):333–45.

19. Barr J, Fraser GL, Puntillo K, et al.; American College of Critical Care Medicine. Clinical practice guidelines for the management of pain, agitation, and delirium in adult patients in the intensive care unit. *Crit Care Med.* 2013;41(1):263–306.

20. Zhang L, Wang X, Ai Y, et al. Epidemiological features and risk factors of sepsis-associated encephalopathy in intensive care unit patients: 2008–2011. *Chin Med J (Engl).* 2012;125(5):828–31.

21. Gofton TE, Young GB. Sepsis-associated encephalopathy. *Nat Rev Neurol.* 2012;8(10):557–66.

22. Wijdicks EF, Stevens M. The role of hypotension in septic encephalopathy following surgical procedures. *Arch Neurol.* 1992;49(6):653–6.

23. Zhang QH, Sheng ZY, Yao YM. Septic encephalopathy: when cytokines interact with acetylcholine in the brain. *Mil Med Res.* 2014;1:20.

24. Sharshar T, Blanchard A, Paillard M, Raphael JC, Gajdos P, Annane D. Circulating vasopressin levels in septic shock. *Crit Care Med.* 2003;31(6):1752–8.

25. Hirasawa H, Oda S, Nakamura M. Blood glucose control in patients with severe sepsis and septic shock. *World J Gastroenterol.* 2009;15(33):4132–6.

26. Maher J, Young GB. Septic encephalopathy. *J Intensive Care Med.* 1993;8(4):177–87.

27. van den Boogaard M, Ramakers BP, van Alfen N, et al. Endotoxemia-induced inflammation and the effect on the human brain. *Crit Care.* 2010;14(3):R81.

28. van den Boogaard M, Kox M, Quinn KL, et al. Biomarkers associated with delirium in critically ill patients and their relation with long-term subjective cognitive dysfunction; indications for different pathways governing delirium in inflamed and noninflamed patients. *Crit Care.* 2011;15(6):R297.

29. Eidelman LA, Putterman D, Putterman C, Sprung CL. The spectrum of septic encephalopathy. Definitions, etiologies, and mortalities. *JAMA.* 1996;275(6):470–3.

30. Bolton C. Neuromuscular abnormalities in critically ill patients. *Intensive Care Med.* 1993;19(6):309–10.

31. Brummel NE, Balas MC, Morandi A, Ferrante LE, Gill TM, Ely EW. Understanding and reducing disability in older adults following critical illness. *Crit Care Med.* 2015;43(6):1265–75.

32. Singer M, Deutschman CS, Seymour CW, et al. The Third International Consensus definitions for sepsis and septic shock (Sepsis-3). *JAMA.* 2016;315(8):801–10.

33. Stone JJ, Childs S, Smith LE, Battin M, Papadakos PJ, Huang JH. Hourly neurologic assessments for traumatic brain injury in the ICU. *Neurol Res.* 2014;36(2):164–9.

34. Young GB, Bolton CF, Archibald YM, Austin TW, Wells GA. The electroencephalogram in sepsis-associated encephalopathy. *J Clin Neurophysiol.* 1992;9(1):145–52.

35. Friedman D, Claassen J, Hirsch LJ. Continuous electroencephalogram monitoring in the intensive care unit. *Anesth Analg.* 2009;109(2):506–23.

36. Abou Khaled KJ, Hirsch LJ. Advances in the management of seizures and status epilepticus in critically ill patients. *Crit. Care Clin.* 2006;22(4):637–59.

37. Oddo M, Carrera E, Claassen J, Mayer SA, Hirsch LJ. Continuous electroencephalography in the medical intensive care unit. *Crit Care Med.* 2009;37(6):2051–6.

38. Claassen J, Mayer SA, Kowalski RG, Emerson RG, Hirsch LJ. Detection of electrographic seizures with continuous EEG monitoring in critically ill patients. *Neurology.* 2004;62(10):1743–8.

39. Hosokawa K, Gaspard N, Su F, Oddo M, Vincent JL, Taccone FS. Clinical neurophysiological assessment of sepsis-associated brain dysfunction: a systematic review. *Crit Care.* 2014;18(6):674.

40. Gilmore EJ, Gaspard N, Choi HA, et al. Acute brain failure in severe sepsis: a prospective study in the medical intensive care unit utilizing continuous EEG monitoring. *Intensive Care Med.* 2015;41(4):686–94.

41. Kurtz P, Gaspard N, Wahl AS, et al. Continuous electroencephalography in a surgical intensive care unit. *Intensive Care Med.* 2014;40(2):228–34.

42. Foreman B, Mahulikar A, Tadi P, et al.; Critical Care EEG Monitoring Research Consortium (CCEMRC). Generalized periodic discharges and "triphasic waves": a blinded evaluation of inter-rater agreement and clinical significance. *Clin Neurophysiol.* 2016;127(2):1073–80.

43. Polito A, Eischwald F, Maho AL, et al. Pattern of brain injury in the acute setting of human septic shock. *Crit Care.* 2013;17(5):R204.

44. Zauner C, Gendo A, Kramer L, et al. Impaired subcortical and cortical sensory evoked potential pathways in septic patients. *Crit Care Med.* 2002;30(5):1136–9.

45. Zauner C, Gendo A, Kramer L, Kranz A, Grimm G, Madl C. Metabolic encephalopathy in critically ill patients suffering from septic or nonseptic multiple organ failure. *Crit Care Med.* 2000;28(5):1310–5.

46. Claassen J, Taccone FS, Horn P, Holtkamp M, Stocchetti N, Oddo M; Neurointensive Care Section of the European Society of Intensive Care Medicine. Recommendations on the use of EEG monitoring in critically ill patients: consensus statement from the neurointensive care section of the ESICM. *Intensive Care Med.* 2013;39(8):1337–51.

47. Piazza O, Cotena S, De Robertis E, Caranci F, Tufano R. Sepsis associated encephalopathy studied by MRI and cerebral spinal fluid S100B measurement. *Neurochem Res.* 2009;34(7):1289–92.

48. Pendlebury WW, Perl DP, Munoz DG. Multiple microabscesses in the central nervous system: a clinicopathologic study. *J Neuropathol Exp Neurol.* 1989;48(3):290–300.

49. Zenaide PV, Gusmao-Flores D. Biomarkers in septic encephalopathy: a systematic review of clinical studies. *Rev Bras Ter Intensiva.* 2013;25(1):56–62.

50. Braman SS, Dunn SM, Amico CA, Millman RP. Complications of intrahospital transport in critically ill patients. *Ann Intern Med.* 1987;107(4):469–73.

51. Waydhas C. Intrahospital transport of critically ill patients. *Crit Care.* 1999;3(5):R83–9.

52. Stubbs DJ, Yamamoto AK, Menon DK. Imaging in sepsis-associated encephalopathy--insights and opportunities. *Nat Rev Neurol.* 2013;9(10):551–61.

53. Ebersoldt M, Sharshar T, Annane D. Sepsis-associated delirium. *Intensive Care Med.* 2007;33(6):941–50.

54. Bozza FA, Garteiser P, Oliveira MF, et al. Sepsis-associated encephalopathy: a magnetic resonance imaging and spectroscopy study. *J Cereb Blood Flow Metab.* 2010;30(2):440–8.

55. Picht T, Krieg SM, Sollmann N, et al. A comparison of language mapping by preoperative navigated transcranial magnetic stimulation and direct cortical stimulation during awake surgery. *Neurosurgery.* 2013;72(5):808–19.

56. Zanotti Cavazzoni S, Dellinger RP. Hemodynamic optimization of sepsis-induced tissue hypoperfusion. *Crit Care.* 2006;10 Suppl 3:S2.

57. Pierrakos C, Antoine A, Velissaris D, et al. Transcranial doppler assessment of cerebral perfusion in critically ill septic patients: a pilot study. *Ann Intensive Care.* 2013;3:28.

58. Vaskó A, Siró P, László I, et al. Assessment of cerebral tissue oxygen saturation in septic patients during acetazolamide provocation—a near infrared spectroscopy study. *Acta Physiol Hung.* 2014;101(1):32–9.

59. Terborg C, Schummer W, Albrecht M, Reinhart K, Weiller C, Röther J. Dysfunction of vasomotor reactivity in severe sepsis and septic shock. *Intensive Care Med.* 2001;27(7):1231–4.

60. Chaudhry N, Duggal A. Sepsis associated encephalopathy. *Adv Med.* 2014;2014:762320.

61. Taccone FS, Scolletta S, Franchi F, Donadello K, Oddo M. Brain perfusion in sepsis. *Curr Vasc Pharmacol.* 2013;11(2):170–86.

62. Taccone FS, Castanares-Zapatero D, Peres-Bota D, Vincent JL, Berre' J, Melot C. Cerebral autoregulation is influenced by carbon dioxide levels in patients with septic shock. *Neurocrit Care.* 2010;12(1):35–42.

63. Bowie RA, O'Connor PJ, Mahajan RP. Cerebrovascular reactivity to carbon dioxide in sepsis syndrome. *Anaesthesia.* 2003;58(3):261–5.

64. Van den Berghe G, Wouters P, Weekers F, et al. Intensive insulin therapy in critically ill patients. *N Engl J Med.* 2001;345(19):1359–67.

65. Krinsley JS, Egi M, Kiss A, et al. Diabetic status and the relation of the three domains of glycemic control to mortality in critically ill patients: an international multicenter cohort study. *Crit Care.* 2013;17(2):R37.

66. Marik PE, Raghavan M. Stress-hyperglycemia, insulin and immunomodulation in sepsis. *Intensive Care Med.* 2004;30(5):748–56.

67. Schortgen F, Clabault K, Katsahian S, et al. Fever control using external cooling in septic shock: a randomized controlled trial. *Am J Respir Crit Care Med.* 2012;185(10):1088–95.

68. Villar J, Slutsky AS. Effects of induced hypothermia in patients with septic adult respiratory distress syndrome. *Resuscitation.* 1993;26(2):183–92.

69. Perman SM, Goyal M, Neumar RW, Topjian AA, Gaieski DF. Clinical applications of targeted temperature management. *Chest.* 2014;145(2):386–93.

70. Riker R, Shehabi Y, Bokesch P, et al.; SEDCOM (Safety and Efficacy of Dexmedetomidine Compared With Midazolam) Study Group. Dexmedetomidine vs midazolam for sedation of critically ill patients: a randomized trial. *JAMA.* 2009;301(5):489–99.

71. Pandharipande PP, Pun BT, Herr DL, et al. Effect of sedation with dexmedetomidine vs lorazepam on acute brain dysfunction in mechanically ventilated patients: the MENDS randomized controlled trial. *JAMA.* 2007;298(22):2644–53.

72. Pandharipande PP, Sanders RD, Girard TD, et al.; MENDS investigators. Effect of dexmedetomidine versus lorazepam on outcome in patients with sepsis: an a priori-designed analysis of the MENDS randomized controlled trial. *Crit Care.* 2010;14(2):R38.

73. Spapen H, Nguyen DN, Troubleyn J, Huyghens L, Schiettecatte J. Drotrecogin alfa (activated) may attenuate severe sepsis-associated encephalopathy in clinical septic shock. *Crit Care.* 2010;14(2):R54.

74. Burkhart CS, Dell-Kuster S, Siegemund M, et al. Effect of n-3 fatty acids on markers of brain injury and incidence of sepsis-associated delirium in septic patients. *Acta Anaesthesiol Scand.* 2014;58(6):689–700.

75. Gao R, Tang YH, Tong JH, Yang JJ, Ji MH, Zhu SH. Systemic lipopolysaccharide administration-induced cognitive impairments are reversed by erythropoietin treatment in mice. *Inflammation.* 2015;38(5):1949–58.

76. Ozcan PE, Senturk E, Orhun G, et al. Effects of intravenous immunoglobulin therapy on behavior deficits and functions in sepsis model. *Ann Intensive Care.* 2015;5(1):62.

77. Wu J, Dong L, Zhang M, et al. Class I histone deacetylase inhibitor valproic acid reverses cognitive deficits in a mouse model of septic encephalopathy. *Neurochem Res.* 2013;38(11):2440–9.

78. Huang YN, Lai CC, Chiu CT, Lin JJ, Wang JY. L-ascorbate attenuates the endotoxin-induced production of inflammatory mediators by inhibiting MAPK activation and NF-κB translocation in cortical neurons/glia cocultures. *PLoS One* 2014;9(7):e97276.

79. National Heart, Lung, and Blood Institute Acute Respiratory Distress Syndrome (ARDS) Clinical Trials Network, Rice TW, Wheeler AP, Thompson BT, et al. Initial trophic vs full enteral feeding in patients with acute lung injury: the EDEN randomized trial. *JAMA.* 2012;307(8):795–803.

80. Needham DM, Dinglas VD, Bienvenu OJ, et al.; NIH NHLBI ARDS Network. One year outcomes in patients with acute lung injury randomised to initial trophic or full enteral feeding: prospective follow-up of EDEN randomised trial. *BMJ.* 2013;346:f1532.

81. Needham DM, Dinglas VD, Morris PE, et al.; NIH NHLBI ARDS Network. Physical and cognitive performance of patients with acute lung injury 1 year after initial trophic versus full enteral feeding EDEN Trial follow-up. *Am J Respir Crit Care Med.* 2013;188(5):567–76.

82. National Heart, Lung, and Blood Institute ARDS Clinical Trials Network, Truwit JD, Bernard GR, Steingrub J,et al. Rosuvastatin for sepsis-associated acute respiratory distress syndrome. *N Engl J Med.* 2014;370(23):2191–200.

83. Needham DM, Colantuoni E, Dinglas VD, et al. Rosuvastatin versus placebo for delirium in intensive care and subsequent cognitive impairment in patients with sepsis-associated acute respiratory distress syndrome: an ancillary study to a randomised controlled trial. *Lancet Respir Med.* 2016;4(3):203–12.

84. Dellinger RP, Levy MM, Rhodes A, et al.; Surviving Sepsis Campaign Guidelines Committee including The Pediatric Subgroup. Surviving Sepsis Campaign: international guidlines for management of severe sepsis and septic shock, 2012. *Crit Care Med.* 2013; ;39(2):165–228.

85. Ely EW, Inouye SK, Bernard GR, et al. Delirium in mechanically ventilated patients: validity and reliability of the confusion assessment method for the intensive care unit (CAM-ICU). *JAMA.* 2001;286(21):2703–10.

86. Bergeron N, Dubois MJ, Dumont M, Dial S, Skrobik Y. Intensive Care Delirium Screening Checklist: evaluation of a new screening tool. *Intensive Care Med.* 2001; 27(5):859–64.

# 14 Neuroprotection for Premature Birth and Neonatal Brain Injury

Eugene Chang

## GENERAL CONSIDERATIONS

Hypoxic-ischemic encephalopathy (HIE) commonly leads to neonatal brain injury both before and after delivery. While perinatal birth asphyxia accounts for a proportion of neonatal brain injury in neonates younger than 37 weeks, preterm birth (PTB) is the more significant risk factor. In fact, data on HIE are scarce in the preterm population. PTB and chorioamnionitis confound the diagnosis of preterm HIE and are the more significant risk factors for perinatal brain injury in preterm infants.[1]

PTB is a leading cause of neonatal morbidity and mortality. While only slight headway has been made in reducing early delivery, care of the preterm neonate has steadily advanced. With modern technology, it is now realistic to expect long-term survival in preterm births extending down to 23 weeks gestation. Given that improvements in survival of preterm neonates have outpaced efforts to prevent PTB, the impact of long-term complications on survivors is increasingly recognized. The neurologic consequences of extreme prematurity range from mild behavioral and cognitive deficits to severe disability.

With respect to perinatal neuroprotection, cerebral palsy (CP) has been the clinical neurologic malady that has been the subject of the greatest degree of investigation. The worldwide prevalence of CP is 1.5–2.5 per 1,000 live births, and its prevalence has remained remarkably stable over time despite increased survival of at-risk preterm infants.[2] Although the overall prevalence of CP has remained stable, the prevalence of CP subtypes has changed over time, reflecting the increased contribution of prematurity to the development of CP.

Although many preterm survivors have neuromotor abnormalities on examination, most are ultimately not diagnosed with CP, which most often manifests as spasticity, weakness, and tremor.[3] Fine motor skill impairments occur in 40–60% of very preterm infants.[4] Developmental coordination disorder occurs in about 18% of children born at earlier than 32 weeks gestation.[5] Other motor abnormalities related to prematurity include mild gross motor delay, persistent neuromotor abnormalities, and functional impairments related to motor planning and/or sensorimotor integration.[3]

Visual and hearing impairment are inversely related to gestational age at delivery and birth weight and are increased in the setting of intraventricular hemorrhage (IVH) and/or periventricular leukomalacia (PVL). A population-based survey of caregivers found that, in children born at less than 28 weeks gestation, 6% had moderate to severe visual impairment and 4% had moderate to severe hearing impairment, whereas children born at 28–32 weeks gestation had a much lower incidence (0.5% for moderate to severe visual impairment, 0.5% for hearing loss).[6] Bilateral isolated hearing loss has been observed to occur in 2.2% of children born at less than 28 weeks gestation at 2 to 3 years of age.[7]

Cognitive and academic impairments may be the most prevalent neurodevelopmental sequelae of prematurity.[3] Sommer et al. observed that at 2 years of age, 54% of infants born at less than 27 weeks gestation had a Griffith Mental Development Quotient more than two standard deviations (SD) below the mean and that only 40% had normal cognitive abilities.[8] Marrett et al. demonstrated that cognitive impairment was the most common disability in children born at 30–34 weeks gestation.[9] Finally, PTB at less than 27 weeks has been associated with a significant increase in the risk of autism spectrum disorders (ASD), with an adjusted hazard ratio of 2.7 (95% confidence interval [CI], 1.5–5.0).[10]

## MECHANISMS OF INJURY

Fetal hypoxia and brain asphyxia were formerly considered to be the main causes of CP.[11] In truth, these account for only a small portion of CP. For the majority of CP cases, there are multiple factors during pregnancy, delivery, and the postnatal period that can act synergistically to lead to the development of this disorder.[11] Germane to this review, PTB may alter normal brain development and lead to a diagnosis of CP.[12]

In preterm survivors, spastic diplegia is the most common type of CP. It is usually seen in the setting of diffuse white matter injury with intraparenchymal hemorrhage and/or cystic PVL.[11] Multiple studies have demonstrated that corticospinal tract injury is the primary location of pathology in CP.[13–15] It has also been demonstrated that both the descending corticomotor tracts and ascending sensorimotor tracts may be involved.[16] Less consistently, it has been demonstrated that the posterior thalamic radiations, which connect the thalamus to the posterior parietal and occipital cortices, show evidence of injury in CP.[16–18] There is also neuronal loss in the subplate zone, a transient fetal layer that lies deep with respect to the cortical plate zone neurons, as well as in the basal ganglia and cerebellum.[11] In an autopsy study, Robinson et al. demonstrated that there is a loss of expression of GABAergic neurons in the subplate zone.[19] Taken together, these studies indicate that in the preterm neonate there are multiple brain regions that are injured and play a role in the clinical manifestations of CP.

PVL is the predominant form of white matter injury in the neonatal brain.[20] There is a component of focal or multifocal necrosis with loss of all cellular elements, as well as a diffuse pattern of loss of developing oligodendrocytes accompanied by astrogliosis and microgliosis. This ultimately leads to either cystic or

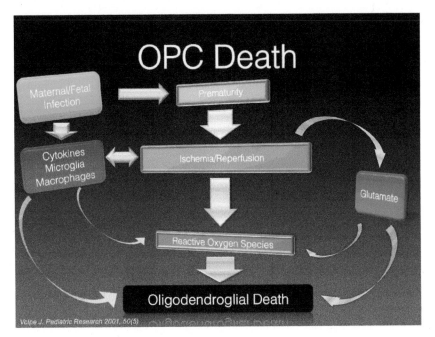

FIGURE 14.1  Summary of the target pathways leading to OPC death and PVL. Adapted from Volpe JJ. Neurobiology of periventricular leukomalacia in the premature infant. Pediatr Res. 2001;50(5):553–62.

noncystic PVL. While the incidence of cystic PVL has decreased over time, non-cystic PVL is seen in about 50% of infants born at less than 1,000 g.[21]

On a cellular level, it appears that developing oligodendrocytes are the main cell type injured in the setting of prematurity (Figure 14.1). Oligodendroglial progenitor cells (OPC) may be particularly vulnerable, as demonstrated in both animal models and human brain.[22–23] These myelin-producing cells are vulnerable during critical periods of development, during which various insults can result in cell death and recognizable white matter injury.[22] It has been demonstrated in mixed glial cultures that lipopolysaccharide exposure leads to a reduction in peroxisomal proliferation in OPCs and prevents their maturation into myelin-forming oligodendrocytes.[24] Consequently, this lineage of cells that plays a critical role in the formation of white matter may be irreparably reduced or damaged prior to birth, thus making antenatal interventions on behalf of the fetus critically important for prevention of long-term neurologic sequelae.

Protection of OPCs is critical for prevention of neurodevelopmental sequelae, and understanding the pathogenesis of injury to these cells is necessary in order to develop neuroprotective interventions. The pathogenesis of PVL is related to three major factors: cerebral ischemia, systemic infection/inflammation, and the vulnerability of OPCs during early development (24–32 weeks).[20]

Cerebral ischemia is a common pathway of neonatal brain injury, in both extra- and intrauterine environments. The resulting temporal sequence is well described and includes reperfusion and partial recovery, typically within 30–60 minutes following the acute insult. Subsequent to this, over the next 1–6 hours, recovery of cerebral oxidative metabolism, inflammation, and programmed cell death characterize the latent phase. Next, excitotoxicity and mitochondrial failure leads to cell death and clinical deterioration in the secondary phase of injury. Finally, over the longer term, there is late cell death, remodeling, and astrogliosis (tertiary phase).[25] These phases of injury and recovery may overlap and are not strictly sequential. Ischemia and inflammation can lead to microglial activation, excitoxicity, and oxidative stress, resulting in injury mainly to OPCs in the preterm brain.[26-27] These mechanisms are areas of potential intervention for neuroprotection.

Experimental models have shown that ischemia and inflammation lead to cell death primarily through oxidative stress. OPCs, unlike mature oligodendrocytes, are sensitive to oxidative stress and vulnerable to attack by reactive oxygen species (ROS) and reactive nitrogen species (RNS).[23,28] Antioxidants may be effective in the prevention of ROS/RNS-mediated damage to OPCs.[23,29]

Cerebral ischemia also leads to glutamate release and results in OPC death due to excitotoxicity.[20] Cell death that results from excess glutamate is both receptor and non–receptor mediated. The key receptors with respect to OPC death in the setting of ischemia/inflammation are the α-amino-3-hydroxy-5-methyl-4-isoxazolepropionic acid/kainate (AMPA/KA) type, which are concentrated on cell somata, and the N-methyl-D-aspartic acid (NMDA) receptor, which is concentrated on oligodendroglial processes.[20] The finding of these receptors on OPCs and their involvement in perinatal brain injury makes NMDA receptors a possible target for neuroprotection.[30] Finally, with non–receptor mediated cell death, excess glutamate leads to blockade of cystine transport, which subsequently leads to depletion of intracellular glutathione, injury from oxidative stress, and cell death.[20,31]

White matter injury is the most common form of tissue damage in the preterm neonate. Perinatal neurologic injury, however, is not limited to white matter. It has been increasingly recognized that significant gray matter injury plays a role as abnormalities of cortical, thalamic, and basal ganglia neurons have been observed. Volpe demonstrated that neuronal/axonal injury often accompanies white matter injury and coined the term "encephalopathy of prematurity" to refer to the complex abnormalities in the neonatal brain in the setting of prematurity.[27] Neuronal-axonal disturbances may underlie neurologic sequelae affecting cognition and behavior, and therefore are also potential targets for intervention in neuroprotection of the preterm infant.

## RISK FACTORS FOR NEUROLOGICAL INJURY

The neurodevelopmental sequelae just described are strongly associated with prematurity. Spontaneous PTB has multiple causes, but it is strongly associated with intra-amniotic infection, ascending intrauterine infection, and systemic infection. The association between PTB and infection has been known for some time, with reports of an association being reported as early as 1950.[32] Positive amniotic fluid cultures have been noted in 20–30% of patients with preterm labor.[33] Moreover, greater than 85% of patients with spontaneous PTB at less than 28 weeks gestation have histologic chorioamnionitis.[34] Romero proposed that vaginal microbes ascend to the membranes and amniotic fluid and incite an inflammatory response that results in either preterm rupture of the membranes or preterm labor.[35-36] Additionally, although less commonly, microbes may be introduced hematologically, as in cases of systemic illness such as pyelonephritis with bacteremia or *Listeria monocytogenes* infections, or directly as in the case of amniocentesis.

More recently, investigators have highlighted the relationship between intra-amniotic inflammation and PTB. In women with spontaneous preterm labor, the presence of intra-amniotic inflammation without infection, as demonstrated by amniotic fluid culture and/or detection of microbial 16S ribosomal DNA, is associated with adverse perinatal outcomes.[37] In the setting of maternal infection or inflammation, the fetus can develop an inflammatory response that can lead to significant neurologic injury through several pathways.

The fetal inflammatory response syndrome has been described as an elevation of interleukin-6 (IL-6) plasma concentration in fetuses in the setting of preterm labor or preterm premature rupture of membranes.[38] It has been demonstrated that fetuses with higher plasma levels of IL-6 (>11 pg/mL), as determined by cordocentesis, have higher rates of severe neonatal morbidity (78% vs. 30%, $P <0.001$). It has also been demonstrated that elevated umbilical cord levels of IL-6 (>400 pg/mL) are associated with periventricular leukomalacia (odds ratio [OR] 6.2, 95% CI 2–19.1).[39]

The major risk factor for ischemic injury of the preterm brain appears to be placental abruption. There are a variety of conditions that acutely decrease perfusion of the placenta and delivery of oxygen, including cord prolapse, uterine rupture, and placental abruption.[25] Of these, placental abruption is a significant cause of PTB. Cord prolapse and uterine rupture are complications that are more typically related to term labor or term premature rupture of membranes. While abruption is a risk factor for fetal hypoxia-ischemia, this is not the sole mechanism for brain injury in the preterm neonate.

## MONITORING FOR NEUROLOGIC INJURY

There are several modalities for monitoring brain injury in the preterm neonate. Cranial ultrasound is readily available and noninvasive, and it has been the mainstay for evaluation of the neonatal brain.[40] It is highly sensitive for detection of hemorrhage and assessment of ventricular size. It can detect severe white matter injury and cystic lesions, but it is not very sensitive for detecting less severe forms of white matter injury.

Magnetic resonance imaging (MRI) is a more sensitive imaging tool for detecting neonatal encephalopathy in both term and preterm neonates.[26] It is rapidly becoming the standard of care at tertiary care centers in the United States. It allows for the detection of a number of central nervous system lesions that are not detected by cranial ultrasound. With respect to HIE in the preterm population, the main sites of injury are the basal ganglia, white matter, brainstem, and cortex. In preterm infants without HIE, diffuse white matter injury is the predominant finding, although differentiating it from the nonmyelinated white matter regions of a normal newborn brain is challenging and requires an experienced radiologist.[40]

Apart from conventional MRI, imaging with diffusion weighted imaging, diffusion tensor imaging (DTI), and magnetic spectroscopy are increasingly being utilized.[26] Acutely, findings on conventional MRI can be normal when spectroscopy and DTI reveal injured tissue. An elevated lactate–to–N-acetyl aspartate ratio in the basal ganglia within the first 48 hours of life can predict long-term neurologic impairment.[25] It is hoped that improved ability to detect neurologic injury earlier in the preterm neonate will allow for more effective hyperacute intervention.

# NEUROPROTECTION STRATEGIES

Currently, there are no distinct postnatal interventions for neuroprotection of the preterm neonate. Hypothermia has become the standard of care for neuroprotection in term infants with hypoxia-ischemia, but it has not been well-studied in preterm neonates. Most of the focus in neuroprotection of the preterm neonate has been on antenatal treatment.

## Corticosteroids

In 1972, it was demonstrated that preterm neonates exposed to corticosteroids prenatally had lower rates of respiratory distress syndrome, leading to its widespread use in obstetrics.[41] Several studies have since demonstrated that antenatal glucocorticoids protect against brain damage, as evidence by a decreased rate of ultrasound-detected IVH.[42] A review of the effects of corticosteroids, which included 13 studies and 2,872 infants, demonstrated a significant decrease in intracranial hemorrhage (RR 0.54, 95% CI, 0.43–0.69).[43] Similarly, several studies have demonstrated a reduction in PVL with the use of corticosteroids.[42]

The reductions in both PVL and IVH observed on imaging lead to the hope that corticosteroid treatment also improves neurodevelopmental outcomes. Pooled data from four randomized trials of antenatal corticosteroid treatment have demonstrated a significant reduction in CP (OR 0.59, 95% CI, 0.35–0.97).[42] One study demonstrated that children born prematurely (birth weight <1,501 g) who were exposed to corticosteroids antenatally had higher IQ scores at 14 years of age than did children who were not exposed to corticosteroids antenatally.[44] These studies support the notion that corticosteroids are clinically effective neuroprotective agents in the setting of prematurity. The National Institutes of Health (NIH) and the American College of Obstetricians and Gynecology (ACOG) jointly recommend antenatal use of corticosteroids to fetuses at risk of preterm delivery for prevention of respiratory distress syndrome, IVH, and neonatal death.[45] Specifically, they recommended a course of corticosteroids (12 mg of betamethasone given intramuscularly 12 hours apart for two doses, or dexamethasone 6 mg intramuscularly for four doses) be given to all fetuses between 24–34 weeks gestation at risk for preterm delivery.

## Magnesium Sulfate

While the antenatal use of corticosteroids to improve neonatal outcomes is clearly warranted in patients at risk for preterm delivery, the benefit of magnesium sulfate ($MgSO_4$) is less clear. There are few studies that directly address the mechanism of action of $MgSO_4$ for fetal neuroprotection. Most of the work cited concerns its action as a noncompetitive antagonist of the NMDA receptor.[46]

While mature oligodendrocytes lack NMDA receptors, the presence of NMDA receptors on OPC processes and AMPA receptors on OPC cell bodies account for their vulnerability to glutamate excitotoxicity.[30,47–49] Prevention of glutamate receptor-mediated excitotoxicity and OPC death by $MgSO_4$ therefore may reduce white matter injury or prevent neuronal cell death. In an animal model of inflammation-induced PTB and fetal brain injury, pregnant mice were randomly assigned to receive intrauterine injection of lipopolysaccharide or saline, followed by intraperitoneal injection of $MgSO_4$ or saline, resulting in four treatment groups.

**Table 14.1** Magnesium Sulfate for Neuroprotection: Summary of the gestational ages, dosing regimens, and findings of the three major prospective trials examining MgSO$_4$ as a neuroprotectant in the setting of preterm birth

| Study | Gestational Age | Dose | CP Findings RR (95% CI) |
|-------|-----------------|------|-------------------------|
| ACTOMgSO4 | <30 weeks | 4 g load, then 1g/h up to 24 h | RR 0.83 (0.64–1.09) |
| PREMAG | <33 weeks | 4 g Bolus | RR 0.63 (0.35–1.15) |
| BEAM | <32 weeks | 6 g load, then 2 g/h for 12 h | RR 0.55 (0.32–0.95) |

Fetal brains were collected for neuronal cultures. MgSO$_4$ ameliorated the neuronal injury induced by lipopolysaccharide.[46]

Nelson and Grether were the first to report that MgSO$_4$ may prevent clinical CP.[50] Among 155,636 children born, they identified very-low-birth weight (<1,500 g) infants surviving to 3 years with moderate or severe congenital CP and compared them to randomly selected very-low-birth weight survivors with respect to whether their mothers received MgSO$_4$. The children with CP were exposed to magnesium sulfate less often than the controls (OR 0.14, 95% CI, 0.05–0.51). This finding subsequently led to three large, randomized placebo-controlled trials (Table 14.1).

In 2003, Crowther et al. reported the results of a multicenter randomized trial in Australia and New Zealand (ACTOMgSO$_4$).[51] A total of 1,062 women at risk of PTB before 30 weeks gestation were randomized to receive either a 4 g load of MgSO$_4$ (0.5 g/mL) or placebo, followed by a maintenance infusion of 2 mL/h for up to 24 hours. The primary outcomes were total pediatric mortality, CP, and the combined outcome of death and CP at 2 years of age. The study was powered to determine whether there was a 50% reduction in CP (reduction from 10% to 5%) and required a sample size of 848 children. This sample size was adjusted upward to 1,250 to account for a predicted mortality rate of 20% and multiple births. A total of 1,062 patients were enrolled, with 535 randomized to MgSO$_4$ and 527 to placebo. There were no significant differences in the primary outcomes. Total pediatric mortality occurred in 14% versus 17% of the MgSO$_4$ and placebo groups, respectively (RR 0.83, 95% CI, 0.64–1.09). CP occurred in 7% versus 8% of the MgSO$_4$ and placebo groups, respectively (RR 0.83, 95% CI, 0.54–1.27). There was a trend for a better combined outcome, as observed in 20% versus 24% of treated and untreated patients, respectively (RR 0.83, 95% CI, 0.66–1.03). Substantial motor dysfunction, a secondary outcome, was significantly decreased, with 3% in the MgSO$_4$ group versus 7% in the placebo–treated group (RR 0.51, 95% CI, 0.29–0.91). While this was essentially a negative study, it was underpowered to detect modest reductions in CP.

Subsequently, the PREMAG randomized trial of MgSO$_4$ for neuroprotection used a different dosing schedule (a single 4 g bolus) and gestational age cutoff (<33 weeks).[52-53] The primary outcome in the 2006 study was neonatal mortality prior to discharge, severe white matter injury, and the combination of these two outcomes. Like Crowther's study, this study was powered to detect a 50% reduction in the primary outcome and required a sample size of 906 patients. A total of 573 women were enrolled and 564 were analyzed.[52] Of these, 286 were randomized to receive MgSO$_4$ and 278 received placebo. The total number of infants in the study was 688 (352 receiving MgSO$_4$ and 336 receiving placebo). In this study, 92% of patients received the full dose of $MgSO_4$ at a mean of 1 hour and 38 minutes (range 5 minutes to 25 hours 5 minutes) before delivery. Like Crowther's study, there were no significant differences in the primary outcomes. Neonatal mortality occurred in 9% versus 10% (OR 0.79, 95% CI, 0.44–1.44). Severe white matter injury occurred in 10 versus 12% (OR 0.78, 95% CI, 0.47–1.31). Finally, the combined outcome occurred in 16% versus 18% (OR 0.86, 95% CI, 0.55–1.34). Similar to Crowther's study, there was a trend toward improvement in severe white matter injury with $MgSO_4$.

In a 2-year follow-up study, long-term clinical outcomes were evaluated in 688 infants.[53] $MgSO_4$ was not associated with significant improvement in CP (OR 0.63, 95% CI 0.35–1.15) or other outcomes, but there were trends toward improvements in gross motor dysfunction (OR 0.65, 95% CI 0.41–1.02); combined death and CP (0.65, 95% CI .42–1.03); death and gross motor dysfunction (OR 0.62, 95% CI 0.41–0.93); and death, CP, and cognitive dysfunction (OR 0.68, 0.47–1.00).

A large multicenter trial in the United States studied 2,241 women at risk for imminent delivery between 24–31 weeks gestation, who were randomized to receive either $MgSO_4$ or placebo.[54] Patients receiving $MgSO_4$ or identical appearing placebo were given a 6 g loading dose followed by a maintenance dose at 2 g per hour for up to 12 hours. If the patient had not delivered, or delivery was no longer felt to be imminent after 12 hours, the infusion was discontinued. $MgSO_4$ (or placebo) was restarted if delivery again became anticipated, and, if more than 6 hours had elapsed since administration, another loading dose was given. The primary outcomes studied were stillbirth, death prior to 1 year of age, and moderate/severe CP as assessed at 2 years of age or later. The study was powered to detect a 30% reduction in the primary outcome. Similar to the previous two studies, there was no significant difference in the primary outcomes. The rate of death or moderate/severe CP was 11.3% versus 11.7% (RR 0.97, 95% CI, 0.77–1.23). There was a nonsignificant increase in deaths with $MgSO_4$, 9.5% versus 8.5% with an RR of 1.12 (0.85–1.47). Contrary to the previous studies, the rate of moderate/severe CP was significantly lower in patients treated with $MgSO_4$, 1.9% versus 3.5% with a RR of 0.55 (0.32–0.95). The investigators concluded that $MgSO_4$ may have a small beneficial effect as a neuroprotectant, with a number needed to treat of 62 to prevent one case of moderate to severe CP.

Several meta-analyses followed the publication of these three trials.[55–56] All three meta-analyses demonstrated similar findings, though the studies they analyzed were slightly differently. Conde-Agudelo and Romero demonstrated significant reductions in CP, moderate-severe CP, and substantial gross motor dysfunction, but no significant difference in total pediatric mortality.[55] Costantine et al. demonstrated a reduction in CP of any severity, moderate-severe CP, and the combined outcome of death or moderate-severe CP if $MgSO_4$ was administered at less than 32–34 weeks.[56] Finally, the Cochrane Database review on $MgSO_4$ for neuroprotection demonstrated reductions in CP and substantial gross motor dysfunction without an increase in the risk of pediatric mortality.[57]

## IMPLICATIONS FOR CLINICAL PRACTICE

The focus for prevention of preterm neonatal brain injury centers on the identification of patients at risk for PTB, prevention of PTB, and administration of therapies that may protect the fetal brain. Prediction and prevention of PTB are beyond the scope of this review; however, it is clearly best practice for obstetricians to evaluate cervical length for identifying patients at risk for PTB and use progesterone supplementation in patients with a prior history of PTB. Beyond prevention of PTB, judicious use of corticosteroids and $MgSO_4$ for preterm delivery is reasonable.

## FUTURE DIRECTIONS

The use of $MgSO_4$ for neuroprotection for premature birth remains controversial, and the research highlights the difficulties in studying neuroprotective agents for prenatal use. While pharmacokinetic and mechanistic studies are ideal, they are very time-consuming, difficult, and expensive to conduct. There are several promising neuroprotective treatments for perinatal birth injury that are currently under investigation, including N-acetylcysteine (NAC), erythropoietin, and stem cells.[29,58–60] NAC is particularly promising for prevention of both PTB and perinatal brain injury, given its antioxidant and anti-inflammatory properties.[29,61] Erythropoietin is also promising because it decreases cell death, is anti-inflammatory, increases neurogenesis, and protects developing oligodendrocytes.[60,62–63] Mesenchymal stem cells are being studied, but only in the preclinical stage at this point. All of these approaches require further investigation. Short-term biomarkers that predict development of neurologic sequelae would be of great benefit, allowing for more efficient translational research in the area of neuroprotection.

PTB is the strongest risk factor for neonatal brain injury. Its prevention remains a challenge worldwide, but little headway has been made in reducing PTB rates. Survival of infants born prematurely, however, has improved greatly. The neurodevelopmental consequences of prematurity have therefore become significant issues, especially in those infants born at less than 32 weeks gestation.

Perinatal asphyxia is a risk factor, but the data suggest that systemic inflammation and other mechanisms that lead to PTB also may play a direct role in causing perinatal brain injury. A better understanding of the role of infection/inflammation in PTB and preterm brain injury therefore is necessary to developing strategies to protect the brain of the preterm neonate.

In order to prevent the neurodevelopmental complications of PTB, the development and use of dedicated neuroprotective medications is necessary. While promising neuroprotectant medications have been identified, they require continued study. At this time, the judicious administration of steroids in those at risk for PTB can reduce neurodevelopmental sequelae and should be administered according to published guidelines. $MgSO_4$ for neuroprotection should be included, and local protocols for administration should address dosing and indications. Continued investigation of other neuroprotectants will hopefully lead to future advances in treatment options.

## REFERENCES

1. Gancia P, Pomero G. Therapeutic hypothermia in the prevention of hypoxic-ischaemic encephalopathy: new categories to be enrolled. *J Matern Fetal Neonatal Med.* 2012;25(Suppl 4);86–8.
2. Oskoui M, Coutinho F, Dykeman J, Jetté N, Pringsheim T. An update on the prevalence of cerebral palsy: a systematic review and meta-analysis. *Dev Med Child Neurol.* 2013;55(6):509–19.

3. Allen MC. Neurodevelopmental outcomes of preterm infants. *Curr Opin Neurol.* 2008;21(2):123–8.

4. Bos AF, Van Braeckel KN, Hitzert MM, TanisJC, Roze E. Development of fine motor skills in preterm infants. *Dev Med Child Neurol.* 2013;55:1–4.

5. Faebo Larsen R, Hvas Mortensen L, Martinussen T, Nybo Andersen AM. Determinants of developmental coordination disorder in 7-year-old children: a study of children in the Danish National Birth Cohort. *Dev Med Child Neurol.* 2013;55(11):1016–22.

6. Schiariti V, Houbè JS, Lisonkova S, Klassen AF, Lee SK. Caregiver-reported health outcomes of preschool children born at 28 to 32 weeks' gestation. *J Dev Behav Pediatr.* 2007;28(1):9–15.

7. Bolisetty, S, Dhawan, A, Abdel-Latif, M, Bajuk, B, Stack, J, Lui, K; New South Wales and Australian Capital Territory Neonatal Intensive Care Units' Data Collection. Intraventricular hemorrhage and neurodevelopmental outcomes in extreme preterm infants. *Pediatrics.* 2014;133(1):55–62.

8. Sommer C, Urlesberger B, Maurer-Fellbaum U, Kutschera J, Müller W. Neuro-developmental outcome at 2 years in 23 to 26 weeks old gestation infants. *Klinische Paediatrie.* 2007;219(1):23–9.

9. Marret S, Ancel PY, Marpeau L, et al.; Epipage Study Group. Neonatal and 5-year out-comes after birth at 30–34 weeks of gestation. *Obstet Gynecol.* 2007;110(1):72–80.

10. Kuzniewicz MW, Wi S, Qian Y, Walsh EM, Armstrong MA, Croen LA. Prevalence and neonatal factors associated with autism spectrum disorders in preterm infants. *J Pediatr.* 2014;164(1):20–5.

11. Marret S, Vanhulle C, Laquerriere A. Pathophysiology of cerebral palsy. *Handb Clin Neurol.* 2013;111:169–76.

12. Livinec F, Ancel P-Y, Marret S, et al.; Epipage Group. Prenatal risk factors for cerebral palsy in very preterm singletons and twins. *Obstet Gynecol.* 2005;105(6):1341–7.

13. Nagae LM, Hoon AH, Stashinko E, et al. Diffusion tensor imaging in children with periventricular leukomalacia: variability of injuries to white matter tracts. *AJNR Am J Neuroradiol.* 2007;28(7):1213–22.

14. Rose S, Guzzetta A, Pannek K, Boyd R. MRI structural connectivity, disruption of primary sensorimotor pathways, and hand function in cerebral palsy. *Brain Connect.* 2011;1(4):309–16.

15. Son SM, Ahn YH, Sakong J, et al. Diffusion tensor imaging demonstrates focal lesions of the corticospinal tract in hemiparetic patients with cerebral palsy. *Neurosci Lett.* 2007;420(1):34–8.

16. Scheck SM, Boyd RN, Rose SE. New insights into the pathology of white matter tracts in cerebral palsy from diffusion magnetic resonance imaging: a systematic review. *Dev Med Child Neurol.* 2012;54(8):684–96.

17. Yoshida S, Hayakawa K, Oishi K, et al. Athetotic and spastic cerebral palsy: anatomic characterization based on diffusion-tensor imaging. *Radiology.* 2011; 260(2):511–20.

18. Yoshida S, Hayakawa K, Yamamoto A, et al. Quantitative diffusion tensor tractography of the motor and sensory tract in children with cerebral palsy. *Dev Med Child Neurol.* 2010;52(10):935–40.

19. Robinson S, Li Q, Dechant A, Cohen ML. Neonatal loss of gamma-aminobutyric acid pathway expression after human perinatal brain injury. *J Neurosurg.* 2006;104(6 Suppl):396–408.

20. Volpe JJ, Kinney HC, Jensen FE, Rosenberg PA. The developing oligodendro-cyte: key cellular target in brain injury in the premature infant. *Intl J Dev Neurosci.* 2011;29(4):423–40.

21. Volpe JJ. *Neurology of the newborn*. New York: Elsevier Health Sciences: 2008.

22. Back SA, Han BH, Luo NL, et al. Selective vulnerability of late oligodendrocyte progenitors to hypoxia-ischemia. *J Neurosci*. 2002;22(2):455–63.

23. Haynes RL, Folkerth RD, Keefe RJ, et al. Nitrosative and oxidative injury to premyelinating oligodendrocytes in periventricular leukomalacia. *J Neuropathol Exp Neurol*. 2003;62(5):441–50.

24. Paintlia MK, Paintlia AS, Khan M, Singh I, Singh AK. Modulation of peroxisome proliferator-activated receptor-alpha activity by N-acetyl cysteine attenuates inhibition of oligodendrocyte development in lipopolysaccharide stimulated mixed glial cultures. *J Neurochem*. 2008;105(3):956–70.

25. Douglas-Escobar M, Weiss MD. Hypoxic-ischemic encephalopathy: a review for the clinician. *JAMA Pediatr*. 2015;169(4):397–403.

26. Jin C, Londono I, Mallard C, Lodygensky GA. New means to assess neonatal inflammatory brain injury. *J Neuroinflammation*. 2015;12:180.

27. Volpe JJ. Brain injury in premature infants: a complex amalgam of destructive and developmental disturbances. *Lancet Neurol*. 2009;8(1):110–24.

28. Back SA, Gan X, Li Y, Rosenberg PA, Volpe JJ. Maturation-dependent vulnerability of oligodendrocytes to oxidative stress-induced death caused by glutathione depletion. *J Neurosci*. 1998;18(16):6241–53.

29. Paintlia MKM, Paintlia ASA, Barbosa EE, Singh II, Singh AKA. N-acetylcysteine prevents endotoxin-induced degeneration of oligodendrocyte progenitors and hypomyelination in developing rat brain. *J Neurosci Res*. 2004;78(3):347–61.

30. Manning SM, Talos DM, Zhou C, et al. NMDA receptor blockade with memantine attenuates white matter injury in a rat model of periventricular leukomalacia. *J Neurosci*. 2008;28(26):6670–8.

31. Murphy TH, Miyamoto M, Sastre A, Schnaar RL, Coyle JT. Glutamate toxicity in a neuronal cell line involves inhibition of cystine transport leading to oxidative stress. *Neuron*. 1989;2(6):1547–58.

32. Knox IC, Hoerner JK. The role of infection in premature rupture of the membranes. *Am J Obstet Gynecol*. 1950;59(1):190–4.

33. Watts DH, Krohn MA, Hillier SL, Eschenbach DA. The association of occult amniotic fluid infection with gestational age and neonatal outcome among women in preterm labor. *Obstet Gynecol*. 1992;79(3):351–7.

34. Yoon BH, Romero R, Park JS, Kim M, Oh SY, Kim CJ, Jun JK. The relationship among inflammatory lesions of the umbilical cord (funisitis):umbilical cord plasma interleukin 6 concentration, amniotic fluid infection, and neonatal sepsis. *Am J Obstet Gynecol*. 2000;183(5):1124–9.

35. Romero R, Mazor M, Munoz H, Gomez R, Galasso M, Sherer DM. The preterm labor syndrome. *Ann N Y Acad Sci*. 1994;734:414–29.

36. Romero R, Sirtori M, Oyarzun E, et al. Infection and labor. V. Prevalence, microbiology, and clinical significance of intraamniotic infection in women with preterm labor and intact membranes. *Am J Obstet Gynecol*. 1989;161(3):817–24.

37. Combs CA, Gravett M, Garite TJ, et al.; ProteoGenix/Obstetrix Collaborative Research Network. Amniotic fluid infection, inflammation, and colonization in preterm labor with intact membranes. *Am J Obstet Gynecol*. 2014;210(2):125.e1–125.e15.

38. Gomez R, Romero R, Ghezzi F, Yoon B, Mazor M, Berry S. The fetal inflammatory response syndrome. *Am J Obstet Gynecol*. 1998;179:194–202.

39. Yoon BH, Romero R, Yang SH, et al. Interleukin-6 concentrations in umbilical cord plasma are elevated in neonates with white matter lesions associated with periventricular leukomalacia. *Am J Obstet Gynecol*. 1996;174(5):1433–40.

40. Cabaj A, Bekiesińska-Figatowska M, Mądzik J. MRI patterns of hypoxic-ischemic brain injury in preterm and full term infants—classical and less common MR findings. *Pol J Radiol.* 2012;77(3):71–6.

41. Liggins GC, Howie RN. A controlled trial of antepartum glucocorticoid treatment for prevention of the respiratory distress syndrome in premature infants. *Pediatrics.* 1972;50(4):515–25.

42. O'Shea TM, Doyle LW. Perinatal glucocorticoid therapy and neurodevelopmental outcome: an epidemiologic perspective. *Semin Neonatol.* 2001;6(4):293–307.

43. Roberts D, Dalziel S. Antenatal corticosteroids for accelerating fetal lung maturation for women at risk of preterm birth. *Cochrane Database Syst Rev.* 2006;(3):CD004454.

44. Doyle LW, Ford GW, Rickards AL, et al. Antenatal corticosteroids and outcome at 14 years of age in children with birth weight less than 1501 grams. *Pediatrics.* 2000;106(1):E2.

45. Gilstrap LC. Effect of corticosteroids for fetal maturation on perinatal outcomes. *JAMA.* 1995;273(5):413.

46. Burd I, Breen K, Friedman A, Chai J, Elovitz MA. Magnesium sulfate reduces inflammation-associated brain injury in fetal mice. *Am J Obstet Gynecol.* 2010;202(3): 292.e1–9.

47. Bakiri Y, Burzomato V, Frugier G, Hamilton NB, Káradóttir R, Attwell D. Glutamatergic signaling in the brain's white matter. *Neuroscience.* 2009;158(1):266–74.

48. Káradóttir R, Cavelier P, Bergersen LH, Attwell D. NMDA receptors are expressed in oligodendrocytes and activated in ischaemia. *Nature.* 2005;438(7071):1162–6.

49. Káradóttir R, Attwell D. Neurotransmitter receptors in the life and death of oligodendrocytes. *Neuroscience.* 2007;145(4):1426–38.

50. Nelson KB, Grether JK. Can magnesium sulfate reduce the risk of cerebral palsy in very low birthweight infants? *Pediatrics.* 1995;95(2):263–9.

51. Crowther CA, Hiller JE, Doyle LW, Haslam RR. Effect of magnesium sulfate given for neuroprotection before preterm birth: a randomized controlled trial. *JAMA.* 2003;290(20):2669–76.

52. Marret S, Marpeau L, Zupan-Simunek V, et al. Magnesium sulphate given before very-preterm birth to protect infant brain: the randomised controlled PREMAG trial. *BJOG.* 2006;114(3):310–8.

53. Marret S, Marpeau L, Follet-Bouhamed C, et al. [Effect of magnesium sulphate on mortality and neurologic morbidity of the very-preterm newborn (of less than 33 weeks) with two-year neurological outcome: results of the prospective PREMAG trial]. *Gynecol Obstet Fertil.* 2008;36(3):278–88.

54. Rouse DJ, Hirtz DG, Thom E, et al. A randomized, controlled trial of magnesium sulfate for the prevention of cerebral palsy. *N Engl J Med.* 2008;359(9):895–905.

55. Conde-Agudelo A, Romero R. Antenatal magnesium sulfate for the prevention of cerebral palsy in preterm infants less than 34 weeks' gestation: a systematic review and meta-analysis. *Am J Obstet Gynecol.* 2009;200(6):595–609.

56. Costantine MM, Weiner SJ. Effects of antenatal exposure to magnesium sulfate on neuroprotection and mortality in preterm infants. *Obstet Gynecol.* 2009;114(2, Part 1):354–64.

57. Doyle LW, Crowther CA, Middleton P, et al. Magnesium sulfate for women at risk of preterm birth for neuroprotection of the fetus. *Cochrane Database Syst Rev.* 2009;(1):CD004661.

58. Jenkins DD, Chang E, Singh I. Neuroprotective interventions: is it too late? *J Child Neurol.* 2009;24(9):1212–9.

59. Castillo-Melendez M, Yawno T, Jenkin G, Miller SL. Stem cell therapy to protect and repair the developing brain: a review of mechanisms of action of cord blood and amnion epithelial derived cells. *Front. Neurosci.* 2013;7(194):1–14.

60. Zhang J, Wang Q, Xiang H, Xin Y, Chang M, Lu H. Neuroprotection with erythropoietin in preterm and/or low birth weight infants. *J Clin Neurosci.* 2014;21(8):1283–7.

61. Chang EY, Zhang J, Sullivan S, Newman R, Singh I. N-acetylcysteine attenuates the maternal and fetal proinflammatory response to intrauterine LPS injection in an animal model for preterm birth and brain injury. *J Maternal Fetal Neonatal Med.* 2011;24(5):732–40.

62. Kumral A, Tugyan K, Gonenc S, et al. Protective effects of erythropoietin against ethanol-induced apoptotic neurodegeneration and oxidative stress in the developing C57BL/6 mouse brain. *Dev Brain Res.* 2005;160(2):146–56.

63. McPherson RJ, Juul SE. Recent trends in erythropoietin-mediated neuroprotection. *Intl J Dev Neurosci.* 2008;26(1):103–11.

# 15 Neuroprotection for Spinal Cord Injury

Christopher S. Ahuja

and Michael Fehlings

## GENERAL CONSIDERATIONS

Traumatic spinal cord injuries (SCI) affect more than 1.4 million North Americans and produce devastating physical, social, and vocational impairments for patients. The direct lifetime costs of SCI are estimated to be $1.1–4.6 million per patient.[1–2] Timely delivery of medical and surgical care can significantly enhance both early and long-term outcomes.[3–4] The pathophysiology of SCI extends beyond the cord and involves systemic changes in the respiratory, cardiovascular, and autonomic nervous systems, necessitating management in a critical care setting. As a result, knowledge of the evidence-based treatments for SCI are vital for intensivists, internists, and surgeons.[5] This chapter outlines the current standard of care and highlights important clinical trials that are likely to influence management of acute SCI in the near future.

## MECHANISMS OF AND RISKS FOR SPINAL CORD INJURY

The major causes of SCI vary by level of injury, but most are attributable to motor vehicle accidents (MVA), work-related accidents, falls, sports-related injuries, and assaults.[1] The trauma results in disruption and/or dislocation of the protective osseous and ligamentous structures of the spinal column. The initial impact on the cord causes injury to cell membranes, axons, and the vulnerable microvasculature. This is quickly followed by a secondary injury cascade that causes further cell death and functional disability. Both surgical and medical neuroprotective interventions target key components of this secondary injury cascade so as to mitigate damage.

In the early post-injury period, cell permeabilization, pro-apoptotic signaling, and ischemia contribute to cell death. Disruption of the blood–spinal cord barrier also allows an influx of pro-inflammatory cytokines and vasoactive peptides.[6] Concurrently, by-products of cellular necrosis (DNA, K+, adenosine triphosphate

[ATP]) activate pro-inflammatory signaling by local microglia.[7-8] These processes result in the recruitment of large numbers of macrophages, polymorphonuclear leukocytes, and additional microglia to the injury site. The inflammatory cells generate oxygen free radicals and cytotoxic molecules that cyclically worsen the harsh post-injury environment.[9] Excessive glutamate release by necrotic cells leads to excitotoxic death of adjacent neurons (Figure 15.1).[10-11]

As parenchyma is lost, cystic cavities form and begin to coalesce. Astrocytes migrate to surround these cavities and create an interwoven lattice-like barrier of cells. Fibroblasts similarly proliferate and begin depositing significant quantities of

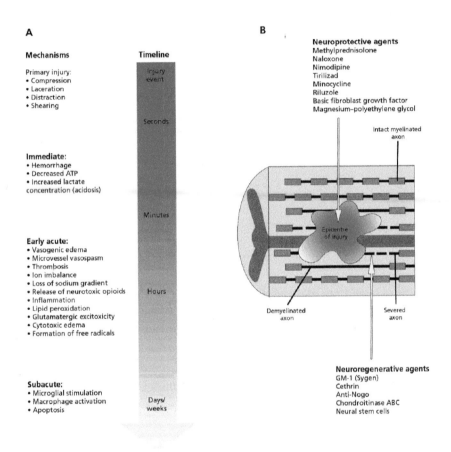

FIGURE 15.1 A. Primary and secondary mechanisms of injury determining the final extent of spinal cord damage. The primary injury event starts a pathobiological cascade of secondary injury mechanisms that unfold in different phases within seconds of the primary trauma and continue for several weeks thereafter. B. Longitudinal section of the spinal cord after injury. The epicenter of the injury progressively expands after the primary trauma as a consequence of secondary injury events. This expansion causes an increased region of tissue cavitation and, ultimately, worsened long-term outcomes. Within and adjacent to the injury epicenter are severed and demyelinated axons. The neuroprotective agents listed act to subvert specific secondary injuries and prevent neural damage, while the neuroregenerative agents act to promote axonal regrowth once damage has occurred. ATP, adenosine triphosphate.

Reprinted with permission from Wilson JR, Forgione N, Fehlings MG. Emerging therapies for acute traumatic spinal cord injury. *CMAJ*. 2013;185(6):485–92.[4]

chondroitin sulfate proteoglycans (CSPGs). Together, these form a highly inhibitory glial scar that acts to prevent regenerative cell migration and neurite outgrowth.

SCI also has profound effects on the cardiovascular and respiratory systems. Sympathetic outflow via the sympathetic trunk (T1–L2) is interrupted, resulting in a loss of peripheral vascular tone. Injuries to the upper thoracic cord and higher levels also result in a loss of cardiac sympathetic chronotropic/inotropic drive. The result is hypotension and bradycardia (neurogenic shock) that can lead to further exacerbation of cord ischemia. Respiratory compromise similarly results from loss of innervation to abdominal muscles (T7–L1), intercostal muscles (T1–T6), and the diaphragm (C3–C5), producing hypercapnia, hypoxia, and impaired secretion clearance.[4,12-13]

## Risk Factors for Spinal Cord Injury

Risk factors for traumatic SCI include male gender, age 16–30 or greater than 65, engaging in risky behaviors (e.g., shallow diving, extreme sports, lack of safety gear), and bone and joint diseases (e.g., osteoporosis, ankylosing spondylitis).[14-15] A critical additional risk factor is pre-existing acquired spinal stenosis (e.g., spondylosis, ossification of the posterior longitudinal ligament [OPLL], ligamentum flavum hypertrophy) or congenital spinal stenosis.[16-17] The degree of impact energy (e.g., high-speed MVA vs. fall from standing) is another important risk factor to consider, but clinicians must be cognizant that low-energy trauma can produce equally severe injuries as high-energy trauma in certain patients. A thorough history and neurologic exam should be the guiding factor in all cases.

## MONITORING FOR INJURY

Early and accurate diagnosis of neurological injury is a critical first step in the appropriate management of patients with SCI.[4-5,18] Whenever possible, the spine should be immobilized during and after airway, breathing, and circulatory stabilization. This represents one of the most important neuroprotective interventions available. A hard cervical collar, flat bed positioning, and coordinated use of a log-roll/spinal board for patient transfers are key immobilization techniques. During airway manipulation, manual in-line cervical spine traction is the ideal method of cervical immobilization.[19]

Once the patient is resuscitated, a detailed neurological exam, such as the American Spinal Injury Association (ASIA) International Standards for Neurological Classification of SCI (ISNCSCI) examination, should be completed. The purpose of the exam is to document baseline function and identify the level of neurologic injury.[20-21] This exam should be repeated frequently during the hospital stay to evaluate changes in status. A computed tomography (CT) scan is recommended for all SCI patients to localize and characterize bony injury and alignment. Plain radiographs are insufficient because they can miss 6% of injuries.[22] Patients with a documented cervical cord injury who have suffered a high-impact injury (e.g., high-speed MVA) should undergo a thoracolumbar spine CT in addition to cervical spine CT to assess for additional spinal injuries that would otherwise be missed. Patients with neurological deficits and normal CT imaging should undergo urgent magnetic resonance imaging (MRI) to rule out spinal cord contusion, soft tissue injuries (e.g., ligamentous disruption, epidural hematomas, critical disc herniations), and ongoing cord compression. MRI is a useful adjunct to CT due to its ability to assess the cord and the extent of ligamentous injury.

MRI also plays an important role in prognostication to determine long-term outcomes after SCI. A novel clinical prediction rule has been developed by Wilson et al., based on individual patient data from two large, prospective, international datasets.[23] Better motor function scores and a higher likelihood of functional independence at 1 year post-injury are predicted by younger age, higher ASIA Impairment Scale grade, higher ASIA motor score at presentation, and favorable MRI signal characteristics. The spectrum of no signal change, presence of edema, or presence of hemorrhage predict progressively worse outcome.

Patients with acute SCI should be cared for in the ICU with continuous cardiac, hemodynamic, and respiratory monitoring. Multiple studies have described lower morbidity and mortality with ICU monitoring and management.[18,24–27] This is largely due to the clinical expertise of the personnel working in these units in managing cardiorespiratory complications. After injury, patients with SCI may have bradycardia, impaired cardiac output, reduced peripheral vascular tone, cardiac arrhythmias, and electrolyte imbalances.[28–29] Respiratory insufficiency also is common after SCI, with patients demonstrating decreased inspiratory capacity and vital capacity that may lead to hypoxemia.[30–31] Early recognition and management of these complications by an expert critical care team can lead to reduced mortality. This was demonstrated in a landmark study by Hachen in 1977.[18] Over a 10-year period, 188 patients with acute SCI were transferred to the ICU directly from the scene of injury. Compared to historical controls, mortality decreased from 32.5% to 6.8% for patients with complete quadriplegia and from 9.9% to 1.4% for patients with incomplete quadriplegia. Importantly, the majority of deaths in this study were attributable to pulmonary complications.

## PHYSIOLOGICAL INTERVENTIONS
### Surgical Decompression

Microvascular injury and cellular necrosis produce hemorrhage and progressive edema. This increases the mechanical pressure on the cord, which cyclically contributes to ischemia and cell death. Surgical removal of surrounding bone and soft tissue effectively decompresses the cord to reduce secondary insult. The Surgical Timing in Acute Spinal Cord Injury Study (STASCIS) prospectively studied 313 cervical SCI patients.[32] Those receiving early decompression (within 24 hours of injury; mean, 14 hours) were twice as likely to demonstrate ASIA Impairment Scale improvement of two or more grades at 6 months post-injury compared with patients receiving late decompression (greater than 24 hours following injury; mean, 48.3 hours).

Another prospective cohort study ($N = 84$) confirmed that early surgical decompression was associated with better outcomes, finding that a greater proportion of patients who underwent early surgery had ASIA Impairment Scale improvements of two or more grades at the time of discharge from the rehabilitation facility compared to the late surgery group.[33] A prospective observational study ($N = 888$) comparing early (within 24 hours of injury) versus late (more than 24 hours after injury) surgical decompression found that patients with ASIA grade A (complete injury) or B (incomplete sensory injury; complete motor injury) injury severity who underwent early surgical decompression had shorter hospital length of stay (LOS).[3] In patients with incomplete injuries (ASIA grades B, C, and D), those who underwent earlier surgery had greater motor recovery.[3] Together, these data have led to the concept of "time is spine," which emphasizes the importance of early diagnosis and intervention in potentiating long-term recovery.[4]

There are efforts under way to assess the efficacy of earlier interventions and interventions targeted to specific SCI patient subpopulations. AOSpine Europe is leading a multicenter, prospective, observational cohort study (SCI-POEM; Clinicaltrials.gov Identifier-NCT01674764) to assess the effect of decompression within 12 hours on long-term outcomes.[34] The Optimal Treatment for Spinal Cord Injury Associated with Cervical Canal Stenosis (OSCIS; NCT01485458) study at Tokyo University is a randomized trial recruiting the specific population of ASIA grade C SCI patients without bony injuries and with pre-existing central canal stenosis.[34] This study compares early (< 24 hour) versus delayed (> 14 day) surgery, with motor and functional outcomes measured up to 1 year post-injury.

## Surgical Decompression for Central Cord Injuries

Traumatic central cord injuries are the most common form of incomplete SCI and tend to occur in patients with pre-existing central canal stenosis. The syndrome is characterized by greater weakness in the upper extremities than the lower extremities, variable sensory loss (with sacral sparing), variable bowel/bladder dysfunction, and, in many patients, rapid early improvements in neurological function. When a bony/ligamentous injury is present, the urgent surgical goals are to decompress, reduce, and stabilize the spine. Patients often present without structural injury, however, and the efficacy and timing of decompression therefore comes into question.

Historically, patients with central cord syndrome were imaged to rule out instability and allowed to plateau in their recovery over weeks before intervention. Emerging evidence now suggests an opportunity to improve long-term outcomes with early surgery may exist for the subgroup of patients with pre-existing central canal stenosis. Analysis of a prospective, international dataset showed that patients receiving early (within 24 hours) surgery had 6-point higher ASIA motor scores and a greater chance of improvement in ASIA grade (OR 2.81) at 12 months post-injury compared to patients receiving late surgery (after 24 hours).[35] A prospective, randomized clinical trial titled Comparing Surgical Decompression Versus Conservative Treatment in Incomplete Spinal Cord Injury (COSMIC; N= 72; NCT01367405) is comparing early decompression (within 24 hours) to conservative treatment.[34]

## Blood Pressure Augmentation

SCI disrupts the sympathetic outflow of the spinal cord and results in a loss of vascular tone below the level of injury. This results in impaired venous return and causes a decrease in cardiac output. With high-thoracic and cervical injuries, sympathetically driven compensatory cardiac chronotropy and inotropy are also lost, resulting in bradycardia and hypotension (neurogenic shock). This is further exacerbated in polytrauma, where hypovolemia is common.

Preclinical SCI data and the clinical traumatic brain injury (TBI) literature suggest that even brief periods of hypotension (systolic blood pressure [SBP] <90 mm Hg) or hypoxia ($PaO_2$ <60 mm Hg) are associated with significantly higher morbidity and mortality rates.[28,36–37] In one study, a single episode of hypotension in TBI was associated with a 150% increase in mortality.[36] While vascular autoregulatory mechanisms in the central nervous system (CNS) are able to maintain perfusion over a wide range of blood pressures, these mechanisms are lost after injury. Furthermore, severe SCI can induce vasospasm and intraluminal thromboses, which further impair parenchymal blood flow and make the cord highly susceptible to secondary ischemia.[4]

Augmentation of blood pressure aims to mitigate ischemia by maintaining a state of normal to slightly increased systemic perfusion. Multiple case series, retrospective studies, and prospective cohort studies have demonstrated that high-normal mean arterial blood pressures (MAPs) of 85–90 mm Hg may enhance SCI outcomes.[25–27] The American Association of Neurological Surgeons (AANS) and Congress of Neurological Surgeons (CNS) suggest MAP targets of 85–90 mm Hg as an option in SCI, to be initiated as early as possible and maintained for the first 7 days following injury.[38] This strategy is increasingly being applied in practice, but the ideal blood pressure target and duration of treatment have not yet been elucidated.

MAP elevation, however, requires the maintenance of a euvolemic or slightly hypervolemic state and often requires an infusion of vasopressors. The clinical interventions to elevate MAP can lead to cardiac stress (e.g., arrhythmias or myocardial ischemia/infarction), peripheral limb ischemia from prolonged use of vasoconstrictors, and pulmonary edema. To assess the efficacy of lower blood pressure targets, a noninferiority trial entitled Mean Arterial Blood Pressure Treatment for Acute Spinal Cord Injury (MAPS; NCT02232165) compares MAP of 65 mm Hg or higher versus MAP of 85 mm Hg or higher and will assess ASIA motor scores at 1 year post-injury.[34] The Canadian Multicenter CSF Monitoring and Biomarker Study (CAMPER; NCT01279811) is examining the effect of spinal cord perfusion pressure (MAP-intrathecal pressure [ITP]) on ASIA Impairment Scale scores and pain at 1 year post-injury, as well as cerebrospinal fluid (CSF) biomarkers as a new assessment technique after SCI.[34]

## Cerebrospinal Fluid Drainage

An additional neuroprotective strategy targeting spinal cord perfusion pressure is to reduce intrathecal pressure through CSF drainage. An indwelling lumbar drain catheter enables continual removal of CSF to achieve a targeted CSF pressure while MAP goals are maintained. This has been shown to reduce the risk of spinal cord ischemia and postoperative neurological deficits during aortic aneurysm surgery, where major radicular branches supplying the cord may be hypoperfused for extended periods of time.

Preclinical experiments have shown a 24% increase in cord blood flow after SCI using a combined treatment of MAP augmentation and CSF drainage.[39] A phase I/II randomized controlled trial (RCT) in patients with acute SCI (N= 22) demonstrated no adverse effects with continual CSF drainage; however, the study was not powered to demonstrate efficacy.[40] A follow-up phase IIB RCT entitled Cerebrospinal Fluid Drainage in Acute Spinal Cord Injury (N = 60; NCT02495545) will compare ISNCSCI motor scores at 180 days post-injury in patients receiving high-target MAP augmentation (MAP 100–110 mm Hg) and CSF drainage (ITP target 10 mm Hg) versus standard MAP augmentation alone (MAP 85–90 mm Hg).[34]

## Hyperbaric Oxygen

Tissue hypoxia, auto-oxidation of amine neurotransmitters, and inflammatory cell activation lead to the generation of hydrogen peroxide, superoxide, and nitric oxide upon reperfusion, all of which damage DNA, proteins, and lipid membranes.[41] An alternative method of preventing hypoxic-ischemia in the cord has been to increase oxygen delivery. Hyperbaric oxygen (HBO) therapy delivers 100% oxygen in a pressurized chamber at 2–3 atmospheres to increase the partial pressure of oxygen in the arterial blood $(PaO_2)$ to supranormal levels. All tissues then receive an increased partial pressure of oxygen, which helps to maintain aerobic metabolism. This has been an effective strategy to improve refractory wound healing.[42] Increased oxygen levels also help to clear nitric oxide, but they increase levels of potentially damaging free radical reactive oxygen species as well. The concomitant increase in free radical scavengers, such as superoxide dismutase and catalase, may ameliorate this potential risk.[43]

The potential benefit or harm of HBO for SCI remains unknown. In preclinical studies, very early (within 4 hours) and early (within 24 hours) HBO in animals with SCI has been shown to reduce necrosis and inflammation in the cord. Clinical trials, however, are lacking, likely due to significant logistical issues in accessing and applying hyperbaric treatments to critically ill patients in the ICU. A small retrospective study ($N= 34$) of patients with cervical SCI without bony injury reported that 75% of patients improved with HBO compared to 65% of patients without HBO therapy, although selection bias may have influenced the findings.[44]

## Therapeutic Hypothermia

Therapeutic hypothermia is an important neuroprotective strategy for many ischemic conditions (e.g., post–cardiac arrest, neonatal hypoxic-ischemic encephalopathy). In the hypothermic state, there is a decrease in the basal metabolic rate of all tissues, particularly the CNS. This reduces oxygen consumption, glucose consumption, CNS blood flow, free radical production (superoxide, hydrogen peroxide, peroxynitrite), neurotoxic neurotransmitter release, pro-apoptotic signaling, inflammation, and blood–spinal cord permeability. Trials in cardiac arrest have shown that a 1°C decrease in core temperature can reduce $O_2$ consumption and $CO_2$ production by approximately 6–10%. This amounts to a 25–40% reduction at therapeutic hypothermia targets of 32–34°C.[45-46]

Cooling is achieved using chilled intravenous fluids, intravascular cooling catheters, and surface cooling (e.g., ice packs, water-cooled blankets). An experienced and well-trained critical care unit is required to safely and rapidly cool patients while addressing common complications such as shivering, pain, peripheral vasoconstriction, coagulopathy, and cardiac arrhythmias. This requires the use of appropriate sedation, analgesia, paralytics, and continuous invasive monitoring.

Several preclinical trials of therapeutic hypothermia for SCI have been conducted and a meta-analysis demonstrated that both systemic and regional hypothermia can improve functional outcomes by approximately 25%.[46] These data led to the development of a prospective pilot study, led by the Miami Project to Cure Paralysis group, that assessed the effect of systemic hypothermia on 1-year functional outcomes in 14 patients with acute SCI.[47] There was a trend toward improved recovery with hypothermia and no increase in adverse events. A follow-up phase II/III study titled Acute Rapid Cooling Therapy for Injuries of the Spinal Cord

(ARCTIC; $N = 200$) addresses the safety and efficacy of hypothermia initiated within 6 hours of injury on a larger scale.[34]

## PHARMACOLOGIC INTERVENTIONS
### Fibroblast Growth Factor

Fibroblast growth factor (FGF) plays a key role in angiogenesis, wound healing, embryological development, and the in vitro maintenance of pluripotency. In SCI animal models, FGF confers neuroprotection from excitotoxicity and secondary injury due to free radicals.[48] A phase I/II RCT ($N= 164$) is comparing the FGF analogue SUN13837 (Edison, New Jersey: Asubio Pharmaceuticals Inc.; once daily for 28 days) versus placebo.[34]

### Magnesium

Magnesium (Mg) is an antagonist of N-methyl-D-aspartate (NMDA) receptors, which bind the excitatory amino acid glutamate. Magnesium also inhibits neutrophil infiltration and free radical generation. These protective properties have been demonstrated in preclinical models of TBI and myocardial infarction (MI). In an animal model of spinal cord contusion injury, Mg administered within 4 hours of injury has been shown to reduce blood–spinal cord barrier damage, reduce lesion size, increase oligodendrocyte survival, decrease neutrophil infiltration, and result in better neurological function.[49]

$MgCl_2$ and $MgSO_4$ are the most common clinical preparations; however, their administration does not result in sufficiently high CNS concentrations to be neuroprotective. By adding an excipient, such as polyethylene glycol (PEG 3350), a higher CSF peak can be obtained. Acorda Therapeutics has conducted a phase I/II RCT ($N= 16$; NCT01750684) of IV AC105 (PEG-Mg; q6h × 30 h).[34]

### Gacyclidine

Another NMDA receptor antagonist, gacyclidine, has been investigated clinically for neuroprotection after SCI. A 1999 phase II trial assessed the efficacy of gacyclidine at three dosing levels versus placebo ($N= 280$). No differences in sensory or motor scores were found at follow-up.[50] No further trials have been registered.

### Granulocyte Colony-Stimulating Factor

Granulocyte colony-stimulating factor (G-CSF; CSF 3) is a glycoprotein that acts as a cytokine and hormone to stimulate granulocyte production, differentiation, and survival. This agent has been used extensively for hematopoietic stimulation after chemotherapy. G-CSF has also been shown to promote survival of ischemic cells in models of MI and stroke.[51-52] After SCI, administration of G-CSF enhances neurogenesis, reduces excitotoxic apoptosis, and decreases expression of tumor necrosis factor-α (TNFα) and interleukin-1β (IL-1β). In a mouse model of compressive SCI, G-CSF treatment resulted in a greater number of surviving long-tract neurons and better functional recovery as assessed by hind limb motor function.[53]

A phase I/IIa trial of low-dose (5 µg/kg/d) versus high-dose (10 µg/kg/d) G-CSF administered intravenously for 5 consecutive days in patients with acute

SCI ($N$ = 16) found no significant adverse events.[54] All patients showed ASIA Impairment Scale score improvements 3 months after injury, and patients receiving high-dose G-CSF had better outcomes. The data must be interpreted cautiously, however, given possible selection bias and the lack of a control group. Another phase I/IIa trial ($N$ = 62) of G-CSF (10 µg/kg/d × 5 days) versus high-dose MPSS found that 17.9% of patients with ASIA B (incomplete sensory; complete motor) and ASIA C (incomplete motor) grade injuries improved by at least two grades with G-CSF treatment.[55] Despite these promising results, the lack of placebo-controlled, appropriately randomized trials of G-CSF is a significant barrier to its clinical acceptance.

### Hepatocyte Growth Factor

Hepatocyte growth factor (HGF) is primarily secreted by mesenchymal cells and promotes cellular growth and motility. It is being investigated in liver regeneration and repair of the heart after myocardial infarction. Laboratory studies have shown HGF to be neuroprotective after SCI by inducing angiogenesis and by maintaining the blood–brain barrier.[56-57] In SCI models, HGF enhances neuron survival, decreases lesion size, reduces oligodendrocyte apoptosis, and improves functional recovery.[57] An important study of cervical SCI in nonhuman primates found that HGF treatment resulted in better functional recovery.[56] A phase I/II trial (NCT02193334; $N$= 48) comparing intrathecal HGF (KP100IT; 0.6 mg weekly × 5 doses) versus placebo is assessing adverse events and ASIA scores up to 24 weeks post-injury.[34]

### Thyrotropin-Releasing Hormone

Thyrotropin-releasing hormone (TRH, TRF), which is produced by the paraventricular nuclei of the hypothalamus, stimulates the release of thyroid-stimulating hormone and prolactin. It also inhibits platelet-activating factor and leukotrienes to reduce the inflammatory response in the CNS. Animal models of TBI and SCI have shown robust improvements in motor scores with TRH treatment shortly after injury. A 1995 phase II RCT ($N$= 20) found significant improvements in motor and sensory function scores for the subgroup of patients with incomplete injuries. Study attrition and small subgroup numbers ($n$ = 6), however, limited the strength of the conclusions.[58] No further trials of TRH have been registered.

### Rho-ROCK Inhibition

Rho and its downstream effector Rho Kinase (ROCK) are potent inhibitors of cell motility and cytoskeleton growth. Rho-ROCK activation results in growth cone collapse and neurite retraction. Cethrin, a subunit of botulinum toxin, is capable of inactivating Rho. Topical application of Cethrin to SCI in experimental studies results in decreased lesion size, increased regeneration of axons through the injury site, and improved behavioral outcomes.[59] A mixed-level phase I/IIa dose-escalation trial ($N$ = 48) assessed VX-210 (Cethrin; Vertex Pharmaceuticals) applied topically as an extradural fibrin sealant. No significant adverse events were observed, and patients with cervical cord injuries demonstrated on average an 18.6 point increase in ASIA motor scores at 12 months post-injury.[60] These exciting results have led to the development of a phase II/III randomized, multicenter trial (NCT02053883) that will selectively focus on patients with ASIA Grade A (complete injury) and B (incomplete sensory; complete motor) C4–C6 injuries.[34] Participants will be given either high-dose Cethrin, low-dose Cethrin, or placebo and assessed by ASIA Impairment Scale, Spinal Cord Independence Measure (SCIM), and Graded Redefined Assessment of Strength, Sensibility and Prehension (GRASSP) scores up to 6 months post-injury.

## Methylprednisolone

Methylprednisolone (MPSS) is a potent glucocorticoid that upregulates anti-inflammatory enzyme transcription, protects against oxidative stress, and interferes with the actions of inflammatory cytokines, cell adhesion molecules, and arachidonic acid metabolites. Experimental studies have shown that MPSS has potent neuroprotective properties in SCI and have formed the basis for multiple large-scale clinical trials over the past 30 years.[60] These trials formed the rationale for AANS/CNS guidelines recommendation of MPSS as a treatment option in acute SCI. The last iteration of the guidelines, however, reversed this position and recommend against MPSS administration, despite there being no new RCT data. Part of the confusion likely stems from the interpretation of the landmark trials and the importance of treatment timing. Here we highlight the most robust prospective data and underscore the critical importance of recognizing subgroups within the heterogeneous SCI patient population.

The 1984 National Acute Spinal Cord Injury Study (NASCIS; $N=330$) was a prospective, randomized, blinded trial of low-dose (100 mg loading + 25 mg q6h) versus high-dose (1000 mg bolus + 250 mg q6h) IV MPSS administered for 10 days post-injury. The study demonstrated no difference in neurologic outcomes for the two regimens. Subsequent laboratory studies, however, showed that the dose in both treatment groups likely failed to produce sufficient serum concentrations to be neuroprotective.[61]

The 1990 NASCIS II ($N = 487$) was a follow-up prospective, blinded, randomized trial that addressed the potential underdosing of NASCIS. A shorter but higher dosing regimen of MPSS (5.4 mg/kg loading + 4.5 mg/kg/h) was compared to naloxone (5.4 mg/kg loading + 4.5 mg/kg/h) and placebo. No difference was observed in overall motor function scores, but sensory function scores were significantly better for patients treated with MPSS. The authors hypothesized a priori that time to initiate treatment likely played a key role in the effect of MPSS. To assess this, a post hoc subgroup analysis of those receiving MPSS within 8 hours of injury (mode time to intervention) was performed; it showed significant improvements in motor and sensory scores.[62]

Parallel preclinical work suggested that longer treatment durations may also be more efficacious. This led to the development of the NASCIS III ($N = 499$), a prospective, randomized, blinded trial of short-course IV MPSS (30 mg/kg loading + 5.4 mg/kg/h × 24 h) versus long-course IV MPSS (30 mg/kg loading + 5.4 mg/kg/h × 48 h) versus tirilizad (nonglucocorticoid lipid peroxidation inhibitor; 2.5 mg/kg q6h × 48 h).[63] The long-duration MPSS treatment group showed no overall difference in neurological outcomes compared to the short-duration MPSS treatment group and showed a trend toward greater respiratory complications (e.g., pneumonia) and severe sepsis. A post hoc subgroup analysis confirmed that

MPSS administered within 3–8 hours of injury was associated with improved (5-point) ASIA motor score recovery compared to MPSS administered after 8 hours post-injury.

A meta-analysis of RCTs by the Cochrane Group found that MPSS administered within 8 hours of injury is associated with a 4-point improvement in motor scores at 6 months post-injury.[64] Despite this being the highest quality of evidence available, the Cochrane meta-analysis was not included in the most recent AANS/CNS guidelines.[38] The 2016 AOSpine guidelines will recommend IV MPSS be administered to patients within 8 hours of injury. These definitive guidelines have been developed by an international group of experts from a diverse range of backgrounds, including physicians, allied care providers, patients, and independent literature/statistical consultants.

## Naloxone

Naloxone is a competitive opioid receptor antagonist that inhibits the activation of microglia. This results in decreased release of inflammatory factors (TNFα, interleukin-1β) and reduced production of harmful superoxides. A 1985 phase I pilot study demonstrated safety, provided dosing data, and showed evidence for neurological improvement with naloxone administration.[65] As part of NASCIS II, naloxone was administered in a randomized, blinded fashion and compared with MPSS and placebo. No change in neurological recovery was found when compared with placebo.[62] No further trials have been registered.

## Riluzole

Riluzole is a benzothiazole antiepileptic drug that acts via sodium channel blockade. It is commonly used in the treatment of amyotrophic lateral sclerosis (ALS). Its role in neuroprotection stems from its ability to mitigate excitotoxicity. Riluzole may also potentiate reuptake of glutamate from the synapse. In preclinical testing, riluzole has been shown to produce dramatic improvements in motor function and electrophysiologic indices.[66-68] These important neuroprotective effects, and existing regulatory approval for ALS, make riluzole a key drug in current clinical trials for SCI.

A collaborative effort by the North American Clinical Trials Network (NACTN), AOSpine, the Rick Hansen Institute, and the Ontario Neurotrauma Foundation has led to the development of a phase II/III RCT (NCT01597518). The Riluzole in Spinal Cord Injury Study (RISCIS; $N = 351$) will compare riluzole (100 mg BID × 24 h then 50 mg BID × 13 days) versus placebo and assess ASIA Impairment Scale, Spinal Cord Independence Measure (SCIM), and brief pain inventory (BPI) scores at 180 days post-injury.[34]

## Minocycline

Minocycline is a broad-spectrum tetracycline antibiotic that is lipid soluble, giving it the ability to cross the blood–brain barrier. It also has potent anti-inflammatory properties and inhibits TNFα, IL-1β, cyclooxygenase-2 (COX-2) and activation of microglia. In animal models of SCI, minocycline has been shown to protect against neuron loss and decrease the size of cord lesions.[69-70] In a mixed-level phase II study, subgroup analysis of cervical SCI patients ($n = 25$) showed an ASIA motor score improvement of 14 points with minocycline treatment compared to placebo.[71] The follow-up phase III Minocycline in Acute Spinal Cord Injury (MASC; NCT01828203; N= 248) RCT will compare IV minocycline (BID as 800 mg × 1, 700 mg × 1, 600 mg × 1, 500 mg × 1, 400 mg × 10) versus placebo and assess ASIA and SCIM scores up to 1 year post injury.[34]

## GM-1

Monosialotetrahexosylganglioside (GM-1) is a ganglioside in the CNS that positively influences neuronal plasticity, survival and repair, and activates neurotrophic factor receptor tyrosine kinases. These effects are further bolstered in the presence of neurotrophins. GM-1 has been successfully used for neuroprotection in animal models of Parkinson disease, Huntington disease, stroke, and SCI.[72] A phase II RCT (N= 37) of GM-1 for SCI showed that daily treatment for 18–32 days improved ASIA motor scores at 1 year post-injury.[73] A follow-up phase III RCT (N= 797) in acute SCI demonstrated a trend toward improved sensory and motor scores.[74] No further studies of GM-1 for SCI have been registered.

## Nimodipine

Nimodipine is a calcium-channel blocker commonly used to prevent post-subarachnoid hemorrhage–related vasospasm. A key mechanism of excitotoxic cell death is the uncontrolled influx of calcium ions, which activates degradation enzymes such as nucleases, proteases, and phospholipases. Calcium-channel blockade has been shown to reduce neuron loss in rodent models of SCI.[75] A phase III RCT (N = 106) of MPSS (30 mg/kg loading + 5.4 mg/kg/h × 23 h) versus nimodipine (0.5 mg/kg/h × 2 h then 0.03 mg/kg/h × 7 days) versus MPSS + nimodipine versus placebo, however, found no differences in ASIA Impairment Scale scores 1 year post-injury.[76]

## IMPLICATIONS FOR CLINICAL PRACTICE
### Current Guidelines

The recommendations of the current AANS/CNS joint guidelines for SCI are summarized in Table 15.1. All recommendations represent either diagnostic or neuroprotective interventions for SCI. Levels of evidence are ranked as level I (well-designed RCTs), level II (nonrandomized cohort studies, case-control studies, or less well-designed randomized studies), or level III (case series, case reports, expert opinions, comparative studies with historical controls, significantly flawed randomized trials).[38]

A key level I recommendation is the use of CT imaging as the primary assessment modality for all patients with SCI. Plain radiographs are insufficient to reliably assess the morphology of bony/ligamentous injuries and frequently miss injuries. Another level I recommendation, that against the use of MPSS for acute SCI, will be changed in the 2017 AOSpine guidelines. The new recommendation will state that MPSS should be administered to patients within 8 hours of injury as a neuroprotective measure.

**Table 15.1** Current Best Practices for Diagnosis and Management of Spinal Cord Injury (SCI)

| Topic | Level of AANS/CNS Recommendation | Guideline/Recommendation |
| --- | --- | --- |
| Hypotension | Level III | Correction of hypotension to systolic blood pressure >90 mm Hg) as soon as possible. |
| | Level III | Maintenance of mean arterial blood pressure between 85 and 90 mm Hg for 7 days. |
| Hypoxia | None | Hypoxia ($PaO_2$ <60 mm Hg or $O_2$ saturation <90%) should be avoided.[3] |
| ICU Monitoring | Level III | SCI patients should be managed in an ICU setting with cardiac, hemodynamic, and respiratory monitoring to detect cardiovascular dysfunction and respiratory insufficiency. |
| Immobilization | Level II | Patients with SCI or suspected SCI (except in penetrating injury) should be immobilized. |
| | Level III | Spinal immobilization should be performed with rigid cervical collar and supportive blocks on a backboard with straps. |
| Specialized Centers | Level III | SCI patients should be transferred expediently to specialized centers of SCI care. |
| Examination | Level II | The ASIA ISNCSCI examination should be performed and documented. |
| Imaging | Level I | No cervical imaging is required in awake trauma patients who have no neck pain/tenderness, normal neurological examination, normal range of motion, and no distracting injuries. |
| | Level I | Computed tomography (CT) is recommended in favor of cervical x-rays. |
| | Level I | CT angiography is recommended in patients who meet the modified Denver screening criteria.[9] |
| Neuroprotection | Level I | Methylprednisolone is not recommended* |
| Spinal Cord Decompression | None | Surgical decompression prior to 24 hours after SCI can be performed safely and is associated with improved neurological outcome.[10] |
| | Level III | Early closed reduction of fracture/dislocation in awake patients without a rostral injury is recommended, and prereduction magnetic resonance imaging (MRI) does not appear to influence outcome. |

The table displays several key recommendations, many of which are from the 2013 updated guidelines from the Joint Section on Disorders of the Spine and Peripheral Nerves of the American Association of Neurological Surgeons and the Congress of Neurological Surgeons. Reprinted with permission from Martin AR, Aleksanderek I, Fehlings MG. Diagnosis and acute management of spinal cord injury: current best practices and emerging therapies. *Curr Trauma Rep.* 2015;1(3):169–81.

*The authors do not agree with this guideline.

Important level II recommendations include the prompt immobilization of all patients with confirmed or potential SCI to prevent further injury and careful documentation of detailed ASIA scoring at baseline and beyond.

Additional neuroprotective measures, classified as level III recommendations, include correction of hypotension (SBP <90 mm Hg) as soon as possible, and maintenance of MAP at 85–90 mm Hg for 7 days post-injury. All patients should be rapidly transferred to a specialized center and managed in an ICU setting with respiratory, cardiac, and hemodynamic monitoring.

The final (unclassified) recommendations discussed in the guidelines are that surgical decompression be performed within 24 hours to improve neurological outcomes and hypoxia ($PaO_2$ <60 mm Hg or $O_2$ saturation <90%) be avoided, even for brief periods.

These guidelines represent a distillation of decades of research in SCI and will continue to evolve as new data become available. It is critical that all practitioners providing care to patients with SCI are well-apprised of the most recent literature because time-sensitive interventions in the acute period can produce lifelong changes for patients.

## FUTURE DIRECTIONS

Early landmark trials in SCI applied broad inclusion criteria in order to recruit high numbers of patients; however, post hoc subgroup analyses revealed the importance of distinguishing specific patient subpopulations. Recognizing the marked heterogeneity of SCI in presentation, pathophysiology, and response to treatment will be a key factor in the success of future trials of neuroprotection for SCI. Several studies, including RISCIS and a trial of intraoperative Cethrin, have incorporated restrictions on ASIA grade and level of injury at presentation for patient participation. This is a critical difference between current and past studies and is likely to provide more robust results and larger effect sizes.

This concept of heterogeneity in SCI needs to extend to individual patient care as well. Neuroprotective therapies must be carefully tailored to specific patients and injury patterns. This requires an in-depth knowledge of the functional and anatomic classification of injuries in patients with SCI. It will also require the development of more robust staging techniques, including advanced MRI techniques and biochemical CSF/serum biomarkers.[77–78] As these evolve, future trials may be able to further stratify patients and identify key niches where significant gains can be made utilizing individual therapies or novel combinatorial strategies.

The completed, ongoing, and upcoming trials described in this chapter represent an exciting body of literature in a field where even small improvements can have tremendous physical, functional, and vocational implications for patients.

## REFERENCES

1. National Spinal Cord Injury Statistical Center. Spinal cord injury facts and figures at a glance. *J Spinal Cord Med.* 2014;37(1):117–8.

2. Christopher & Dana Reeve Foundation. One degree of separation: paralysis and spinal cord injury in the United States. 2010. Available from: http://www.christopherreeve.org/site/c.ddJFKRNoFiG/b.5091685/k.58BD/One_Degree_of_Separation.htm.

3. Dvorak MF NV, Fallah N, Fisher CG, et al. The influence of time from injury to surgery on motor recovery and length of hospital stay in acute traumatic spinal cord injury: an observational Canadian cohort study. *J Neurotrauma.* 2015;32(9):645.

4. Wilson JR, Forgione N, Fehlings MG. Emerging therapies for acute traumatic spinal cord injury. *CMAJ.* 2013;185(6):485–92.

5. Tator CH, Duncan EG, Edmonds VE, Lapczak LI, Andrews DF. Complications and costs of management of acute spinal cord injury. *Paraplegia.* 1993;31(11):700–14.

6. Tator CH, Fehlings MG. Review of the secondary injury theory of acute spinal cord trauma with emphasis on vascular mechanisms. *J Neurosurg.* 1991;75(1):15–26.

7. Whetstone WD, Hsu JY, Eisenberg M, Werb Z, Noble-Haeusslein LJ. Blood-spinal cord barrier after spinal cord injury: relation to revascularization and wound healing. *J Neurosci Res.* 2003;74(2):227–39.

8. Mautes AE, Weinzierl MR, Donovan F, Noble LJ. Vascular events after spinal cord injury: contribution to secondary pathogenesis. *Phys Ther.* 2000;80(7):673–87.

9. Waxman SG. Demyelination in spinal cord injury. *J Neurologic Sci.* 1989;91(1-2):1–14.

10. Li S, Mealing GA, Morley P, Stys PK. Novel injury mechanism in anoxia and trauma of spinal cord white matter: glutamate release via reverse Na+-dependent glutamate transport. *J Neurosci.* 1999;19(14):RC16.

11. Li S, Stys PK. Mechanisms of ionotropic glutamate receptor-mediated excitotoxity in isolated spinal cord white matter. *J Neurosci.* 2000;20(3):1190–8.

12. Boggan JE. Pathophysiology of spinal cord injury. *J Neurosurg.* 1979;50(6):840.

13. Tator CH. Acute spinal cord injury: a review of recent studies of treatment and pathophysiology. *Can Med Assoc J.* 1972;107(2):143–5 passim.

14. Adams J. *Emergency medicine.* New York: Saunders Elsevier; 2013.

15. Spinal trauma. *The Merck Manuals*; 2015. Available from: http://www.merckmanuals.com/professional/injuries-poisoning/spinal-trauma/spinal-trauma.

16. Aebli N, Wicki AG, Ruegg TB, Petrou N, Eisenlohr H, Krebs J. The Torg-Pavlov ratio for the prediction of acute spinal cord injury after a minor trauma to the cervical spine. *Spine J.* 2013;13(6):605–12.

17. Aebli N, Ruegg TB, Wicki AG, Petrou N, Krebs J. Predicting the risk and severity of acute spinal cord injury after a minor trauma to the cervical spine. *Spine J.* 2013;13(6):597–604.

18. Hachen HJ. Idealized care of the acutely injured spinal cord in Switzerland. *J Trauma.* 1977;17(12):931–6.

19. Ahn H, Singh J, Nathens A, et al. Pre-hospital care management of a potential spinal cord injured patient: a systematic review of the literature and evidence-based guidelines. *J Neurotrauma.* 2011;28(8):1341–61.

20. ASIA. International Standards for the Classification of Spinal Cord Injury—Key Sensory Points. 2008. Available from: http://lms3.learnshare.com/Images/Brand/120/ASIA/Key%20Sensory%20Points.pdf.

21. ASIA. International Standards for the Classification of Spinal Cord Injury—Motor Exam Guide. 2008. Available from: http://lms3.learnshare.com/Images/Brand/120/ASIA/Motor%20Exam%20Guide.pdf.

22. Ryken TC, Hadley MN, Walters BC, et al. Radiographic assessment. *Neurosurgery.* 2013;72 Suppl 2:54–72.

23. Wilson JR, Grossman RG, Frankowski RF, et al. A clinical prediction model for long-term functional outcome after traumatic spinal cord injury based on acute clinical and imaging factors. *J Neurotrauma.* 2012;29(13):2263–71.

24. Gschaedler R, Dollfus P, Mole JP, Mole L, Loeb JP. Reflections on the intensive care of acute cervical spinal cord injuries in a general traumatology centre. *Paraplegia.* 1979;17(1):58–61.

25. Tator CH, Rowed DW, Schwartz ML, et al. Management of acute spinal cord injuries. *Can J Surg.* 1984;27(3):289–93, 296.

26. Levi L, Wolf A, Belzberg H. Hemodynamic parameters in patients with acute cervical cord trauma: description, intervention, and prediction of outcome. *Neurosurgery*. 1993;33(6):1007–16; discussion 1016–7.

27. Vale FL, Burns J, Jackson AB, Hadley MN. Combined medical and surgical treatment after acute spinal cord injury: results of a prospective pilot study to assess the merits of aggressive medical resuscitation and blood pressure management. *J Neurosurg*. 1997;87(2):239–46.

28. Amar AP, Levy ML. Pathogenesis and pharmacological strategies for mitigating secondary damage in acute spinal cord injury. *Neurosurgery*. 1999;44(5):1027–39; discussion 1039–40.

29. Lehmann KG, Lane JG, Piepmeier JM, Batsford WP. Cardiovascular abnormalities accompanying acute spinal cord injury in humans: incidence, time course and severity. *J Am Coll Cardiol*. 1987;10(1):46–52.

30. McMichan JC, Michel L, Westbrook PR. Pulmonary dysfunction following traumatic quadriplegia. Recognition, prevention, and treatment. *JAMA*. 1980;243(6):528–31.

31. Mansel JK, Norman JR. Respiratory complications and management of spinal cord injuries. *Chest*. 1990;97(6):1446–52.

32. Fehlings MG, Vaccaro A, Wilson JR, et al. Early versus delayed decompression for traumatic cervical spinal cord injury: results of the Surgical Timing in Acute Spinal Cord Injury Study (STASCIS). *PLoS One*. 2012;7(2):e32037.

33. Wilson JS, Craven C, Verrier M, et al. Early versus late surgery for traumatic spinal cord injury: the results of a prospective Canadian cohort study. *Spinal Cord*. 2012;50(11):840.

34. Clinical Trials.gov. 2015. Available from: https://clinicaltrials.gov/.

35. Lenehan B, Fisher CG, Vaccaro A, Fehlings M, Aarabi B, Dvorak MF. The urgency of surgical decompression in acute central cord injuries with spondylosis and without instability. *Spine (Phila Pa 1976)*. 2010;35(21 Suppl):S180–6.

36. Chesnut RM, Marshall LF, Klauber MR, et al. The role of secondary brain injury in determining outcome from severe head injury. *J Trauma*. 1993;34(2):216–22.

37. King BS, Gupta R, Narayan RK. The early assessment and intensive care unit management of patients with severe traumatic brain and spinal cord injuries. *Surg Clin North Am*. 2000;80(3):855–70, viii–ix.

38. Resnick DK. Updated guidelines for the management of acute cervical spine and spinal cord injury. *Neurosurgery*. 2013;72 Suppl 2:1.

39. Martirosyan NL, Kalani MY, Bichard WD, et al. Cerebrospinal fluid drainage and induced hypertension improve spinal cord perfusion after acute spinal cord injury in pigs. *Neurosurgery*. 2015;76:461–8; discussion 468–9.

40. Kwon BK, Curt A, Belanger LM, et al. Intrathecal pressure monitoring and cerebrospinal fluid drainage in acute spinal cord injury: a prospective randomized trial. *J Neurosurg Spine*. 2009;10:181–93.

41. Hall ED. Antioxidant therapies for acute spinal cord injury. *Neurotherapeutics*. 2011;8(2):152–67.

42. Goldman RJ. Hyperbaric oxygen therapy for wound healing and limb salvage: a systematic review. *PM R*. 2009;1(5):471–89.

43. Huang HXL, Zhang X, Weng Q, et al. Hyperbaric oxygen therapy provides neuroprotection following spinal cord injury in a rat model. *Int J Clin Exp Pathol*. 2013;6(7):1337.

44. Falavigna AT, Velho M, Kleber F. Effects of hyperbaric oxygen therapy after spinal cord injury: systematic review. *Coluna*. 2009;8(3):330.

45. Seder DB, Van der Kloot TE. Methods of cooling: practical aspects of therapeutic temperature management. *Crit Care Med*. 2009;37:S211–22.

46. Batchelor PS, Antonic A, Willis T, et al. Systematic review and meta-analysis of therapeutic hypothermia in animal models of spinal cord injury. *PLoS ONE.* 2013;8(8):e71317.

47. Levi AD, Green BA, Wang MY, et al. Clinical application of modest hypothermia after spinal cord injury. *J Neurotrauma.* 2009;26:407–15.

48. Siddiqui AM, Khazaei M, Fehlings MG. Translating mechanisms of neuroprotection, regeneration, and repair to treatment of spinal cord injury. *Prog Brain Res.* 2015;218:15–54.

49. Kaptanoglu E, Beskonakli E, Solaroglu I, Kilinc A, Taskin Y. Magnesium sulfate treatment in experimental spinal cord injury: emphasis on vascular changes and early clinical results. *Neurosurg Rev.* 2003;26:283–7.

50. Hawryluk GK, Fehlings, M. Protection and repair of the injured spinal cord: A review of completed, ongoing, and planned clinical trials for acute spinal cord injury. *Neurosurg Focus.* 2008;25(5):E14.

51. Kanellakis P, Slater NJ, Du XJ, Bobik A, Curtis DJ. Granulocyte colony-stimulating factor and stem cell factor improve endogenous repair after myocardial infarction. *Cardiovasc Res.* 2006;70(1):117–25.

52. Kollmar R, Henninger N, Urbanek C, Schwab S. G-CSF, rt-PA and combination therapy after experimental thromboembolic stroke. *Exp Transl Stroke Med.* 2010;2:9.

53. Nishio Y, Koda M, Kamada T, et al. Granulocyte colony-stimulating factor attenuates neuronal death and promotes functional recovery after spinal cord injury in mice. *J Neuropathol Exp Neurol.* 2007;66(8):724–31.

54. Takahashi H, Yamazaki M, Okawa A, et al. Neuroprotective therapy using granulocyte colony-stimulating factor for acute spinal cord injury: a phase I/IIa clinical trial. *Eur Spine J.* 2012;21(12):2580–7.

55. Kamiya K, Koda M, Furuya T, et al. Neuroprotective therapy with granulocyte colony-stimulating factor in acute spinal cord injury: a comparison with high-dose methylprednisolone as a historical control. *Eur Spine J.* 2015;24(5):963–7.

56. Kitamura K, Fujiyoshi K, Yamane J, et al. Human hepatocyte growth factor promotes functional recovery in primates after spinal cord injury. *PLoS One.* 2011;6:e27706.

57. Kitamura K, Iwanami A, Fujiyoshi K, et al. Recombinant human hepatocyte growth factor promotes functional recovery after spinal cord injury. In: Uchida KNM, Ozawa H, Katoh S, Toyama Y, editors. *Neuroprotection and regeneration of the spinal cord.* Tokyo: Springer Japan; 2014:147–67.

58. Pitts LH, Ross A, Chase GA, Faden A. Treatment with thyrotropin-releasing hormone (TRH) in patients with traumatic spinal cord injuries. *J Neurotrauma.* 1995;12(3):235.

59. Fehlings MG, Theodore N, Harrop J, et al. A phase I/IIa clinical trial of a recombinant Rho protein antagonist in acute spinal cord injury. *J Neurotrauma.* 2011;28(5):787–96.

60. Fehlings M, Wilson J, Cho N. Methylprednisolone for the treatment of acute spinal cord injury: counterpoint. *Neurosurgery.* 2015;61(1):36.

61. Bracken MB, Collins WF, Freeman DF, et al. Efficacy of methylprednisolone in acute spinal cord injury. *JAMA.* 1984;251(1):45–52.

62. Bracken MB, Shepard MJ, Collins WF, et al. A randomized, controlled trial of methylprednisolone or naloxone in the treatment of acute spinal-cord injury. Results of the Second National Acute Spinal Cord Injury Study. *N Engl J Med.* 1990;322(20):1405–11.

63. Bracken MB, Shepard MJ, Holford TR, et al. Administration of methylprednisolone for 24 or 48 hours or tirilazad mesylate for 48 hours in the treatment of acute spinal cord injury. Results of the Third National Acute Spinal Cord Injury Randomized Controlled Trial. National Acute Spinal Cord Injury Study. *JAMA.* 1997;277(20):1597–604.

64. Bracken M. Steroids for acute spinal cord injury. *Cochrane Database Syst Rev.* 2012; CD001046.

65. Flamm ES, Young W, Collins WF, Piepmeier J, Clifton GL, Fischer B. A phase I trial of naloxone treatment in acute spinal cord injury. *J Neurosurg.* 1985;63:390–7.

66. Nogradi A, Szabo A, Pinter S, Vrbova G. Delayed riluzole treatment is able to rescue injured rat spinal motoneurons. *Neuroscience.* 2007;144(2):431–8.

67. Schwartz G, Fehlings MG. Evaluation of the neuroprotective effects of sodium channel blockers after spinal cord injury: improved behavioral and neuroanatomical recovery with riluzole. *J Neurosurg.* 2001;94(2 Suppl):245–56.

68. Stutzmann JM, Pratt J, Boraud T, Gross C. The effect of riluzole on post-traumatic spinal cord injury in the rat. *Neuroreport.* 1996;7(2):387–92.

69. Wells JE, Hurlbert RJ, Fehlings MG, Yong VW. Neuroprotection by minocycline facilitates significant recovery from spinal cord injury in mice. *Brain.* 2003;126(Pt 7): 1628–37.

70. Festoff BW, Ameenuddin S, Arnold PM, Wong A, Santacruz KS, Citron BA. Minocycline neuroprotects, reduces microgliosis, and inhibits caspase protease expression early after spinal cord injury. *J Neurochem.* 2006;97(5):1314–26.

71. Casha S, Zygun D, McGowan MD, Bains I, Yong VW, Hurlbert RJ. Results of a phase II placebo-controlled randomized trial of minocycline in acute spinal cord injury. *Brain.* 2012;135:1224–36.

72. Imanaka T, Hukuda S, Maeda T. The role of GM1-ganglioside in the injured spinal cord of rats: an immunohistochemical study using GM1-antisera. *J Neurotrauma.* 1996;13(3):163–70.

73. Geisler FH, Dorsey FC, Coleman WP. Recovery of motor function after spinal-cord injury: a randomized, placebo-controlled trial with GM-1 ganglioside. *Engl J Med.* 1991;324(26):1829–38.

74. Geisler FH, Coleman WP, Grieco G, Poonian D; Sygen Study Group. The Sygen multicenter acute spinal cord injury study. *Spine.* 2001;26(24 Suppl):S87–98.

75. Winkler T, Sharma HS, Stalberg E, Badgaiyan RD, Gordh T, Westman J. An L-type calcium channel blocker, nimodipine influences trauma induced spinal cord conduction and axonal injury in the rat. *Acta Neurochir Suppl.* 2003;86:425–32.

76. Petitjean ME, Pointillart V, Dixmerias F, et al. [Medical treatment of spinal cord injury in the acute stage]. *Ann Fr Anesth Reanim.* 1998;17(2):114–22.

77. Pouw MH, Hosman AJ, van Middendorp JJ, Verbeek MM, Vos PE, van de Meent H. Biomarkers in spinal cord injury. *Spinal Cord.* 2009;47(7):519–25.

78. Cadotte DW, Fehlings MG. Will imaging biomarkers transform spinal cord injury trials? *Lancet Neurol.* 2013;12(9):843–4.

# PART IV
# PERI-OPERATIVE
# NEUROPROTECTION

# 16 Neuroprotection for Valvular and Coronary Artery Bypass Grafting Surgery

Karsten Bartels

and G. Burkhard Mackensen

## GENERAL CONSIDERATIONS

Neurological injury after valvular and coronary artery bypass grafting surgery (CABG) encompasses a broad spectrum (Figure 16.1).[1] Postoperative cognitive dysfunction (POCD) is extremely common after CABG surgery; it can be detected in up to 50% of patients at the time of hospital discharge and 25% of patients 6 months postoperatively.[2] Overt stroke after cardiac surgery is much less common, with an incidence ranging from 1.2% to 3.4% after cardiac surgery involving cardiopulmonary bypass (CPB), although more contemporary studies often report lower stroke rates.[3–5] Stroke remains among the most devastating complications in open heart surgery and interventional cardiology because it is associated with high morbidity and mortality. Patients undergoing minimally invasive percutaneous transcatheter aortic valve implantation (TAVI) with currently available delivery systems are at even higher risk for stroke than patients undergoing surgical aortic valve replacement (AVR). Within 1 year after TAVI, stroke rates range from 8.3% to 8.8%.[6–7]

In addition to inducing morbidity and mortality in patients, stroke is associated with significant health care costs for patients and their families.[8] POCD also exerts a negative impact on patients' lives and is associated with limited improvement in quality of life after CABG surgery.[9]

## MECHANISMS OF AND RISKS FOR NEUROLOGICAL INJURY
### Risk Factors for Perioperative Neurological Injury

Patient- and procedure-related variables contribute to the likelihood for perioperative neurologic injury and POCD. Predictors of perioperative neurological injury and POCD after cardiac surgery are summarized in Box 16.1.

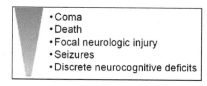

- Coma
- Death
- Focal neurologic injury
- Seizures
- Discrete neurocognitive deficits

FIGURE 16.1 Spectrum of neurologic injury after cardiac surgery.

## Cerebral Embolism

Aortic atherosclerotic disease is associated with stroke after cardiac surgery. A high burden of thoracic aortic atheromatous disease, as detected by perioperative transesophageal echocardiography, has been associated with intraoperative cerebral embolic burden as assessed by transcranial Doppler (TCD) ultrasonography.[10] Although technically challenging, insonation of the middle cerebral artery (MCA) with TCD not only reliably quantifies high-intensity transient signals (HITS) reflecting embolic events, but it also quantifies relative changes in cerebral blood flow (CBF). These relative changes are associated with alterations in MCA flow velocity during conditions under which MCA diameter remains constant.[11-13]

Embolization of particulate and gaseous material into the cerebral microvasculature that results in focal areas of cerebral ischemia has been well studied. Evidence of a direct association between cerebral microembolic load and POCD, however, has been inconsistent.[12,14] This might be explained by our inability to differentiate less harmful gaseous emboli from the more dangerous particulate emboli using TCD.

Magnetic resonance imaging (MRI) is extremely sensitive for detecting ischemic brain injury caused by emboli. Multiple studies have shown new hyperintensities on diffusion-weighted MRI after cardiac surgery in both clinical and experimental contexts.[15-18] In one study, new lesions were detected in three-quarters of the 19 patients enrolled, although these patients did not

---

**Box 16.1** Risk Factors for Perioperative Neurologic Injury and POCD After Cardiac Surgery

**Patient variables:**

Age

History of cerebrovascular disease

Thoracic aortic atheromatous disease

Baseline cognitive function

Education

Delirium

Genetic predisposition

**Procedural variables:**

CPB time

Emergency surgery

Procedure type

Fast rewarming from hypothermia (4–6°C difference between nasopharyngeal and CPB perfusate temperature)

exhibit overt clinical stroke.[15] Importantly, lesions that are detected have not been shown to consistently correlate with POCD.[19] Functional MRI has been proposed to be a more appropriate imaging modality for the evaluation of postoperative changes to brain connectivity.[20] Whether or not functional MRI offers any tangible clinical benefits remains to be seen.

The most obvious causes for cerebral embolism are particulate debris that may be dislodged during aortic cross-clamping or by a "sand-blast" effect of the turbulent flow emerging from the aortic CPB cannula on a severely atheromatous aorta. During TAVI, embolic material is often dislodged to the brain at time of deployment of the valve into a calcified aortic annulus. One study reported that HITS reflecting emboli en route to the brain detected with TCD ultrasound were observed in all 83 of the patients who underwent TAVI.[11] The extremely high incidence (77–84%) of cerebral restrictive diffusion foci documented by MRI following TAVI supports the concept that neurological injury, likely embolic, is more common following TAVI than surgical AVR.[11]

Stroke related to cardiac surgery most often occurs after an initially lucid interval and is referred to as "delayed stroke."[4] The onset of delayed stroke peaks on postoperative days 2 and 3 and has been associated with concurrently occurring atrial fibrillation in some studies.[21] Large retrospective cohort series, however, have generally not confirmed the association between stroke and postoperative atrial fibrillation, especially in patients with normal cardiac output.[3-4] It may be that a pro-inflammatory milieu that peaks on postoperative days 2–4 serves as a driver that promotes stroke and atrial fibrillation independently in this vulnerable postoperative period. This notion is supported by wide-ranging evidence suggesting a role for inflammation in various phases of the pathophysiology of stroke. There is increasing recognition that inflammatory events outside the brain have a significant impact on stroke susceptibility and outcome, possibly by amplification of pathways activated in stroke.[22-23]

## Hypotension

Cerebral perfusion pressure is autoregulated in the healthy brain and permits appropriate CBF across a range of blood pressures. When the cerebral perfusion pressure falls beneath the lower limit of autoregulation, hypoperfusion in watershed areas of the brain and subsequent ischemia can ensue. Indeed, a mean arterial pressure (MAP) that decreases 30% or more from the baseline value has been associated with postoperative stroke after general surgery.[24] In another prospective clinical trial in which patients were randomized to a MAP of 50–60 mm Hg or a high MAP of 80–100 mm Hg during CPB, the incidence of combined cardiac and neurological complications was significantly lower in the high pressure group (4.8% vs. 12.9%).[25]

A relationship between cerebral perfusion pressure and POCD after cardiac surgery has also been documented in a prospective randomized study of 92 patients, with better postoperative Mini-Mental State Examination scores observed in patients maintained with higher blood pressures during CPB (80–90 mm Hg), as compared to patients maintained with lower blood pressures (60–70 mm Hg).[26]

## Systemic Inflammatory Responses

Systemic inflammation exerts effects on the central nervous system that can lead to neuronal damage. The interplay of inflammation with hypoxia can induce acute perioperative organ injury in all vital organs through a host of pathways.[27] Perioperative neuronal injury during CPB, for example, can stem from disruption of the blood–brain barrier.[18,28] While CPB has previously been thought to be the major driver of perioperative inflammation in cardiac surgery, this hypothesis has not been supported by experimental and clinical data. In a rodent model of CPB, levels of the pro-inflammatory cytokine tumor necrosis factor-α (TNFα) and degree of postoperative neurological dysfunction did not differ between animals treated with CPB versus sham operation.[29] Another study comparing CPB versus sham operation (cannula placement) in rodents also showed no difference in cognitive and behavioral markers of cerebral function.[30] These experimental data are consistent with the results from multiple major randomized clinical trials comparing off-pump to on-pump CABG surgery, which essentially have shown little to no tangible difference in relevant clinical outcomes.[31–34]

## Genetic Predisposition

The risk of stroke after cardiac surgery is associated with variants of C-reactive protein (CRP) and the inflammatory cytokine interleukin-6 (IL-6) genes.[35] Such relationships have also been found for POCD. In a prospective cohort study of 513 patients undergoing CABG, single nucleotide polymorphisms for CRP and P-selectin were associated with a lower likelihood of POCD at 6 weeks postoperatively.[36] The apolipoprotein E4 genotype (APOE4), which is a known risk factor for Alzheimer disease, vascular dementia, and worse outcomes following traumatic brain injury, has been inconsistently associated with POCD following cardiac surgery. A study of 282 CABG patients found no association between APOE4 genotype and POCD at 3 or 12 months.[37] A study of 233 CABG and valve surgery patients found that those with the APOE4 genotype had less favorable cognitive outcomes 5 years after cardiac surgery compared to both cardiac surgical patients without the allele and non–cardiac surgical patients with the allele.[38]

## MONITORING FOR NEUROLOGICAL INJURY

While cerebral autoregulation was traditionally thought to occur for cerebral perfusion pressures from 50 mm Hg to 150 mm Hg, individual patients in fact may have quite different low or high inflection points of the CBF autoregulation curve (Figure 16.2).[39–40] A major aim of perioperative monitoring devices is guiding the clinician toward optimization of tissue perfusion according to the specific needs of each patient. Monitors that target the brain and can assist in identifying states where cerebral injury is imminent or occurring and guide intraoperative management include near-infrared spectroscopy (NIRS) to assess cerebral oxygenation and perfusion, TCD to assesses cerebral arterial blood flow, the electroencephalogram (EEG), and the bispectral index (BIS), which is a processed form of the EEG.

NIRS cerebral oximetry devices can help detect the lower inflection point of an individual patient's cerebral autoregulation curve.[22–23] Such individualized approaches permit tailored blood pressure management during cardiac surgery (Figure 16.2). Determining the lower limits of cerebral autoregulation for a given patient (e.g., using NIRS) permits individualized blood pressure management during CPB.[13,41] Cerebral oximetry is widely utilized in daily cardiac anesthesia practice, routinely for surgeries requiring circulatory arrest, and for other elective CABG and

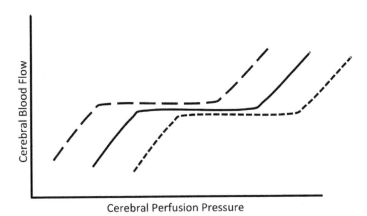

FIGURE 16.2 Cerebral blood flow is autoregulated. The window of autoregulation was classically thought to occur at a cerebral perfusion pressure between 50 and 150 mm Hg (*continuous black line* in figure). Individual patients, however, may have lower (*long dashes*) or higher (*short dashes*) inflection points of the cerebral autoregulation curve.

valve replacement/repair surgeries in some institutions.[42–45] Despite its widespread use, controversy still exists in its interpretation and ability to guide neuroprotective strategies or optimize cerebral outcome after cardiac surgery. A recent systematic literature review of 13 case reports, 27 observational studies, and 2 prospective randomized intervention trials investigated the merits of NIRS use in cardiac surgery.[46] The review concluded that there is only low-level evidence linking low cerebral oxygen saturation during cardiac surgery to postoperative neurological complications, and insufficient data to conclude that interventions to improve desaturation prevent stroke or POCD. Key unanswered questions concern the absolute saturation value at which adverse clinical outcomes increase, the saturation threshold associated with poor prognosis, and whether the trend is of value in predicting postoperative deterioration.[43,45,47] A recent pilot study by Murkin et al. demonstrated the potential that a new ultrasound-tagged near-infrared (UT-NIR) device could detect cerebral autoregulation and thereby identify the lower limit of cerebral autoregulation in comparison to TCD.[48]

Changes in the EEG signal, such as increased δ activity or burst suppression, can be signs of ischemic injury. The occurrence of such changes, however, is nonspecific with regard to the underlying cause. EEG also is not very sensitive to ischemia in that a normal EEG does not ensure a well-perfused brain.[49] Although an association between low BIS and mortality during cardiac surgery has been demonstrated, this relationship is thought to be a manifestation of other relevant patient- and procedure-related factors.[49] The value of EEG for prevention of perioperative ischemic brain injury has yet to be definitively established.

## Clinical Diagnosis of Perioperative Neurological Injury

Stroke has been defined as "Rapidly developed clinical signs of focal or global disturbance of cerebral function, lasting more than 24 h or until death, with no apparent non-vascular cause."[50] Diagnosis therefore requires a physical exam, and the most rigorously validated tool for this purpose is the National Institute of Health Stroke Scale (NIHSS) (Box 16.2). Diagnosing a stroke in the immediate perioperative period is challenging because many of the items on the NIHSS may be impaired due to

**Box 16.2** NIH Stroke Scale Items

1a. Level of Consciousness
1b. Level of Consciousness Questions
1c. Level of Consciousness Commands
2. Best Gaze
3. Visual
4. Facial Palsy
5. Motor Arm
6. Motor Leg
7. Limb Ataxia
8. Sensory
9. Best Language
10. Dysarthria
11. Extinction and Inattention

anesthetic, sedative, or analgesic drug effects rather than stroke. Similarly, invasive monitors such as indwelling catheters can preclude rigorous testing of items such as strength and ataxia.

When perioperative stroke is suspected, the initial primary diagnostic imaging modality of choice is noncontrast computed tomography (CT), combined with CT angiography as indicated. Note that CT imaging only detects early (within 6 hours) correlates of ischemic stroke in 60% of cases. Diffusion-weighted magnetic resonance imaging (MRI) is much more sensitive and detects ischemic stroke in more than 90% of cases (Figure 16.3). The presence of devices such as pacing wires or mechanical assist devices, however, often prevents use of MRI in the acute post cardiac surgery setting.

Measurement of more subtle POCD is usually only performed as part of clinical research using standardized tests that assess distinct cognitive domains.[1] Despite attempts to develop consensus guidelines, definitions of POCD are not

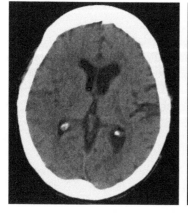 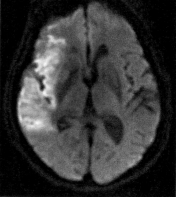

FIGURE 16.3 Brain noncontrast CT (*left*) and diffusion-weighted MRI (*right*) in a patient after acute stroke in the right middle cerebral artery territory. The loss of gray and white matter differentiation on noncontrast CT is quite subtle but can be easily detected using diffusion-weighted MRI.

standardized, thus making the differentiation of cognitive dysfunction due to a distinct perioperative insult versus a consequence of aging and progression of coexisting diseases difficult.[51] For clinical trials on POCD, inclusion of nonsurgical controls is therefore of critical importance.[52]

## NEUROPROTECTION STRATEGIES
### Pharmacologic Interventions

The principle of effective pharmacologic neuroprotection has suffered greatly from lack of translation of seemingly promising animal experimental studies into successful clinical trials.[53] While more than 1,000 substances have been shown to have neuroprotective effects in experimental ischemia, none has proved efficacious in more than 280 clinical trials (see also Chapter 4).[54-55] Promising interventions that have failed to improve outcomes after cardiac surgery include 17-β-estradiol, magnesium, lidocaine, piracetam, and dexamethasone.[56-60] The practicing clinician is left with intellectually appealing pharmacologic concepts for neuroprotection but prospective clinical studies that have thus far not shown any tangible benefits.[61]

### Mechanical Interventions

The 2013 American Heart Association/American Stroke Association (AHA/ASA) guidelines report intravenous recombinant tissue plasminogen activator (r-tPA) use after major surgery as a relative contraindication, and it is therefore rarely considered as a therapeutic option for perioperative stroke after cardiac surgery.[62] Catheter-directed lysis in large prospective clinical trials of nonsurgical populations has failed to exceed the efficacy of systemic r-tPA.[63-64] The recent advent of mechanical thrombectomy as a powerful treatment for stroke due to large vessel occlusion (LVO) makes it the most appealing and useful treatment option for post–cardiac surgery patients.[65-68] Demonstration of LVO is the crucial diagnostic trigger for pursuing endovascular mechanical thrombectomy.

### Atheromatous Disease Management

Emboli from atherosclerotic disease in the aorta frequently lead to intraoperative embolic events during conventional cardiac surgery and TAVI.[10,16-17] While off-pump CABG has not been associated with significant improvements in neurocognitive outcomes, substantial efforts have been made to capture the embolic burden released to the brain at the time of expansion of transcatheter aortic valves.[31,69] While large clinical trials are ongoing, preliminary results using a filter shield of the upper aortic arch vessels deployed at the time of TAVI have shown reductions in ischemic brain lesions from 26.9% to 11.5%, and a reduction of neurological deficits from 15.4% to 3.1%.[70]

### Temperature Management

Therapeutic hypothermia ranging from 32°C to 34°C improves neurological outcomes in survivors of cardiac arrest.[71-72] Encouraged by these landmark studies, therapeutic hypothermia has been adopted as a neuroprotective strategy in perioperative medicine.[73] A trial of hypothermic cardiopulmonary bypass in CABG patients, however, did not confer significant neurological protection.[74] In contrast, avoidance of postoperative hyperthermia has been associated with better cognitive outcomes after CABG.[75] Limiting the rate of rewarming to 2°C (nasopharyngeal versus CPB blood temperature), as compared to a larger temperature difference of 4–6°C, has also been associated with better cognitive outcomes following cardiac surgery.[76]

Whether hypothermia per se or avoidance of hyperthermia is the most appropriate neuroprotective strategy remains to be determined. This is likely to depend on the clinical scenario. Current evidence does not support the use of hypothermia for neuroprotection in this clinical setting, based on a trial in which no significant difference in clinical outcomes was observed in cohorts randomized to 33°C versus 36°C CPB.[77] Recent guidelines by the American Society of Cardiovascular Anesthesiologists, The Society of Thoracic Surgeons, and The American Society of Extra-Corporeal Technology comprehensively summarize recommended temperature management strategies for surgical procedures requiring CPB.[78]

## IMPLICATIONS FOR CLINICAL PRACTICE

Prevention of neurological injury is key to improved neurological outcomes after cardiac surgery because efficacy of therapeutic strategies is limited. The nonpharmacological strategies that can be recommended on the basis of current evidence include (1) optimal temperature management and (2) ultrasound-guided assessment of the (potentially) atheromatous ascending aorta, with appropriate modification of aortic cannulation, clamping, or anastomotic technique. Diagnosis of perioperative neurological injury relies on physical examination, highlighting the need to minimize long-acting sedative drugs in the perioperative period. Diffusion-weighted MRI should be considered in patients with a high suspicion for perioperative ischemic brain injury, even if CT of the brain was negative for stroke.

## FUTURE DIRECTIONS

With the persistent failure of pharmacologic approaches for neuroprotection in clinical trials, great care needs to be taken when evaluating results of animal experimental data for translation to clinical trials. Rigor in study design, appropriate experimental models, as well as replication in different laboratories, is encouraged. More research is needed to establish whether genetic risk factors play a role in determining which patients have adverse neurological outcomes and, if so, whether such associations can be elevated to an approach for personalized perioperative medicine. Individualized approaches, such as goal-directed blood pressure management during CPB, are recommended for further study. Overall, it appears that approaches designed to prevent injury, rather than those designed to ameliorate injury once present, are most likely to lead to tangible clinical benefits in the near future.

## ACKNOWLEDGMENTS

Both Dr. Karsten Bartels as well as Dr. Mackensen have co-authored several review articles on the topics associated with perioperative neurological injury.[1,27,79–81] Concepts outlined in these articles are therefore also found in this book chapter.

# REFERENCES

1. Bartels K, McDonagh DL, Newman MF, Mathew JP. Neurocognitive outcomes after cardiac surgery. *Curr Opin Anaesthesiol.* 2013;26(1):91–7.

2. Newman MF, Kirchner JL, Phillips-Bute B, et al. Longitudinal assessment of neurocognitive function after coronary-artery bypass surgery. *N Engl J Med.* 2001;344(6):395–402.

3. Tarakji KG, Sabik JF 3rd, Bhudia SK, Batizy LH, Blackstone EH. Temporal onset, risk factors, and outcomes associated with stroke after coronary artery bypass grafting. *JAMA.* 2011;305(4):381–90.

4. Hogue CW Jr, Murphy SF, Schechtman KB, Davila-Roman VG. Risk factors for early or delayed stroke after cardiac surgery. *Circulation.* 1999;100(6):642–7.

5. Almassi GH, Sommers T, Moritz TE, et al. Stroke in cardiac surgical patients: determinants and outcome. *Ann Thorac Surg.* 1999;68(2):391–7; discussion 397–8.

6. Smith CR, Leon MB, Mack MJ, et al. Transcatheter versus surgical aortic-valve replacement in high-risk patients. *N Engl J Med.* 2011;364(23):2187–98.

7. Adams DH, Popma JJ, Reardon MJ, et al. Transcatheter aortic-valve replacement with a self-expanding prosthesis. *N Engl J Med.* 2014;370(19):1790–8.

8. Jennum P, Iversen HK, Ibsen R, Kjellberg J. Cost of stroke: a controlled national study evaluating societal effects on patients and their partners. *BMC Health Serv Res.* 2015;15(1):466.

9. Phillips-Bute B, Mathew JP, Blumenthal JA, et al. Association of neurocognitive function and quality of life 1 year after coronary artery bypass graft (CABG) surgery. *Psychosom Med.* 2006;68(3):369–75.

10. Mackensen GB, Ti LK, Phillips-Bute BG, Mathew JP, Newman MF, Grocott HP. Cerebral embolization during cardiac surgery: impact of aortic atheroma burden. *Br J Anaesth.* 2003;91(5):656–61.

11. Kahlert P, Al-Rashid F, Dottger P, et al. Cerebral embolization during transcatheter aortic valve implantation: a transcranial Doppler study. *Circulation.* 2012;126(10):1245–55.

12. Rodriguez RA, Rubens FD, Wozny D, Nathan HJ. Cerebral emboli detected by transcranial Doppler during cardiopulmonary bypass are not correlated with postoperative cognitive deficits. *Stroke.* 2010;41(10):2229–35.

13. Ono M, Brady K, Easley RB, et al. Duration and magnitude of blood pressure below cerebral autoregulation threshold during cardiopulmonary bypass is associated with major morbidity and operative mortality. *J Thorac Cardiovasc Surg.* 2014;147(1):483–9.

14. Neville MJ, Butterworth J, James RL, Hammon JW, Stump DA. Similar neurobehavioral outcome after valve or coronary artery operations despite differing carotid embolic counts. *J Thorac Cardiovasc Surg.* 2001;121(1):125–36.

15. Merino JG, Latour LL, Tso A, et al. Blood-brain barrier disruption after cardiac surgery. *AJNR Am J Neuroradiol.* 2013;34(3):518–23.

16. Barber PA, Hach S, Tippett LJ, Ross L, Merry AF, Milsom P. Cerebral ischemic lesions on diffusion-weighted imaging are associated with neurocognitive decline after cardiac surgery. *Stroke.* 2008;39(5):1427–33.

17. Fairbairn TA, Mather AN, Bijsterveld P, et al. Diffusion-weighted MRI determined cerebral embolic infarction following transcatheter aortic valve implantation: assessment of predictive risk factors and the relationship to subsequent health status. *Heart.* 2012;98(1):18–23.

18. Bartels K, Ma Q, Venkatraman TN, et al. Effects of deep hypothermic circulatory arrest on the blood brain barrier in a cardiopulmonary bypass model—a pilot study. *Heart Lung Circ.* 2014;23(10):981–4.

19. Gerriets T, Schwarz N, Bachmann G, et al. Evaluation of methods to predict early long-term neurobehavioral outcome after coronary artery bypass grafting. *Am J Cardiol.* 2010;105(8):1095–101.

20. Lombard FW, Mathew JP. Neurocognitive dysfunction following cardiac surgery. *Semin Cardiothorac Vasc Anesth.* 2010;14(2):102–10.

21. Hedberg M, Boivie P, Engstrom KG. Early and delayed stroke after coronary surgery—an analysis of risk factors and the impact on short- and long-term survival. *Eur J Cardiothorac Surg.* 2011;40(2):379–87.

22. Ng JL, Chan MT, Gelb AW. Perioperative stroke in noncardiac, nonneurosurgical surgery. *Anesthesiology.* 2011;115(4):879–90.

23. Krishnamoorthy V, Mackensen GB, Gibbons EF, Vavilala MS. Cardiac dysfunction after neurologic injury: What do we know and where are we going? *Chest.* 2016;149(5):1325–31.

24. Bijker JB, Persoon S, Peelen LM, et al. Intraoperative hypotension and perioperative ischemic stroke after general surgery: a nested case-control study. *Anesthesiology.* 2012;116(3):658–64.

25. Gold JP, Charlson ME, Williams-Russo P, et al. Improvement of outcomes after coronary artery bypass. A randomized trial comparing intraoperative high versus low mean arterial pressure. *J Thorac Cardiovasc Surg.* 1995;110(5):1302–11.

26. Siepe M, Pfeiffer T, Gieringer A, et al. Increased systemic perfusion pressure during cardiopulmonary bypass is associated with less early postoperative cognitive dysfunction and delirium. *Eur J Cardiothorac Surg.* 2011;40(1):200–7.

27. Bartels K, Karhausen J, Clambey ET, Grenz A, Eltzschig HK. Perioperative organ injury. *Anesthesiology.* 2013;119(6):1474–89.

28. Bartels K, Meissner K. Morphine and the Blood-Brain Barrier—Diffusion, Uptake, or Efflux? *Can J Anesth.* Epub Date: July 18, 2017.

29. Jungwirth B, Kellermann K, Qing M, Mackensen GB, Blobner M, Kochs EF. Cerebral tumor necrosis factor alpha expression and long-term neurocognitive performance after cardiopulmonary bypass in rats. *J Thorac Cardiovasc Surg.* 2009;138(4):1002–7.

30. Jungwirth B, Eckel B, Blobner M, Kellermann K, Kochs EF, Mackensen GB. The impact of cardiopulmonary bypass on systemic interleukin-6 release, cerebral nuclear factor-kappa B expression, and neurocognitive outcome in rats. *Anesth Analg.* 2010;110(2):312–20.

31. Shroyer AL, Grover FL, Hattler B, et al. On-pump versus off-pump coronary-artery bypass surgery. *N Engl J Med.* 2009;361(19):1827–37.

32. Houlind K, Kjeldsen BJ, Madsen SN, et al. On-pump versus off-pump coronary artery bypass surgery in elderly patients: results from the Danish on-pump versus off-pump randomization study. *Circulation.* 2012;125(20):2431–9.

33. Kozora E, Kongs S, Collins JF, et al. Cognitive outcomes after on- versus off-pump coronary artery bypass surgery. *Ann Thorac Surg.* 2010;90(4):1134–41.

34. Diegeler A, Borgermann J, Kappert U, et al. Off-pump versus on-pump coronary-artery bypass grafting in elderly patients. *N Engl J Med.* 2013;368(13):1189–98.

35. Grocott HP, White WD, Morris RW, et al. Genetic polymorphisms and the risk of stroke after cardiac surgery. *Stroke.* 2005;36(9):1854–8.

36. Mathew JP, Podgoreanu MV, Grocott HP, et al. Genetic variants in P-selectin and C-reactive protein influence susceptibility to cognitive decline after cardiac surgery. *J Am Coll Cardiol.* 2007;49(19):1934–42.

37. Silbert BS, Evered LA, Scott DA, Cowie TF. The apolipoprotein E epsilon4 allele is not associated with cognitive dysfunction in cardiac surgery. *Ann Thorac Surg.* 2008;86(3):841–7.

38. Bartels K, Li YJ, Li YW, et al. Apolipoprotein epsilon 4 genotype is associated with less improvement in cognitive function five years after cardiac surgery: a retrospective cohort study. *Can J Anaesth.* 2015;62(6):618–26.

39. van Beek AH, Claassen JA, Rikkert MG, Jansen RW. Cerebral autoregulation: an overview of current concepts and methodology with special focus on the elderly. *J Cereb Blood Flow Metab.* 2008;28(6):1071–85.

40. Aries MJ, Elting JW, De Keyser J, Kremer BP, Vroomen PC. Cerebral autoregulation in stroke: a review of transcranial Doppler studies. *Stroke.* 2010;41(11):2697–704.

41. Ono M, Zheng Y, Joshi B, Sigl JC, Hogue CW. Validation of a stand-alone near-infrared spectroscopy system for monitoring cerebral autoregulation during cardiac surgery. *Anesth Analg.* 2013;116(1):198–204.

42. Cho H, Nemoto EM, Yonas H, Balzer J, Sclabassi RJ. Cerebral monitoring by means of oximetry and somatosensory evoked potentials during carotid endarterectomy. *J Neurosurg.* 1998;89(4):533–8.

43. Grocott HP, Davie SN. Future uncertainties in the development of clinical cerebral oximetry. *Front Physiol.* 2013;4:360.

44. Guarracino F. Cerebral monitoring during cardiovascular surgery. *Curr Opin Anaesthesiol.* 2008;21(1):50–4.

45. Fischer GW, Lin HM, Krol M, et al. Noninvasive cerebral oxygenation may predict outcome in patients undergoing aortic arch surgery. *J Thorac Cardiovasc Surg.* 2011;141(3):815–21.

46. Zheng F, Sheinberg R, Yee MS, Ono M, Zheng Y, Hogue CW. Cerebral near-infrared spectroscopy monitoring and neurologic outcomes in adult cardiac surgery patients: a systematic review. *Anesth Analg.* 2013;116(3):663–76.

47. Murkin JM, Adams SJ, Novick RJ, et al. Monitoring brain oxygen saturation during coronary bypass surgery: a randomized, prospective study. *Anesth Analg.* 2007;104(1):51–8.

48. Murkin JM, Kamar M, Silman Z, Balberg M, Adams SJ. Intraoperative cerebral autoregulation assessment using ultrasound-tagged near-infrared-based cerebral blood flow in comparison to transcranial doppler cerebral flow velocity: a pilot study. *J Cardiothorac Vasc Anesth.* 2015;29(5):1187–93.

49. Kertai MD, Whitlock EL, Avidan MS. Brain monitoring with electroencephalography and the electroencephalogram-derived bispectral index during cardiac surgery. *Anesth Analg.* 2012;114(3):533–46.

50. The World Health Organization. MONICA Project (monitoring trends and determinants in cardiovascular disease): a major international collaboration. WHO MONICA Project Principal Investigators. *J Clin Epidemiol.* 1988;41(2):105–14.

51. Uysal S, Reich DL. Neurocognitive outcomes of cardiac surgery: a review. *J Cardiothorac Vasc Anesth.* 2013;27(5):958–71.

52. Selnes OA, Gottesman RF, Grega MA, Baumgartner WA, Zeger SL, McKhann GM. Cognitive and neurologic outcomes after coronary-artery bypass surgery. *N Engl J Med.* 2012;366(3):250–7.

53. Hoerauf JM, Moss AF, Fernandez-Bustamante A, Bartels K. Study Design Rigor in Animal-Experimental Research Published in Anesthesia Journals. *Anesth Analg.* Epub Date: Feb 8, 2017.

54. Young AR, Ali C, Duretete A, Vivien D. Neuroprotection and stroke: time for a compromise. *J Neurochem.* 2007;103(4):1302–9.

55. Macrez R, Ali C, Toutirais O, et al. Stroke and the immune system: from pathophysiology to new therapeutic strategies. *Lancet Neurol.* 2011;10(5):471–80.

56. Hogue CW Jr, Freedland K, Hershey T, et al. Neurocognitive outcomes are not improved by 17beta-estradiol in postmenopausal women undergoing cardiac surgery. *Stroke.* 2007;38(7):2048–54.

57. Mathew JP, White WD, Schinderle DB, et al. Intraoperative magnesium administration does not improve neurocognitive function after cardiac surgery. *Stroke.* 2013;44(12):3407–13.

58. Mathew JP, Mackensen GB, Phillips-Bute B, et al. Randomized, double-blinded, placebo controlled study of neuroprotection with lidocaine in cardiac surgery. *Stroke.* 2009;40(3):880–7.

59. Holinski S, Claus B, Alaaraj N, et al. Cerebroprotective effect of piracetam in patients undergoing open heart surgery. *Ann Thorac Cardiovasc Surg.* 2011;17(2):137–42.

60. Ottens TH, Dieleman JM, Sauer AC, et al.; DExamethasone for Cardiac Surgery (DECS) Study Group. Effects of dexamethasone on cognitive decline after cardiac surgery: a randomized controlled trial. *Anesthesiology.* 2014;121(3):492–500.

61. Hogue CW Jr, Palin CA, Arrowsmith JE. Cardiopulmonary bypass management and neurologic outcomes: an evidence-based appraisal of current practices. *Anesth Analg.* 2006;103(1):21–37.

62. Jauch EC, Saver JL, Adams HP Jr, et al. Guidelines for the early management of patients with acute ischemic stroke: a guideline for healthcare professionals from the American Heart Association/American Stroke Association. *Stroke.* 2013;44(3):870–947.

63. Ciccone A, Valvassori L, Nichelatti M, et al. Endovascular treatment for acute ischemic stroke. *N Engl J Med.* 2013;368(10):904–13.

64. Broderick JP, Palesch YY, Demchuk AM, et al.; Interventional Management of Stroke (IMS) III Investigators. Endovascular therapy after intravenous t-PA versus t-PA alone for stroke. *N Engl J Med.* 2013;368(10):893–903.

65. Fukuda I, Imazuru T, Osaka M, Watanabe K, Meguro K, Wada M. Thrombolytic therapy for delayed, in-hospital stroke after cardiac surgery. *Ann Thorac Surg.* 2003;76(4):1293–5.

66. Katzan IL, Masaryk TJ, Furlan AJ, et al. Intra-arterial thrombolysis for perioperative stroke after open heart surgery. *Neurology.* 1999;52(5):1081–4.

67. Moazami N, Smedira NG, McCarthy PM, et al. Safety and efficacy of intraarterial thrombolysis for perioperative stroke after cardiac operation. *Ann Thorac Surg.* 2001; 72(6):1933–7; discussion 1937–9.

68. Chalela JA, Katzan I, Liebeskind DS, et al. Safety of intra-arterial thrombolysis in the postoperative period. *Stroke.* 2001;32(6):1365–9.

69. Lamy A, Devereaux PJ, Prabhakaran D, et al. Effects of off-pump and on-pump coronary-artery bypass grafting at 1 year. *N Engl J Med.* 2013;368(13):1179–88.

70. Lansky AJ, Schofer J, Tchetche D, et al. A prospective randomized evaluation of the TriGuard HDH embolic DEFLECTion device during transcatheter aortic valve implantation: results from the DEFLECT III trial. *Eur Heart J.* 2015;36(31):2070–8.

71. Bernard SA, Gray TW, Buist MD, et al. Treatment of comatose survivors of out-of-hospital cardiac arrest with induced hypothermia. *N Engl J Med.* 2002;346(8):557–63.

72. Hypothermia After Cardiac Arrest Study Group. Mild therapeutic hypothermia to improve the neurologic outcome after cardiac arrest. *N Engl J Med.* 2002;346(8):549–56.

73. Mackensen GB, McDonagh DL, Warner DS. Perioperative hypothermia: use and therapeutic implications. *J Neurotrauma.* 2009;26(3):342–58.

74. Grigore AM, Mathew J, Grocott HP, et al. Prospective randomized trial of normothermic versus hypothermic cardiopulmonary bypass on cognitive function after coronary artery bypass graft surgery. *Anesthesiology.* 2001;95(5):1110–9.

75. Grocott HP, Mackensen GB, Grigore AM, et al. Postoperative hyperthermia is associated with cognitive dysfunction after coronary artery bypass graft surgery. *Stroke.* 2002;33(2):537–41.

76. Grigore AM, Grocott HP, Mathew JP, et al. The rewarming rate and increased peak temperature alter neurocognitive outcome after cardiac surgery. *Anesth Analg.* 2002; 94(1):4–10.

77. Nielsen N, Wetterslev J, Cronberg T, et al. Targeted temperature management at 33 degrees C versus 36 degrees C after cardiac arrest. *N Engl J Med.* 2013;369(23):2197–206.

78. Engelman R, Baker RA, Likosky DS, et al. The Society of Thoracic Surgeons, the Society of Cardiovascular Anesthesiologists, and the American Society of ExtraCorporeal Technology: clinical practice guidelines for cardiopulmonary bypass--temperature management during cardiopulmonary bypass. *J Cardiothorac Vasc Anesth.* 2015;29(4):1104–13.

79. Graber LC, Quillinan N, Marrotte EJ, McDonagh DL, Bartels K. Neurocognitive outcomes after extracorporeal membrane oxygenation. *Best Pract Res Clin Anaesthesiol.* 2015;29(2):125–35.

80. Newman MF, Mathew JP, Grocott HP, et al. Central nervous system injury associated with cardiac surgery. *Lancet.* 2006;368(9536):694–703.

81. Conlon N, Grocott HP, Mackensen GB. Neuroprotection during cardiac surgery. *Expert Rev Cardiovasc Ther.* 2008;6(4):503–20.

# 17 Neuroprotection for Aortic Surgery and Stenting

Jared W. Feinman

and John G. Augoustides

## GENERAL CONSIDERATIONS

Aortic disease encompasses a wide array of pathologies, all of which may have differing implications for perioperative neuroprotection of the brain and/or spinal cord. The clinical approach to aortic surgery and stenting for diseases of the aorta is based on understanding the anatomical extent and etiology of the particular aortic lesion.

### Anatomy of the Aorta: Understanding the Pathology of the Lesion

The thoracic aorta can be divided into three sections: the ascending aorta, aortic arch, and descending thoracic aorta (Figure 17.1).[1] The ascending aorta begins at the level of the aortic valve, extends to just before the origin of the brachiocephalic artery, and encompasses the aortic root as well.[1] The aortic arch is the aortic segment that typically includes the major arterial branches to the head, neck, and upper extremities. In the normal arrangement, the aortic arch begins with the origin of the brachiocephalic artery and ends with the origin of the left subclavian artery.[1] Although this normal arrangement is the most common, variations in the branches of the aortic arch do occur and can be clinically significant in the individual patient.[1-2] The descending thoracic aorta (DTA) begins just distal to the origin of the left subclavian artery and continues all the way to the diaphragm, at which point the abdominal aorta begins.[1,3] The abdominal aorta ends at its bifurcation into right and left common iliac arteries. The abdominal aorta has two major segments related to the origin of the renal arteries: the suprarenal segment above their origin and the infrarenal segment below their origin.[1,3]

The aortic wall throughout the entire extent of the aorta has three histological layers.[1,3] The inner layer, known as the intima, is composed of endothelium. The middle layer, known as the media, is comprised of concentric layers of elastic and collagen fibers as well as smooth muscle.[1,3] The outer layer of the aortic wall, known

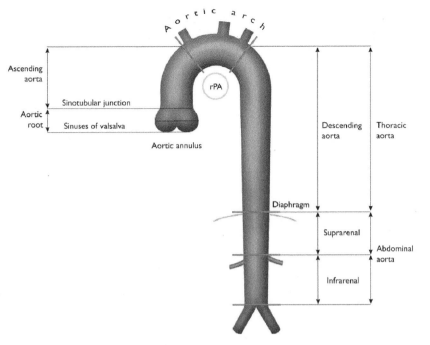

FIGURE 17.1 Segments of the thoracic and abdominal aorta. *rPA*, right pulmonary artery.
From Erbel R, Aboyans V, Boileau C, et al. 2014 ESC guidelines on the diagnosis and treatment of aortic diseases: document covering acute and chronic aortic diseases of the thoracic and abdominal aorta of the adult. *Eur Heart J.* 2014;35(41):2873–926.

as the adventitia, consists of collagen, vasa vasorum, and lymphatics.[1,3] The localization of an aortic disease process to one or more of these aortic segments and/or layers has implications for perioperative management and possible neurological injury that will be highlighted in this chapter.[1–3]

## Etiology of Aortic Disease: Understanding the Cause and Surgical Treatment of the Lesion

Aortic disease is a leading cause of death worldwide.[1,3–4] While a variety of pathologies can affect the aorta, including infectious processes, trauma, and inflammatory illnesses, by far the most common are aneurysmal disease and aortic dissection.[1,3–4] Thus, this chapter will focus predominately on the perioperative management of these two pathological conditions.

An aortic aneurysm is defined as dilation of the aorta to a size greater than 150% of normal, with all three layers of the aortic wall still intact.[1,3] Aortic dilation less than this degree is termed *aortic ectasia*. In healthy adults, normal aortic diameters typically do not exceed 40 mm, with that number diminishing distally as there is a gradual downstream tapering of the aorta. Aortic diameters are influenced by multiple factors, including age, gender, body surface area, and blood pressure.[1,3] As a clinical guide, aortic aneurysms tend to progress in size at an average rate of 1–2 mm per year of life.[5] Risk factors for aneurysm formation include age, hypertension, hypercholesterolemia, smoking history, and bicuspid aortic valve that is frequently associated with an aortopathy.[6] Inherited aortopathies are an important

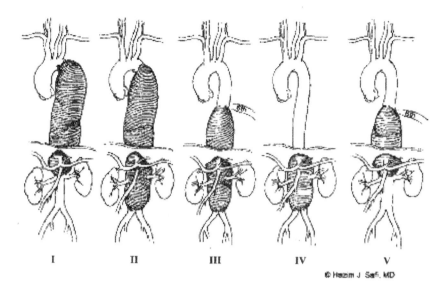

FIGURE 17.2 Modified Crawford classification of thoracoabdominal aneurysm. Extent I: From distal to the left subclavian artery to above the renal arteries. Extent II: From distal to the left subclavian artery to the aortic bifurcation (entire thoracoabdominal aorta). Extent III: From the 6th intercostal space to the aortic bifurcation. Extent IV: From the diaphragm to the aortic bifurcation (entire abdominal aorta). Extent V: From the 6th intercostal space to above the renal arteries. From Puchakayala MR, Lau WC. Descending thoracic aortic aneurysms. *Cont Educ Anaesth Crit Care Pain.* 2006;6:54–9.

genetic etiology in aortic aneurysms and include both familial clusters of aneurysmal disease as well as connective tissue disorders like Marfan and Loeys-Dietz syndromes.[1,3] Furthermore, many of the risk factors for aortic aneurysms are the same as those for atherosclerotic disease since aortic atheroma is a major etiology for aneurysm.[1,3]

Aortic aneurysms are classified by their location and extent. In the DTA, aneurysm extent is classified as follows: extent A involves the proximal third, extent B involves the middle third, and extent C involves the distal third.[1,3] In the thoracoabdominal aorta (TAA), aneurysm extent is described according to the modified Crawford classification (Figure 17.2: extent I through extent V).[1,3]

The timing of surgical intervention for an aortic aneurysm is based on factors such as location, size, rate of progression, symptoms, and patient comorbidities.[1,3] Surgical intervention is generally elective, except in cases of life-threatening aneurysm complications, such as rupture or dissection. In general, aneurysms of the ascending aorta and arch require intervention when the diameter exceeds 55 mm, with earlier intervention indicated in the ascending aorta at diameters of 45–50 mm in patients with risk factors such as Marfan syndrome and bicuspid aortic valve.[1,3,7] Aneurysms of the DTA and/or the TAA typically require consideration for intervention when the aortic diameter exceeds 50–55 mm.[1,3,7]

Aortic dissection results from an intimal tear that allows blood to exit the true lumen, dissect the intima from the aortic wall, and create a false lumen that may breach the adventitia (aortic wall) to cause rupture.[1,3] The dissection process can propagate across aortic segments in a proximal and/or distal fashion.[7–8] Furthermore, it may also involve major aortic branches, causing compression of the true lumen that interrupts distal blood supply and produces regional malperfusion.[1,3,7] The Penn classification has characterized the clinical presentations of

**Table 17.1** Penn Classification of Clinical Presentations in Acute Aortic Dissection

| Clinical Presentation | Definition |
|---|---|
| **Class A** (uncomplicated) | Absence of ischemia<br>No regional ischemia from branch vessel malperfusion<br>No generalized ischemia from cardiovascular collapse |
| **Class B** (complicated) | Branch vessel malperfusion with regional ischemia<br>e.g., acute stroke syndrome due to extensive carotid dissection; spinal cord ischemia presenting with acute paraplegia due to extensive descending thoracic aortic dissection |
| **Class C** (complicated) | Cardiovascular collapse with generalized ischemia due to circulatory shock<br>e.g., pump failure; aortic rupture |
| **Class BC** (complicated) | Branch-vessel malperfusion combined with Cardiovascular collapse resulting in both regional and generalized ischemia |

Adapted from Augoustides JG, Szeto WY, Desai ND, et al. Classification of acute type A dissection: focus on clinical presentation and extent. *Eur J Cardiothoracic Surg.* 2011;39:519–22; and Augoustides JG, Szeto WY, Woo EY, Andritsos M, Fairman RM, Bavaria JE. The complications of uncomplicated acute type B dissection: the introduction of the Penn classification. *J Cardiothorac Vasc Anesth.* 2012;26:1139–44.

acute aortic dissection from an ischemic perspective as follows: class a (absence of ischemia), class b (regional ischemia from branch vessel malperfusion), and class c (generalized ischemia from cardiovascular collapse) (Table 17.1).[9–10] Aortic dissections are also categorized according to extent by both the DeBakey and Stanford classifications (Box 17.1 and Figure 17.3).[1,3] Regardless of clinical presentation, acute dissection of the ascending aorta (Stanford type A; DeBakey types

---

**Box 17.1** Classification of Aortic Dissection by Extent

### DeBakey Classification

**Type I**: The majority of the aorta is dissected (the ascending aorta, aortic arch, descending thoracic aorta, and abdominal aorta).

**Type II**: The dissection is confined to the ascending aorta.

**Type III**: The dissection has originated in the descending thoracic aorta.

**Type IIIA**: The primary intimal tear originated in the descending thoracic aorta with distal extension to the diaphragm or proximal extension to the aortic arch.

**Type IIIB**: The primary intimal tear originated in the descending thoracic aorta with distal extension below the diaphragm.

### Stanford Classification

**Type A**: The dissection includes the ascending aorta regardless of the distal extent.

**Type B**: The dissection is confined to the descending thoracic aorta regardless of distal extent.

Adapted from Erbel R, Aboyans V, Boileau C, et al. 2014 ESC guidelines on the diagnosis and treatment of aortic diseases: document covering acute and chronic aortic diseases of the thoracic and abdominal aorta of the adult. *Eur Heart J.* 2014;35:2873–2926.

| De Bakey | Type I | Type II | Type III |
|---|---|---|---|
| Stanford | Type A | Type A | Type B |

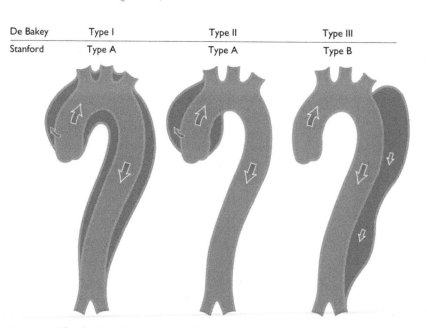

FIGURE 17.3   Classification of aortic dissection by extent.

From Erbel R, Aboyans V, Boileau C, et al. 2014 ESC guidelines on the diagnosis and treatment of aortic diseases: document covering acute and chronic aortic diseases of the thoracic and abdominal aorta of the adult. *Eur Heart J.* 2014;35:2873–926.

I and II) is considered a surgical emergency since immediate intervention significantly reduces mortality.[1,3,9] The management for acute dissection of the DTA (Stanford type B; DeBakey type III) depends on clinical presentation as outlined by the Penn classification.[1,3,10] In the setting of class a (uncomplicated) presentations, the primary management is medical, with emerging indications for endovascular intervention in patients at high risk for downstream complications.[1,3,10] In the setting of class b and class c complicated presentations, the primary management is interventional, with thoracic endovascular aortic repair (TEVAR) preferred over open repair.[1,3,10–11]

The traditional surgical treatment of both aortic aneurysm and dissection consists of open resection of the diseased aortic segments and subsequent replacement with synthetic graft material.[1,3,7] For aortic disease confined to the ascending aorta, surgical replacement of the ascending aorta and/or root is performed on cardiopulmonary bypass (CPB). If the aortic arch is also involved, then aortic arch replacement is performed with CPB with systemic hypothermic circulatory arrest (HCA) and cerebral perfusion adjuncts to facilitate the surgery by creating a bloodless field while simultaneously protecting the brain from ischemic injury.[1,3,12] Open surgical repair for aortic disease involving the DTA or the TAA is typically performed with CPB in the contemporary era with specialized techniques such as HCA and left heart bypass to maximize neural protection in the setting of major proximal or distal extent.[1,3,13] In current practice, TEVAR has become the treatment of choice for amenable pathologies of the DTA and the abdominal aorta.[1,3] Furthermore, in high-risk patients, endovascular stenting has increasingly been applied for ascending aortic repair and hybrid aortic arch replacement, in combination with brachiocephalic vessel translocation for selected cases (Figure 17.4).[1,3,14–15]

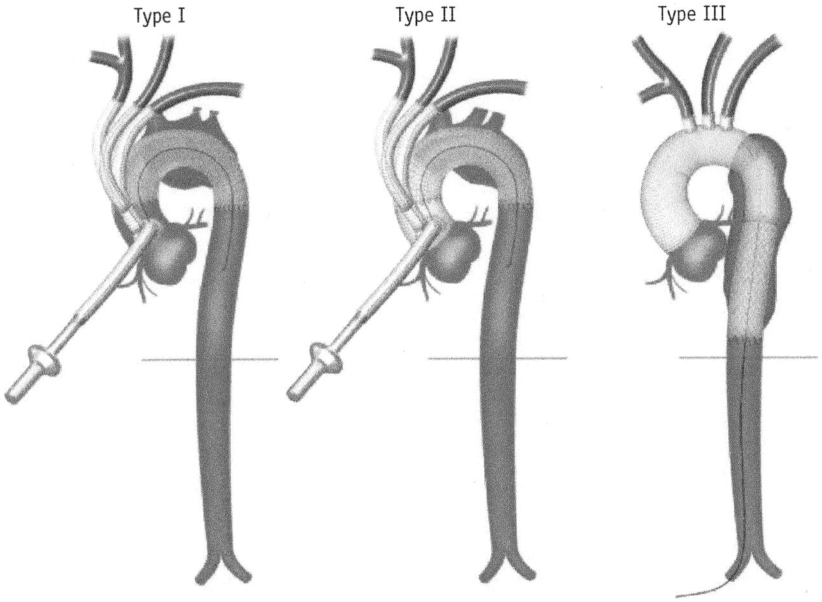

FIGURE 17.4  Classification of hybrid aortic arch repair. Type I: Total arch debranching with thoracic endovascular aortic repair (TEVAR). Type II: Ascending aorta replacement with total arch debranching and TEVAR in setting of proximal disease extension. Type III: Total arch replacement with ascending aortic replacement and elephant trunk for both proximal and distal extension of disease.

From Erbel R, Aboyans V, Boileau C, et al. 2014 ESC guidelines on the diagnosis and treatment of aortic diseases: document covering acute and chronic aortic diseases of the thoracic and abdominal aorta of the adult. *Eur Heart J.* 2014;35(41):2873–926.

## MECHANISMS OF AND RISKS FOR NEUROLOGICAL INJURY
### Embolic Stroke

Thoracic aortic surgery with or without CPB has a significant risk of delivering cerebral embolism consisting of both microemboli and macroemboli.[1,3,7] Microemboli often consist of microbubbles of air, lipid particles, and platelet aggregates that often lead to the occlusion of small arterioles and capillaries.[7] Although these microemboli typically occur in the majority of patients undergoing thoracic aortic surgery, their clinical effects are not always apparent and may require detailed neuropsychological testing and/or brain imaging for detection and delineation.[7,16] Macroemboli, on the other hand, are sizeable aortic plaque fragments that embolize after maneuvers, such as cannulation, clamping, unclamping, and stent deployment.[1,3,7,17] These macroemboli may occlude flow to larger cerebral vessels, leading to a focal neurological deficit that may present as a transient ischemic attack or a clinical stroke.[17–18]

### Ischemic Stroke During Aortic Arch Repair

Surgical aortic pathologies that involve the aortic arch require the temporary cessation of blood flow to the brain to allow aortic arch reconstruction and reimplantation of the head vessels to the new arch graft.[1,3,12] To minimize cerebral ischemia and stroke risk in this setting, aortic arch reconstruction has traditionally been conducted with HCA since hypothermia is a major neuroprotective strategy in these procedures.[12] While there is some variance in the temperature at which HCA is conducted, the physiologic premise is that by reducing cerebral metabolic rate and oxygen consumption through hypothermia, the safe period for circulatory arrest can be extended, allowing aortic arch repair to occur more safely.[1,3,7,12,19–20] Moderate and deep levels of hypothermia significantly reduce cerebral metabolism and oxygen demand but do not confer complete ischemic protection.[12,21] Cerebral perfusion adjuncts, such as anterograde or retrograde cerebral perfusion, may extend the safe period for HCA, but the risk of ischemic stroke during aortic arch surgery remains in the 3% to 5% range, even in centers of excellence.[21–24]

## Spinal Cord Ischemia

Paraparesis and paraplegia due to spinal cord ischemia (SCI) is a major source of morbidity and mortality, particularly after repair of the DTA and TAA.[7,13,25] In the 1980s and 1990s, open TAA aneurysm repair carried a significant risk for SCI, especially for large-extent disease such as Crawford type I and type II TAA aneurysms (15–30% risk).[13,25] While the risk of SCI has fallen significantly in the contemporary era due to multimodal interventions (addressed later in this chapter), it remains a clinically important adverse outcome.[25–28]

The etiology of SCI in DTA and TAA interventions is best explained by understanding the anatomy of the arterial network that forms the blood supply to the spinal cord (Figure 17.5).[7,13,25] The single anterior spinal artery and the paired

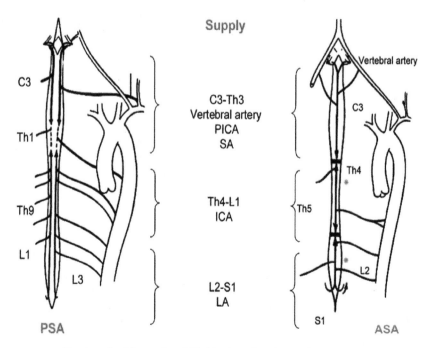

FIGURE 17.5 Blood supply of the spinal cord. The blood supply to the spinal cord consists of an arterial network. The single anterior spinal artery (*right*) and the paired posterior spinal arteries (*left*) derive cranially from the vertebral arteries. This arterial network (*center*) is then augmented by segmental input at the cervical, thoracic (top red star), and lumbosacral levels (bottom red star). *PICA*, posterior inferior cerebellar artery; *SA*, subclavian artery; *ICA*, intercostal arteries; *LA*, lumbar arteries.

From Etz CD, Weigang E, Hartert M, et al. Contemporary spinal cord protection during thoracic and thoracoabdominal aortic surgery and endovascular aortic repair: a position paper of the vascular domain of the European Association for Cardiothoracic Surgery. *Eur J Cardiothorac Surg.* 2015;47(6):943–57.

posterior spinal arteries derive cranially from both vertebral arteries. This spinal cord arterial network (SCAN) subsequently receives segmental arterial input at the cervical, thoracic, lumbar, and sacral levels (Figure 17.5). The sacral augmentation to the SCAN is derived from branches on the internal iliac arteries bilaterally.[7,13] A major thoracolumbar contributor to the SCAN is the artery of Adamkiewicz, which most commonly arises from intercostal and lumbar arteries from the T8 –L2 levels.[7,13,25] Although it may have important thoracolumbar input for the SCAN, it has proved difficult to identify preoperatively due to substantial anatomical variation, and its clinical significance has accordingly been integrated as part of the SCAN concept.[7,13,25] The SCAN can also be conceptualized as having intraspinal and paraspinal compartments (Figure 17.6).[13,25,29] These compartments, through their extensive arterial connections, provide vascular reserve within the SCAN for protection against SCI both in an immediate and delayed fashion.[13,25,29]

SCI after aortic interventions occurs primarily via two mechanisms: (1) intraoperative ischemia due to interruption of blood supply of sufficient duration to cause irreversible damage to nerve tissue, and (2) a reduction in blood supply from the sacrifice of segmental input to the SCAN at the thoracolumbar levels that is

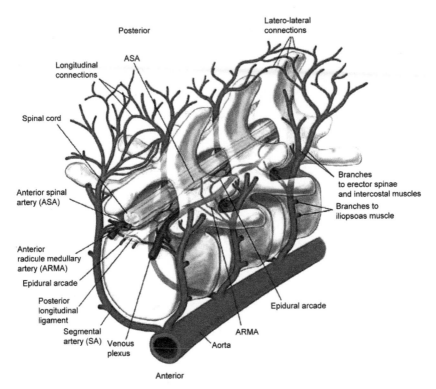

FIGURE 17.6 The compartments of the spinal cord arterial network (SCAN). The SCAN has an intraspinal compartment with epidural arterial arcades that are extensively interconnected to provide immediate vascular reserve for protection against spinal cord ischemia. The SCAN also has a paraspinal compartment that primarily supplies the paraspinal musculature but that also can provide extensive vascular reserve in a sustainable fashion for protection against spinal cord ischemia. *ASA*, anterior spinal artery; *SA*, segmental artery; *ARMA*, anterior radiculomedullary arteries; *LA*, lumbar arteries.

From Etz CD, Weigang E, Hartert M, et al. Contemporary spinal cord protection during thoracic and thoracoabdominal aortic surgery and endovascular aortic repair: a position paper of the vascular domain of the European Association for Cardiothoracic Surgery. *Eur J Cardiothorac Surg.* 2015;47:943–57.

insufficient for cord viability.[13,25] The former typically presents as SCI on emergence from anesthesia, and the latter often presents as delayed SCI after emergence from anesthesia.[13,25] While TEVAR can typically avoid this first mechanism for SCI, the coverage and occlusion of segmental arterial input to the SCAN still occurs.[1,13] The risk of paraplegia is still present with TEVAR at a rate of generally less than 5% (which is much lower than with open repair of the DTA and TAA), even in high-risk patients.[13,25,30]

## Risk Factors for Stroke

### Aortic Atheroma

The ascending aorta and aortic arch are the major sources of embolic stroke during aortic interventions.[1,3] Direct aortic manipulation required for surgical exposure, cannulation, clamping, and grafting are events that may dislodge plaque from the aortic wall.[1,3,31] During TEVAR, cerebral embolization of aortic atheroma may occur during passage of hardware, such as wires, balloons, and stents.[32-33] Severe aortic atheromatous disease, defined as plaque larger than 4 mm or a mobile component, is common in patients undergoing aortic surgery and stenting because atheromatous disease is a major risk factor for aortic aneurysm.[1,3] Severe aortic atheroma is also a risk factor for extensive thoracic aortic calcification, also known as *porcelain aorta*. This condition is a major risk factor for procedural stroke, and it requires careful planning to mitigate this risk.[34]

### Duration of Hypothermic Circulatory Arrest

While hypothermia reduces the risk of stroke during circulatory arrest for aortic arch repair, this risk is still present and increases with the duration of HCA.[21] A period of HCA greater than 25 minutes is a risk factor for neurocognitive dysfunction, and beyond 40 minutes is a significant risk factor for stroke. The safe duration of HCA can be extended with cerebral perfusion adjuncts, as discussed later.[12,21,35]

### Risk Factors for Spinal Cord Ischemia

The risk factors for SCI in aortic surgery and stenting (Table 17.2) are logical due to their known effects on the SCAN and spinal cord perfusion.[13,35] A major determinant for SCI in aortic surgery and stenting is the extent of acute compromise of the SCAN, as reflected by the number of intercostal and lumbar spinal arteries sacrificed during the operation.[25] The extent of collateral arterial sacrifice is a function of the extent and clinical presentation of the aortic pathology, including aneurysm and dissection (Figures 17.2 and 17.3; Tables 17.1 and 17.2; Box 17.1). Extensive aneurysm of the TAA, such as types I and II, consequently have a higher risk for SCI than types III and IV that begin more distally in the TAA.[25,27-28] Although reimplantation of thoracolumbar arteries may ameliorate the acute compromise of the SCAN, this procedure also has competing risks, such as blood loss and hypotension, that may predispose to SCI.[25]

When TEVAR is performed, an important determinant of SCI risk is the extent of segmental spinal artery coverage, including inputs from the subclavian artery, intercostal arteries, lumbar arteries, and internal iliac arteries (Table 17.2).[25] The extent of this vascular coverage (and occlusion of segmental arterial flow) determines the

| Risk Factor | Effect |
| --- | --- |
| Aortic Dissection | Branch vessel malperfusion |
| Previous Aortic Surgery | Compromise of the SCAN with loss of vascular reserve |
| Severe PVD | Chronic reduction of distal inflow to the SCAN |
| Aortic Clamping | Acute loss of spinal cord perfusion |
| Systemic Hypotension | Acute decrease in spinal cord perfusion pressure |
| Increases in CSF Pressure | Decreases spinal cord perfusion pressure (compartment syndrome) |
| Sacrifice of SSA | Acute loss of SCAN (surgical occlusion) |
| Coverage of SSA | Acute loss of SCAN (stent coverage) |
| Poor Distal Perfusion | Insufficient inflow into distal part of SCAN (on pump/no pulsatile perfusion) |
| Arterial Steal | Loss of spinal cord perfusion pressure due to bleeding from patent SSA after surgical incision of the aortic segment for replacement (e.g., aneurysm sac) |
| Reperfusion Injury | Spinal cord edema from ischemia and reperfusion |
| Thrombosis of SSA | Postoperative loss of SCAN |

*SCAN,* spinal cord arterial network; *PVD,* peripheral vascular disease; *CSF,* cerebrospinal fluid; *SSA,* spinal segmental arteries, such as intercostal and lumbar arteries.

Adapted from Etz CD, Weigang E, Hartert M, et al. Contemporary spinal cord protection during thoracic and thoracoabdominal aortic surgery and endovascular aortic repair: a position paper of the vascular domain of the European Association for Cardiothoracic Surgery. *Eur J Cardiothorac Surg.* 2015;47:943–57.

degree of perfusion compromise to the SCAN.[13] Recent literature suggests that although coverage and occlusion of the left subclavian artery is common to achieve an adequate proximal seal and avoid endoleaks, this technique increases the risk for SCI.[7,13,25,36] The risk factors for neurological injury in aortic surgery and stenting provide a clinical framework for minimizing this injury (as discussed later).

## MONITORING FOR NEUROLOGICAL INJURY
### Intraoperative Monitoring

### Electroencephalography for Aortic Arch Repair

While continuous intraoperative electroencephalography (EEG) is not a standard of care for aortic arch repair requiring HCA, it is utilized by many institutions to guide the conduct of hypothermia, monitor for neurological injury, and assess the adequacy of cerebral perfusion adjuncts (see Chapter 5 for full details about EEG and neuroprotection).[20–21] During cooling, the EEG initially remains similar to baseline, until around 30°C (±3°C) when periodic complexes appear unilaterally or bilaterally in approximately 65% of patients.[37] These periodic complexes were initially thought to be epileptic but are more likely related to gray and white matter dysfunction.[37] As the brain continues to cool, these periodic complexes disappear and the EEG amplitude decreases and finally enters burst-suppression at a nasopharyngeal temperature of approximately 24°C (±4°C).[37–39] If cooling continues, isoelectricity is achieved at an average nasopharyngeal temperature of 17.8°C (±4°C).[38] There is a great deal of variability, however, in the temperature at which isoelectricity occurs, so cooling to the physiologic endpoint of an isoelectric EEG (as opposed to a fixed temperature) may have some benefit.[38-39]

On average, burst suppression reappears 19 minutes (±9 minutes) after the restoration of anterograde blood flow to the brain, and continuous EEG activity returns after 47 minutes (±27 minutes).[40] A delayed return to continuous EEG activity, or return that occurs at a higher than average temperature, may herald associated postoperative neurological injury.[37,40] Furthermore, EEG may be especially useful when cerebral perfusion adjuncts are utilized during HCA with mild to moderate hypothermia.[38,40] Changes in the EEG signal pattern and amplitude may indicate ischemia and be used to guide efforts to restore cerebral perfusion with respect to flow and pressure.[37-40]

## Cerebral Near-Infrared Spectroscopy

Cerebral near-infrared spectroscopy (NIRS) is noninvasive as it monitors oxygen content of cerebral tissue via adhesive pads applied to the forehead of the patient (see Chapter 5).[41] The role of NIRS for cerebral monitoring during HCA with anterograde cerebral perfusion has proved feasible, safe, and effective.[41-42] In this setting, it can detect cerebral ischemia and prompt intraoperative interventions to restore adequacy of cerebral perfusion, whether unilateral or bilateral.[7,41-42]

## Monitoring for Spinal Cord Ischemia

Intraoperative neurophysiologic monitoring of the spinal cord via somatosensory evoked potentials (SSEPs) and/or motor evoked potentials (MEPs) will frequently detect SCI during reconstruction of the DTA and TAA, including TEVAR (see Chapter 5 for full details related to SSEP and MEP).[13,25,37] Both modalities facilitate early detection of SCI at a point when prompt interventions to restore spinal cord perfusion can prevent infarction.[25] In general, decreased signal amplitude in either SSEPs or MEPs at the appropriate neural level correlates with SCI.[13,25] The SSEPs primarily monitor the dorsal spinal cord that mediates proprioception and vibration, although they also monitor the spinocerebellar tracts that lie more anteriorly within the cord.[25,37] A relative blind spot for SSEPs is the anterior spinal cord motor tracts that are at high risk during DTA interventions.[25,37] A classic clinical presentation of SCI in this setting is paraparesis with sensory sparing.[25] Since MEPs primarily monitor the anterior spinal cord, they may at times be more sensitive to SCI during DTA/TAA reconstruction due to the fact that surgical intervention is more likely to compromise flow to the anterior spinal artery than the posterior spinal arteries.[37] A decrement in MEP amplitude of 75% is frequently a sign of critical SCI that necessitates aggressive intraoperative maneuvers to restore spinal cord perfusion.[37] Both SSEP and MEP require moderation of anesthetic techniques to minimize anesthetic agents' interference with monitoring of evoked potentials.[7,13,37]

## Postoperative Monitoring

The postoperative physical exam is the gold standard for detecting neurological injury after aortic interventions.[13] Routine comprehensive neurological assessment is essential in the postoperative period.[7,13] Concerning findings can be further investigated with neurological consultation and specialized testing, such as neuraxial imaging, as indicated.[7,13]

## NEUROPROTECTION STRATEGIES
### Interventions to Reduce Embolic Load

### Epiaortic Ultrasound for Atheroma Detection

As previously described, significant atheroma is a major risk factor for embolic stroke in proximal thoracic aortic reconstruction.[7,16–18] Traditionally, atheroma extent and severity has been assessed perioperatively by techniques such as computed axial tomography, transesophageal echocardiography (TEE), and manual palpation.[31,34] A blind spot for TEE is the distal ascending aorta due to the presence of the air–filled trachea.[43–44] This is a major limitation for TEE in this setting because this aortic segment undergoes major manipulations, such as cannulation and clamping.[43–44]

Epiaortic imaging is a complementary ultrasonic modality that is accomplished by placing an ultrasound probe directly on the aortic segments of interest to assess the burden of aortic atheroma.[43–44] A comprehensive epiaortic ultrasound exam has been described by the American Society of Echocardiography and the Society of Cardiovascular Anesthesiologists.[43] The recommended imaging sequence consists of five long- and short-axis views of the ascending aorta and arch.[43] This imaging modality is important since multiple trials have demonstrated its superiority to both TEE and manual palpation for assessment of atheroma in proximal thoracic aortic segments.[43] While there are no large-scale, randomized trials that have rigorously tested epiaortic ultrasound for stroke reduction in this setting, clinical trials have demonstrated that patients whose cardiac surgical procedure was changed based on epiaortic imaging had a lower stroke rate than expected.[43–45]

### Embolic Protection Devices

Given the role of atheromatous embolization in stroke, various embolic protection devices to filter and remove intraaortic debris have been investigated.[45–46] The Embol-X cannula (Edwards Lifesciences, Irvine, California) is an aortic cannula with a built-in embolic capture device in the form of a retractable mesh filter that is positioned above the aortic clamp site to trap aortic debris.[45–46] Clinical trials have demonstrated that this aortic cannula design captures debris almost all the time and that it can reduce stroke risk.[45–46] This initial design failed to gain widespread surgical acceptance, however, and a refined device has been designed and tested in a pilot clinical trial.[47] A second aortic cannula with embolic protection properties, the Cardiogard cannula (Cardiogard Medical, Or Yehuda, Israel), has recently received commercial approval.[45] The design of this cannula includes two lumens: the first for the passage of oxygenated blood to the ascending aorta and the second for continuous return of blood from the ascending aorta at flows of about 1 L per minute to the CPB circuit for embolic filtration.[48–49] Pilot trials have demonstrated significant reductions in cerebral embolic burden and protection from stroke.[48–49] Given these favorable data, the Cardiothoracic Surgical Trials Network is currently conducting a large, multicenter, randomized trial to assess whether these two embolic protection cannulae significantly reduce the risk of stroke as defined by clinical and radiographic criteria. For full details of this landmark trial, consult the trials registry at www.clinicaltrials.gov with trial identifier NCT02389894. This trial will be completed in 2017 and will likely have an important impact on the conduct of aortic cannulation in adult cardiac surgery.

## Choice of Arterial Cannulation Site for Aortic Surgery

There has been controversy regarding the femoral artery as an arterial cannulation option for thoracic aortic surgery due to concerns about retrograde cerebral atheroembolism.[50–51] The role of TEE for atheroma grading in the DTA has recently been highlighted in enhancing the safety of this cannulation strategy. In the setting of severe atheroma in the DTA, a central cannulation choice, such as the axillary artery, should be considered.[50–51] Recent meta-analysis has suggested that central arterial cannulation (e.g., axillary artery, innominate artery) as a routine for thoracic aortic surgery provides superior clinical outcomes both in the elective and emergency settings.[51–52] Recent literature reviews have also highlighted that although central cannulation significantly reduces the risks of atheroembolism and malperfusion, femoral cannulation remains a life-saving option for emergency CPB.[53–54] The innominate artery also provides convenient arterial access for central cannulation in thoracic aortic surgery that also can be utilized for anterograde cerebral perfusion during aortic arch repair (discussed in the next section).[55]

## Neuroprotective Interventions During Circulatory Arrest for Aortic Arch Repair

### Cerebral Perfusion Strategies

Although hypothermia is a major neuroprotective strategy in aortic arch surgery, the practice of HCA frequently includes selective cerebral perfusion as an adjunct to facilitate aortic arch repair and reduce the risk of clinical neurological dysfunction.[1,3,12] In recent surveys of aortic arch surgery practice in Europe, the minority of arch repairs were performed with HCA alone.[19] The options available for cerebral perfusion include retrograde cerebral perfusion (RCP) and anterograde cerebral perfusion (ACP), either in a unilateral or bilateral fashion.[21–23]

The conduct of RCP involves retrograde perfusion of the brain via the superior vena cava cannula to achieve a pressure of 15–20 mm Hg as measured at the right internal jugular vein.[21–23] While outcomes using RCP have been reasonable, the contribution of RCP to cerebral metabolism is likely quite low.[21,56–58] Instead, RCP aids in maintaining cerebral hypothermia, prevents air and debris microemboli from reaching the terminal vessels in the cerebral circulation, and washes out metabolites.[58] RCP has been shown to have a protective effect against stroke during HCA.[56–58]

In the contemporary era, the common modality for selective cerebral perfusion is ACP, employed either unilaterally (via the axillary artery, innominate artery, or right carotid artery) or bilaterally (via the innominate and left carotid arteries).[19–21] Unlike RCP, ACP maintains the physiologic direction of flow and likely provides metabolic support.[21] The practice of ACP varies between institutions, but pressures are typically targeted to 50–70 mm Hg, with flow rates in the range of 10 mL/kg/min.[1,3,21,59] While the neuroprotective advantages of ACP may not be readily apparent in the setting of deep hypothermia, they have allowed the practice of HCA to evolve safely toward moderate hypothermia.[13,21–22,60–61] Unilateral and bilateral ACP appear clinically equivalent in the setting of adequate neuromonitoring; however, a recent meta-analysis indicates that, in the setting of prolonged HCA duration, clinical outcomes appear to be superior with bilateral ACP.[13,60–61]

## Degree of Hypothermia

An international consensus has defined four ranges of hypothermia during HCA: profound (≤14°C), deep (14.1–20°C), moderate (20.1–28°C) and mild (28.1–34°C).[62] Traditionally, adult aortic arch repair with HCA was conducted with either profound or deep HCA to maximize the neuroprotective effects from hypothermia.[21,62–63] In the contemporary era, the requirement for deep hypothermia has been challenged.[12,62–63] Despite excellent neuroprotection, deep hypothermia increases the risks of coagulopathy, an exaggerated systemic inflammatory response, and end-organ dysfunction.[21,63] The adoption of ACP has allowed for the conduct of HCA at more moderate levels of hypothermia than was previously feasible.[12] Multiple trials have demonstrated the safety and improved clinical outcomes of ACP with moderate HCA due to avoidance of deep hypothermia.[64–66]

## Interventions to Reduce Spinal Cord Ischemia During Thoracic Aorta Surgery

### Cerebrospinal Fluid Drainage in Open DTA and TAA Repairs

Proximal aortic clamping in DTA and TAA procedures leads to a rise in cerebrospinal fluid (CSF) pressure.[13,25] Since spinal cord perfusion pressure is defined as the difference between mean arterial pressure and CSF pressure, increases in CSF pressure compromise spinal cord perfusion throughout the SCAN.[13,25] The aim of CSF drainage is to reduce the CSF pressure below a goal of 10–15 mm Hg to maximize spinal cord perfusion pressure.[13,25] This is achieved via placement of a flexible drainage catheter into the intrathecal space at a low lumbar interspace (often at L4–L5). Complications of this procedure occur in 1% of patients and include intracranial hypotension, subdural or intracerebral hematoma, spinal headache, persistent CSF leak, intraspinal hematoma, meningitis, and catheter fracture.[13,25] These risks can be minimized with a perioperative protocol that includes monitoring of CSF pressure, intermittent rather than continuous CSF drainage, limiting drainage volume of 25 mL/h, and routine monitoring of coagulation function at the times of drain insertion and removal.[13,25,67]

There have been multiple trials evaluating the effectiveness of CSF drainage in reducing SCI during open DTA and TAA repair.[13,25,68] A key trial randomized 145 patients undergoing extent I or II TAA repairs to perioperative CSF drainage or not. This intervention was associated with an 80% relative risk reduction in clinical SCI.[68] A subsequent updated meta-analysis found that 10 of 13 qualifying studies showed a reduction in SCI with CSF drainage.[68] The three studies that failed to show a reduction in SCI risk frequently had patients with CSF pressures higher than 15 mm Hg, likely indicating ineffective drainage.[68] CSF drainage is a class I recommendation for patients undergoing open thoracoabdominal aortic aneurysm (TAAA) repair in both the latest European and North American aortic guidelines.[1,3,25]

## Reimplantation of Spinal Segmental Arteries

The decision to reimplant the segmental supply to the SCAN provided by inter-costal and lumbar arteries during open DTA and TAA reconstruction remains a debated strategy to prevent SCI.[13,25] In almost 25% of patients, the majority of the segmental spinal arteries are occluded due to the primary aortic pathology. Furthermore, reimplantation lengthens the duration of aortic clamping, worsens intraoperative hypotension due to back bleeding, and a substantial portion of reim-planted spinal arteries likely thrombose early in the postoperative period.[25] Despite these concerns, there is evidence that this intervention can reduce SCI in certain high-risk scenarios.[13,25]

## Further Interventions to Reduce SCI During Open TAAA Repair

Based on the outlined equation for spinal cord perfusion pressure, maintenance and/or augmentation of the systemic mean arterial pressure can prevent SCI by increasing blood supply throughout the SCAN. This "permissive hypertension" is a cornerstone of perioperative management and frequently requires interventions such as acute volume expansion, maintenance of hemoglobin, and systemic vaso-pressor titration.[13,25] Furthermore, left heart bypass during open DTA and TAA reconstructions facilitates precise control of mean arterial pressure both proximal and distal to the clamped aortic segments to optimize perfusion of the SCAN for protection against SCI.[13,25]

Epidural cooling has been proposed to reduce SCI during open DTA and TAA reconstruction by reducing spinal cord oxygen demand and thus increasing spinal cord tolerance of ischemia.[13,25,69] This can be accomplished by the insertion of a low thoracic epidural catheter through which iced (4°C) saline is infused to achieve an intraoperative CSF temperature of 25–28°C. While epidural cooling has been associated with reduced SCI compared with historical controls, its application has raised concerns about contamination and spinal cord edema following the cessation of active cooling.[69] Although this technique has undergone further investigation, it has not been adopted by the majority of centers and is not strongly recommended in the most current aortic guidelines.[1,3,13,25]

In contrast, the performance of open DTA and TAA reconstructions with HCA and deep hypothermia has proved clinically effective for minimizing SCI.[70–71] Recent clinical trials in high-risk patients have documented a risk of SCI with this deep hypothermic technique in the 2.5% to 5.0% range.[70–71] Although the risks of HCA with deep hypothermia include significant coagulopathy, as outlined earlier, this technique is a reasonable alternative in experienced aortic centers.[70–71]

## Reducing SCI Risk During TEVAR

While the benefit of CSF drainage in open DTA and TAA repairs is already estab-lished in clinical guidelines, its role for reducing SCI risk in TEVAR is less well established. This is partly explained by the observation that TEVAR has a signifi-cantly lower risk of perioperative SCI than equivalent open aortic procedures.[1,3,72] Although stent deployment in the aorta sacrifices the segmental spinal arteries, it avoids the back bleeding, vascular steal, effects of cross-clamping, and systemic hypotension and anemia that are associated with open repair.[13,25] A recent meta-analysis failed to establish a definitive reduction in SCI risk from CSF drainage during TEVAR.[72] Nevertheless, CSF drainage and permissive hypertension are the mainstays of rescue therapy for SCI associated with TEVAR and may be indicated prophylactically in high-risk patients.[1,3,13,25,73–74]

A further management issue during TEVAR is an adequate proximal landing zone for the planned stent and whether the origin of the left subclavian artery (LSA) can be covered despite the higher risk of SCI due to loss of input to the SCAN, as outlined earlier.[1,3,13,25,75] Blood flow to the LSA can be maintained, however, by performing either transposition of this artery to the left carotid artery or carotid-to-subclavian bypass grafting with coil embolization of the LSVA stump.[75] Preoperative revascularization of the LSCA is listed as a class II recommendation for patients undergoing TEVAR by the European Association for Cardiothoracic Surgery.[1,25]

## Pharmacologic Interventions

A wide variety of pharmacologic adjuncts have been considered for perioperative neuroprotection of the brain and spinal cord during aortic surgery and stenting.[1,3,7,12–13,25] The supporting evidence for these agents is limited.[76–77] One of the most commonly employed classes of medications used during aortic surgery is barbiturates, predominately thiopental.[76–77] Although thiopental reduces cerebral metabolic activity, strong evidence of clinically relevant neuroprotection is lacking, and its adverse effects include delayed anesthetic emergence and myocardial depression. Propofol has also been tested in this setting, although the evidence is weaker than currently exists for the barbiturates.[76–78]

Corticosteroids have been employed during extensive aortic procedures, such as aortic arch repair and DTA/TAA reconstructions for neuroprotection.[12–13] Clinical data, however, have been conflicting. A recent large registry trial in acute type A aortic dissection ($N = 2,137$) suggested that steroids may reduce the incidence of postoperative delirium (odds ratio 0.5; 95% CI 0.24–0.96; $P = 0.049$).[78]

A single-center trial involving 330 patients examined intrathecal papaverine as part of a multimodal spinal cord protection strategy during open DTA and TAA repair.[79] Papaverine is a vasodilator and may increase spinal cord perfusion, especially in the low thoracic region of the spinal cord.[79] The study found a reduced incidence of permanent paraplegia (3.6% vs. 7.5%, $P = 0.01$) and paraparesis (1.6% vs. 6.3%, $P = 0.01$) in the intrathecal papaverine group when compared to controls. While promising, these findings need to be confirmed in adequately powered randomized clinical trials.[79]

## IMPLICATIONS FOR CLINICAL PRACTICE
### Surgery on the Ascending Aorta

A significant risk factor for neurological injury during surgery on the ascending aorta is cerebral atheroembolism.[1,3,7] Epiaortic scanning is safe, effective, and reliable for intraoperative assessment of atheroma severity to guide surgical aortic manipulation.[43–44] It is reasonable to perform epiaortic ultrasound in this setting, especially in high-risk patients with a significant atheroma burden suggested by clinical assessment including perioperative TEE.[1,3,43–45] Although embolic protection with specially designed aortic cannulae appears effective, adequately powered randomized clinical trials are required to determine whether their ability to reduce atheroembolism results in significant outcome benefits, such as reduced mortality and protection from stroke.[45] Multiple meta-analyses have also suggested that an axillary arterial cannulation strategy for complex aortic surgery significantly reduces mortality and stroke.[51–54]

## Aortic Arch Repair with Hypothermic Circulatory Arrest

The conduct of aortic arch reconstruction with HCA, including the choice of cerebral perfusion adjuncts, remains institution- and surgeon-dependent, given the paucity of adequate randomized trials to inform practice.[1,3,12,21] The cumulative evidence thus far suggests that ACP (unilateral or bilateral) with moderate hypothermia and adequate monitoring is the perfusion strategy that offers the best clinical outcomes, including mortality, neurological injury, and coagulopathy.[12] Given that this perfusion strategy has largely supplanted deep hypothermia, it is probable that it will become the standard technique for the conduct of aortic arch procedures.[1,3,12,61–66] As for the commonly employed pharmacologic adjuncts, the evidence supporting their outcome benefits remains weak, and there is a need for high-quality trials.[21]

## Surgery on the Descending Thoracic and Thoracoabdominal Aorta

The development of SCI with paraplegia remains a devastating complication of surgical reconstruction of the DTA and TAA. As such, the surgical procedure should be planned carefully to minimize the risk of SCI, with a focus on the current concepts of the SCAN and spinal cord perfusion pressure.[1,3,13,25] The perioperative roles of neuromonitoring, permissive hypertension, and CSF drainage are essential for spinal cord protection and rescue from an evolving ischemic insult.[13,25] Surgical strategies to minimize the risk of SCI in this setting include TEVAR, preservation of arterial segmental supply to the SCAN, left heart bypass, and hypothermia.[13,25] The role of pharmacologic adjuncts in reducing SCI remains an area for further study. Given the reduced risk of SCI associated with TEVAR, it is likely that this surgical strategy will disseminate even further throughout perioperative aortic practice, especially with advances in stent design.[1,3,13,25]

## FUTURE DIRECTIONS

Aortic surgery and stenting for an array of pathologies has undergone clinical maturation, prompting rigorous clinical guidelines that also serve as a foundation for further inquiry and innovation.[1,3,25] The advances in stent design have established TEVAR as a therapeutic option for diseases of the TAA, DTA, and aortic arch. The advent of transcatheter aortic valve replacement has further inspired efforts to advance stenting techniques as a management option for diseases of the aortic root and ascending aorta.[1,3,80–81] Although continuous innovation will advance the practice of aortic surgery and stenting, protection of the brain and spinal cord will remain a clinical priority that requires further high-quality randomized trials to inform optimal neuroprotective strategies in the future.[1,3,12–13,25,45–46,80–82]

## REFERENCES

1. Erbel R, Aboyans V, Boileau C, et al.; ESC Committee for Practice Guidelines. 2014 ESC guidelines on the diagnosis and treatment of aortic diseases: document covering acute and chronic aortic diseases of the thoracic and abdominal aorta of the adult. *Eur Heart J.* 2014;35(41):2873–926.

2. Maxwell BG, Harrington KB, Beygui RE, Oakes DA. Congenital anomalies of the aortic arch in acute type A aortic dissection: implications for monitoring, perfusion strategy, and surgical repair. *J Cardiothorac Vasc Anesth.* 2014;28(3):467–72.

3. Hiratzka LF, Bakris GL, Beckman JA, et al. 2010 ACCF/AHA/AATS/ACR/ASA/SCA/SCAI/SIR/STS/SVM Guidelines for the diagnosis and management of patients with thoracic aortic disease. A Report of the American College of Cardiology Foundation/American Heart Association Task Force on Practice Guidelines, American Association for Thoracic Surgery, American College of Radiology, American Stroke Association, Society of Cardiovascular Anesthesiologists, Society for Cardiovascular Angiography and Interventions, Society of Interventional Radiology, Society of Thoracic Surgeons, and Society for Vascular Medicine. *J Am Coll Cardiol.* 2010;55:e27–e129.

4. Svensson LG, Kouchoukos NT, Miller DC, et al.; Society of Thoracic Surgeons Endovascular Surgery Task Force. Expert consensus document on the treatment of descending thoracic aortic disease using endovascular stent-grafts. *Ann Thorac Surg.* 2008;85(1 Suppl):S1–41.

5. Elefteriades JA, Zigansjin BA, Rizzo JA, et al. Indications and imaging for aortic surgery: size and other matters. *J Thorac Cardiovasc Surg.* 2015;149(2 Suppl):S10–3.

6. Della Corte A, Body SC, Bocher Am, et al.; International Bicuspid Aortic Valve Consortium (BAVCon) Investigators. Surgical treatment of bicuspid aortic valve disease: knowledge gaps and research perspectives. *J Thorac Cardiovasc Surg.* 2014;147(6):1749–57.

7. Hershberger R, Cho JS. Neurologic complications of aortic diseases and aortic surgery. *Handb Clin Neurol.* 2014;119:223–38.

8. Baliga RR, Nienaber CA, Bossone E, et al. The role of imaging in aortic dissection and related syndromes. *JACC Cardiovasc Imaging.* 2014;7(4):406–24.

9. Augoustides JG, Szeto WY, Desai ND, et al. Classification of acute type A dissection: focus on clinical presentation and extent. *Eur J Cardiothoracic Surg.* 2011;39(4):519–22.

10. Augoustides JG, Szeto WY, Woo EY, Andritsos M, Fairman RM, Bavaria JE. The complications of uncomplicated acute type B dissection: the introduction of the Penn classification. *J Cardiothorac Vasc Anesth.* 2012;26(6):1139–44.

11. Mousa AY, Abu-Haliman S, Gill G, et al. Current treatment strategies for acute type B aortic dissection. *Vasc Endovasc Surg.* 2015;49(1-2):30–6.

12. Gutsche JT, Ghadimi K, Patel PA, et al. New frontiers in aortic therapy: focus on deep hypothermic circulatory arrest. *J Cardiothorac Vasc Anesth.* 2014;28(4):1171–5.

13. Augoustides JG, Stone ME, Drenger B. Novel approaches to spinal cord protection during thoracoabdominal aortic interventions. *Curr Opin Anaesthesiol.* 2014;27(1):98–105.

14. Vallabhajosyula P, Gottret JP, Bavaria JE, Desai ND, Szeto WY. Endovascular repair of the ascending aorta in patients at high risk for open repair. *J Thorac Cardiovasc Surg.* 2015;149(2 Suppl):S144–50.

15. Bavaria J, Vallabhajosyula P, Moeller P, Szeto W, Desai N, Pochettino A. Hybrid approaches in the treatment of aortic arch aneurysms: postoperative and midterm outcomes. *J Thorac Cardiovasc Surg.* 2013;145(3 Suppl):S85–90.

16. Uysal S, Reich DL. Neurocognitive outcomes of cardiac surgery. *J Cardiothorac Vasc Anesth.* 2013;27(5):958–71.

17. Bartels K, McDonagh DL, Newman MF, Mathew JP. Neurocognitive outcomes after cardiac surgery. *Curr Opin Anaesthesiol.* 2013;26(1):91–7.

18. Messe SR, Acker MA, Kasner SE, et al.; Determining Neurologic Outcomes from Valve Operations (DeNOVO) Investigators. Stroke after aortic valve surgery: results from a prospective cohort. *Circulation.* 2014;129(22):2253–61.

19. Gutsche JT, Feinman J, Silvay G, et al. Practice variations in the conduct of hypothermic circulatory arrest for adult aortic arch repair: focus on an emerging European paradigm. *Heart Lung Vessel.* 2014;6(1):43–51.

20. Augoustides JG, Patel P, Ghadimi K, Choi J, Yue Y, Silvay G. Current conduct of deep hypothermic circulatory arrest in China. *HSR Proc Intensive Care Cardiovasc Anesth.* 2013;5(1):25–32.

21. Svyatets M, Tolani K, Zhang M, Tulman G, Charchaflieh J. Perioperative management of deep hypothermic circulatory arrest. *J Cardiothorac Vasc Anesth.* 2010;24(4):644–55.

22. Angeloni E, Benedetto U, Takkenberg JJM, et al. Unilateral versus bilateral antegrade cerebral protection during circulatory arrest in aortic surgery: a meta-analysis of 5100 patients. *J Thorac Cardiovasc Surg.* 2014;147(1):60–7.

23. Appoo JJ, Augoustides JG, Pochettino A, et al.; Improving Clinical Outcomes through Clinical Research Investigators. Perioperative outcome in adults undergoing elective deep hypothermic circulatory arrest with retrograde cerebral perfusion in proximal aortic arch repair: evaluation of protocol-based care. *J Cardiothorac Vasc Anesth.* 2006;20(1):3–7.

24. Andersen ND, Ganapathi AM, Hanna JM, Williams JB, Gaca JG, Hughes GC. Outcomes of acute type a dissection repair before and after implementation of a multidisciplinary thoracic aortic surgery program. *J Am Coll Cardiol.* 2014;63(17):1796–803.

25. Etz CD, Weigang E, Hartert M, et al. Contemporary spinal cord protection during thoracic and thoracoabdominal aortic surgery and endovascular aortic repair: a position paper of the vascular domain of the European Association for Cardiothoracic Surgery. *Eur J Cardiothorac Surg.* 2015;47(6):943–57.

26. LeMaire SA, Price MD, Green SY, Zarda S, Coselli JS. Results of open thoracoabdominal aortic aneurysm repair. *Ann Cardiothorac Surg.* 2012;1(3):286–92.

27. Frederick JR, Woo YJ. Thoracoabdominal aortic aneurysm. *Ann Cardiothorac Surg.* 2012;1(3):277–85.

28. Ziganshin BA, Elefteriades JA. Surgical management of thoracoabdominal aneurysms. *Heart.* 2014;100(20):1577–82.

29. Meffert P, Bischoff MS, Brenner R, Siepe M, Beyersdorf F, Kari FA. Significance and function of different spinal collateral compartments following thoracic aortic surgery: immediate versus long-term flow compensation. *Eur J Cardiothorac Surg.* 2014;45(5):799–804.

30. Zipfel B, Buz S, Redlin M, Hullmeine D, Hammerschmidt R, Hetzer R. Spinal cord ischemia after thoracic stent-grafting: causes apart from intercostal artery coverage. *Ann Thorac Surg.* 2013;96(1):31–8.

31. Seco M, Edelman JB, Van Boxtel B, et al. Neurologic injury and protection in adult cardiac and aortic surgery. *J Cardiothorac Vasc Anesth.* 2015;29(1):185–95.

32. Kahjert P, Eggebrecht H, Janosi RA, et al. Silent cerebral ischemia after thoracic endovascular aortic repair: a neuroimaging study. *Ann Thorac Surg.* 2014;98(1):53–8.

33. Gutsche JT, Cheung AT, McGarvey ML, et al. Risk factors for stroke after thoracic endovascular aortic repair. *Ann Thorac Surg.* 2007;84(4):1195–200.

34. Abramowitz Y, Jilaihawi H, Chakravarty T, Mack MJ, Makkar RR. Porcelain aorta: a comprehensive review. *Circulation.* 2015;131(9):827–36.

35. Reich DL, Uysal S, Sliwinski M, et al. Neuropsychologic outcome after deep hypothermic circulatory arrest in adults. *J Thorac Cardiovasc Surg.* 1999;117(1):156–63.

36. Rizvi AZ, Murad MH, Fairman RM, Erwin PJ, Montori VM. The effect of left subclavian artery coverage on morbidity and mortality in patients undergoing endovascular thoracic aortic interventions: a systematic review and meta-analysis. *J Vasc Surg.* 2009;50(5):1159–69.

37. Sloan TB, Edmonds HL, Koht A. Intraoperative electrophysiologic monitoring in aortic surgery. *J Cardiothorac Vasc Anesth.* 2013;27(6):1364–73.

38. Stecker MM, Cheung AT, Pochettino A, et al. Deep hypothermic circulatory arrest: I. Effects of cooling on electroencephalogram and evoked potentials. *Ann Thorac Surg.* 2001;71(1):14–21.

39. James ML, Andersen ND, Swaminathan M, et al. Predictors of electrocerebral inactivity with deep hypothermia. *J Thorac Cardiovasc Surg.* 2014;147(3):1002–7.

40. Stecker MM, Cheung AT, Pochettino A, et al. Deep hypothermic circulatory arrest: II. Changes in electroencephalogram and evoked potentials during rewarming. *Ann Thorac Surg.* 2001;71(1):22–8.

41. Bevan PJ. Should cerebral near-infrared spectroscopy be standard of care in adult cardiac surgery? *Heart Lung Circ.* 2015;24(6):544–50.

42. Urbanski PP, Lenos A, Kolowca M, et al. Near-infrared spectroscopy for neuromonitoring of unilateral cerebral perfusion. *Eur J Cardiothorac Surg.* 2013;43(6):1140–4.

43. Glas KE, Swaminathan M, Reeves ST, et al. Guidelines for the performance of a comprehensive intraoperative epiaortic ultrasonographic examination: recommendations of the American Society of Echocardiography and the Society of Cardiovascular Anesthesiologists–endorsed by the Society of Thoracic Surgeons. *J Am Soc Echocardiogr.* 2007;20(11):1227–35.

44. Marshall WG, Barzilai B, Kouchoukos NT, Saffitz J. Intraoperative ultrasonic imaging of the ascending aorta. *Ann Thorac Surg.* 1989;48(3):339–44.

45. Engelman RM, Engelman DT. Strategies and devices to minimize stroke in adult cardiac surgery. *Semin Thorac Cardiovasc Surg.* 2015;27(1):24–9.

46. Mack M. Can we make stroke during cardiac surgery a never event? *J Thorac Cardiovasc Surg.* 2015;149(4):965–7.

47. Ye J, Webb JG. Embolic capture with updated intra-aortic filter during coronary artery bypass grafting and transaortic transcatheter aortic valve implantation: first in-human experience. *J Thorac Cardiovasc Surg.* 2014;148(6):2905–10.

48. Shani L, Cohen O, Beckerman Z, et al. A novel emboli protection cannula during cardiac surgery: in vitro results. *J Thorac Cardiovasc Surg.* 2014;148(2):668–75.

49. Bolotin G, Huber CH, Shani L, et al. Novel emboli protection system during cardiac surgery: a multi-center, randomized, clinical trial. *Ann Thorac Surg.* 2014;98(5):1627–33; discussion 1633–4.

50. Augoustides JG, Harris H, Pochettino A. Direct innominate artery cannulation in acute type A dissection and severe thoracic aortic atheroma. *J Cardiothorac Vasc Anesth.* 2007;21(5):727–9.

51. Benedetto U, Raja SG, Amrani SG, et al. The impact of arterial cannulation strategy on operative outcomes in aortic surgery: evidence from a comprehensive meta-analysis of comparative studies on 4476 patients. *J Thorac Cardiovasc Surg.* 2014; 148(6):2936–43.

52. Benedetto U, Mohamed H, Vitulli P, Petrou M. Axillary versus femoral arterial cannulation in type A acute aortic dissection: evidence from a meta-analysis of comparative studies and adjusted risk estimates. *Eur J Cardiothorac Surg.* 2015;48(6):953–9.

53. Patris V, Toufektzian L, Field M, Argiriou M. Is axillary superior to femoral artery cannulation for acute type A aortic dissection surgery? *Interact Cardiovasc Thorac Surg.* 2015;21(4):515–20.

54. Ren Z, Wang Z, Hu R, et al. Which cannulation (axillary cannulation or femoral cannulation) is better for acute type A aortic dissection repair? A meta-analysis of nine clinical studies. *Eur J Cardiothorac Surg.* 2015;47(3):408–15.

55. Augoustides JG, Desai ND, Szeto WY, Bavaria JE. Innominate artery cannulation: the Toronto technique for antegrade cerebral perfusion in aortic arch reconstruction—a clinical trial opportunity for the International Aortic Arch Surgery Study Group. *J Thorac Cardiovasc Surg.* 2014;148(6):2924–6.

56. Okita Y, Miyata H, Motomura N, Takamoto S; Japan Cardiovascular Surgery Database Organization. A study of brain protection during total arch replacement comparing antegrade cerebral perfusion versus hypothermic circulatory arrest, with or without retrograde cerebral perfusion: analysis based on the Japan Adult Cardiovascular Surgery Database. *J Thorac Cardiovasc Surg.* 2015;149(2 Suppl):S65–73.

57. Safi HJ, Miller CC 3rd, Lee TY, Estrera AL. Repair of ascending and transverse aortic arch. *J Thorac Cardiovasc Surg.* 2011;142(3):630–3.

58. Bavaria JE, Pochettino A. Retrograde cerebral perfusion (RCP) in aortic arch surgery: efficacy and possible mechanisms of brain protection. *Semin Thorac Cardiovasc Surg.* 1997;9(3):222–32.

59. Halkos ME, Kerendi F, Myung R, Kilgo P, Puskas JD, Chen EP. Selective antegrade cerebral perfusion via right axillary artery cannulation reduces morbidity and mortality after proximal aortic surgery. *J Thorac Cardiovasc Surg.* 2009;138(5):1081–9.

60. Hu Z, Wang Z, Ren Z, et al. Similar cerebral protective effectiveness of antegrade and retrograde cerebral perfusion combined with deep hypothermia circulatory arrest in aortic arch surgery: a meta-analysis and systematic review of 5060 patients. *J Thorac Cardiovasc Surg.* 2014;148(2):544–60.

61. Angeloni E, Melina G, Refice SK, et al. Unilateral versus bilateral antegrade cerebral protection during aortic surgery: an updated meta-analysis. *Ann Thorac Surg.* 2015;99(6):2024–31.

62. Yan TD, Bannon PG, Bavaria J, et al. Consensus on hypothermia in aortic arch surgery. *Ann Cardiothorac Surg.* 2013;2(2):163–8.

63. Luehr M, Bachet J, Mohr FW, Etz CD. Modern temperature management in aortic arch surgery: the dilemma of moderate hypothermia. *Eur J Cardiothorac Surg.* 2014;45(1):27–39.

64. Tian DH, Wan B, Bannon PG, et al. A meta-analysis of deep hypothermic circulatory arrest versus moderate hypothermic circulatory arrest with selective antegrade cerebral perfusion. *Ann Cardiothorac Surg.* 2013;2(2):148–58.

65. Vallabhajosyula P, Jassar AS, Menon RS, et al. Moderate versus deep hypothermic circulatory arrest for elective aortic transverse hemiarch reconstruction. *Ann Thorac Surg.* 2015;99(5):1511–7.

66. Leshnower BG, Thourani VH, Halkos ME, et al. Moderate versus deep hypothermia with unilateral selective antegrade cerebral perfusion for acute type A dissection. *Ann Thorac Surg.* 2015;100(5):1563–8; discussion 1568–9.

67. Hobbs RD, Ullery BW, Mentzer AR, Cheung AT. Protocol for prevention of spinal cord ischemia after thoracoabdominal surgery. *Vascular.* 2016;24(4):430–4.

68. Khan SN, Stansby G. Cerebrospinal fluid drainage for thoracic and thoracoabdominal aortic aneurysm surgery. *Cochrane Database Syst Rev.* 2012;10:CD003635.

69. Cambria RP, Davison JK, Carter C, et al. Epidural cooling for spinal cord protection during thoracoabdominal aneurysm repair: a five-year experience. *J Vasc Surg.* 2000;31(6):1093–102.

70. Kouchoukos NT, Kulik A, Castner CF. Outcomes after thoracoabdominal aortic aneurysm repair using hypothermic circulatory arrest. *J Thorac Cardiovasc Surg.* 2013;145(3 Suppl):S139–41.

71. Fabbro M, Gregory A, Gutsche JT, Ramakrishna H, Szeto WY, Augoustides JG. Case 11-2014: successful open repair of an extensive descending thoracic aortic aneurysm in a complex patient. *J Cardiothorac Vasc Anesth.* 2014;28(5):1397–402.

72. Wong CS, Healy D, Canning C, Coffey JC, Boyle JR, Walsh SR. A systematic review of spinal cord injury and cerebrospinal fluid drainage after thoracic aortic endografting. *J Vasc Surg.* 2012;56(5):1438–47.

73. Arora H, Ullery BW, Kumar PA, Cheung AT. Pro: patients at risk for spinal cord ischemia after thoracic aortic repairs should receive prophylactic cerebrospinal fluid drainage. *J Cardiothorac Vasc Anesth.* 2015;29(5):1376–80.

74. Isaak RS, Furman W. Con: patients at risk for spinal cord ischemia after thoracic aortic repairs should receive prophylactic cerebrospinal fluid drainage. *J Cardiothorac Vasc Anesth.* 2015;29(5):1381–3.

75. Patterson BO, Holt PJ, Nienaber C, Fairman RM, Heijmen RH, Thompson MM. Management of the left subclavian artery and neurologic complications after thoracic endovascular aortic repair. *J Vasc Surg.* 2014;60(6):1491–7.

76. Dewhurst AT, Moore SJ, Liban JB. Pharmacological agents as cerebral protectants during deep hypothermic circulatory arrest in adult thoracic aortic surgery. *Anaesthesia.* 2002;57(10):1016–21.

77. Al-Hashimi S, Zaman W, Waterworth P, Bilal H. Does the use of thiopental provide added cerebral protection during deep hypothermic circulatory arrest? *Interact Cardiovasc Thorac Surg.* 2013;17:392–7.

78. Krüger T, Hoffmann I, Blettner M, Borger MA, Schlensak C, Weigang E; GERAADA Investigators. Intraoperative neuroprotective drugs without beneficial effects? Results of the German Registry for Acute Aortic Dissection Type A (GERAADA). *Eur J Cardiothorac Surg.* 2013;44(5):939–46.

79. Lima B, Nowick ER, Blackstone EH, et al. Spinal cord protective strategies during descending and thoracoabdominal aortic aneurysm repair in the modern era: the role of intrathecal papaverine. *J Thorac Cardiovasc Surg.* 2012;143(4):945–52.

80. Dudzinski DM, Isselbacher EM. Diagnosis and management of thoracic aortic disease. *Curr Cardiol Rep.* 2015;17(12):106.

81. Appoo JJ, Tsa LW, Pozeg ZI, et al. Thoracic aortic frontier: review of current applications and directions of thoracic endovascular aortic repair (TEVAR). *Can J Cardiol.* 2014;30(1):52–63.

82. Von Aspern K, Luehr M, Mohr FW, Etz CD. Spinal cord protection in open and endovascular thoracoabdominal aortic aneurysm repair: critical review of current concepts and future perspectives. *J Cardiovasc Surg (Torino).* 2015;56(5):745–9.

# 18 Neuroprotection for Carotid Endarterectomy and Carotid Artery Stenting

## Zirka H. Anastasian and Eric J. Heyer

## GENERAL CONSIDERATIONS

Carotid endarterectomy (CEA) and carotid artery stenting (CAS) are offered to symptomatic patients (i.e., with nondisabling stroke or transient ischemic attack [TIA]) with carotid atherosclerotic disease to prevent fatal or disabling strokes. These procedures, however, carry a risk of perioperative stroke, with an incidence of approximately 5% with CEA and approximately 4–8% with CAS.[1–3] Both procedures also are associated with cognitive dysfunction early in the postprocedure period in approximately 25% of patients.[4–6]

### Description of the Procedures

During CEA, an incision is made on the neck medial to the sternocleidomastoid muscle. The common, internal, and external carotid arteries are identified and dissected free from the surrounding tissue; vessel loops are placed around them. These arteries, as well as the superior thyroid artery, are then clamped sequentially (internal, common, and external carotid artery). Prior to clamping, anesthesiologists should increase the mean arterial pressure (MAP) to 20% or more over the baseline value to optimize collateral cerebral blood flow (CBF) and reduce the risk of hypoperfusion injury.[7] After vessel clamping proximal and distal to the surgical site, the lumen of the internal carotid artery (ICA) is opened with a longitudinal incision, and the atheromatous plaque substance is excised. The artery is sutured closed either by patching the carotid artery or primary closure. Hemostasis is then achieved, and the overlying layers are closed with suture. An alternative surgical approach is the eversion technique, in which the ICA is transected from the common carotid artery, the plaque is removed, and the ICA is reimplanted into the carotid bulb.

After clamping of the carotid artery, a shunt may be placed with catheter tips proximal to the common carotid artery (CCA) clamp and distal to the ICA clamp, bypassing the surgical field so that blood flow to the ipsilateral hemisphere is partially or completely preserved. This management strategy, however, is applied variably. A review of practice in the Northeast showed that one-third of CEA cases are done with routine shunting, one-third with no shunting, and one-third with selective shunting.[8]

An alternative treatment for carotid artery stenosis is CAS. This involves insertion of a catheter into the stenotic lumen of the ICA, typically via the femoral artery. Primary insertion of a stent is placed after balloon angioplasty, which involves dilation of a balloon mounted to the catheter tip.

The benefits of CAS over CEA include avoidance of an incision in the neck and the associated risks of cranial and cutaneous nerve damage, reduced general surgical complications such as neck hematoma and myocardial infarction, and shorter hospital stay. Additionally, lesions that lie beyond the carotid bifurcation can be treated. Stenting, however, does not remove the plaque and may itself produce emboli by disrupting the atherosclerotic plaque.

## Patient Selection

Current practice guidelines recommend that symptomatic patients (i.e., with non-disabling ischemic stroke or transient cerebral ischemic symptoms) who are at average or low surgical risk should undergo CEA if (1) the ICA lumen diameter is reduced by more than 70% as documented by noninvasive imaging, or by more than 50% as documented by catheter angiography; and (2) the anticipated rate of perioperative stroke or mortality is less than 6%.[9] For symptomatic patients with moderate level of stenosis (i.e., 50–69%), decision-making must take into account the fact that CEA has less benefit in this patient group compared to symptomatic patients with a higher degree of stenosis (70–99%).[10] Symptomatic patients with stenosis of less than 50% do not benefit from CEA.[11]

CAS is an alternative to CEA that has the advantage of being less invasive. Trials have shown that both procedures are effective for patients with a high risk of stroke or stroke-related death, each of which may prove to be more beneficial to specific subgroups of patients.[12]

The selection of asymptomatic patients for carotid revascularization should take into consideration comorbid conditions, life expectancy, and other individual factors, and should include a thorough discussion of the risks and benefits of the procedure with an understanding of patient preferences.[9] An index for determining risk of complications (perioperative stroke, myocardial infarction, and death) from CEA performed in asymptomatic patients with carotid artery stenosis has been developed that includes age, dyspnea on exertion or rest, previous peripheral revascularization or amputation, chronic obstructive pulmonary disease, recent angina, and functional status as predictors.[13]

## Perioperative Management

Current guidelines recommend that aspirin be started before CEA.[9] Beyond the first month after CEA, aspirin, clopidogrel, or the combination of low-dose aspirin plus extended-release dipyridamole should be administered for long-term prophylaxis against ischemic cardiovascular events. After CEA, patch angioplasty can be beneficial for closure of arteriotomy. The administration of HMG-CoA reductase inhibitors ("statins") or equivalent alternatives in patients with statin-related side effects is reasonable irrespective of serum lipid levels.

Current guidelines recommend dual antiplatelet therapy with aspirin plus clopidogrel before CAS and for a minimum of 30 days after CAS.[9]

## MECHANISMS OF AND RISKS FOR NEUROLOGICAL INJURY
### Perioperative Stroke

CEA may result in perioperative ischemic stroke due to either dislodged emboli or inadequate collateral blood flow during cross-clamping of the carotid artery. During CEA, placement of clamps can dislodge plaque, and thrombus can form on the endarterectomized surface, on suture lines, or on residual plaque. Because there is a high likelihood of significant stenosis within one or more of the major vessels that provide collateral blood flow, ischemic stroke may occur with low CBF due to temporary vessel occlusion in combination with insufficient collateral circulation. Maintaining normal to elevated arterial perfusion pressure is critical to ensure adequate collateral CBF during cross-clamping. Neuromonitoring is the primary technique used to verify that CBF is adequate during the CEA procedure.

With CAS, embolic stroke accounts for the majority of the neurological risk because thrombus or plaque material may be dislodged during the stenting.[14]

### Risk Factors for Perioperative Stroke

Established risk factors for perioperative stroke related to CEA and CAS include increased age and preoperative hypertension.[15] The increased risk in patients aged 75 years and older is not large and therefore age should not be regarded as a contraindication to surgery.[16] The association between preoperative systolic hypertension (>180 mm Hg) and risk of operative stroke and death during CEA has been demonstrated in a systematic literature review.[16] In the International Carotid Stenting Study (ICSS), 8.3% of patients undergoing CEA experienced postprocedural hypertension, which was associated with higher baseline blood pressure.[17–18]

Other factors that increase the risk for perioperative stroke in patients undergoing CEA include peripheral vascular disease and angiographic findings such as occlusion of the contralateral ICA, stenosis of the ipsilateral internal carotid siphon, or stenosis of the ipsilateral external carotid artery.[16,19] These risk factors are likely to be predictors of more diffuse cerebrovascular disease and an associated risk of insufficient collateral blood flow during surgery.

Female gender has also been identified as a risk factor for perioperative stroke, but it is unclear why.[15] One potential explanation is that women tend to be smaller and, on average, have a smaller carotid artery diameter, increasing the risk of procedural stroke due to in-situ thrombosis following more technically demanding surgery.[16] In several studies female gender was not an independent predictor of risk in multivariable analyses, suggesting that differences between male and female patients in other characteristics could account for the increased operative risk in women.[20]

The optimal timing of CEA and CAS after symptoms of a stroke or TIA is a topic of debate.[21] If the carotid intervention is performed urgently or within the first few days of symptom onset, the risk of periprocedural stroke has to be weighed against the risk of early stroke recurrence. The Swedish Vascular Registry reported that when CEA was performed < 48 hours of symptom onset, there was an 11.5%

incidence of death or stroke within 30 days of CEA, but when CEA was performed >48 hours after symptom onset the incidence was less than 5%.[22] Two other studies reported no excess procedural risk when CEA was performed <48 hours of symptom onset.[23–24] Early CAS may be an option for minimizing the risk of recurrent early stroke and the overall risk of perioperative complications.

## Postoperative Cognitive Decline

Since carotid revascularization procedures carry a risk for cerebral ischemic injury, many studies have examined neurocognitive outcomes in this patient population. Cognitive decline following CEA and CAS is believed to reflect perioperative neurological injury that is milder in severity than that producing stroke. Indeed, CEA patients with early cognitive dysfunction have significantly elevated biomarkers of neuronal injury, as well as asymmetric CBF on magnetic resonance perfusion brain scans.[25–26]

CEA and CAS both introduce microemboli into the cerebral circulation. Studies examining perioperative microemboli detected by transcranial Doppler (TCD) monitoring have found that CAS has a higher incidence of high-intensity transient signals (HITS) compared with CEA, even with the use of distal protection devices.[27–28] The relationship between number of microemboli entering the cerebral circulation during CAS and CEA and neurocognitive outcome, however, is unclear.[29–30] Variability in type (gaseous vs. particulate) and size of emboli, which TCD cannot discriminate, may be a factor.

Both CEA and CAS are associated with risk for new ischemic lesions apparent on diffusion-weighted magnetic resonance imaging (DW-MRI), with CAS having a higher incidence than CEA (37% vs. 10%).[31] Numerous studies, however, have failed to find a relationship between the number or volume of new lesions and cognitive outcome.[32] The lack of relationship may be due to DW-MRI not capturing all of the damage underlying cognitive decline and that some DW-MRI lesions may be of no functional significance.

There is no evidence, however, that CEA and CAS differ with respect to neurocognitive outcomes. A systematic review of 37 studies (18 examining CEA, 12 examining CAS, and 7 comparing CEA to CAS) showed that CEA was associated with cognitive decline in 10–15% of patients, and that CEA and CAS did not differ with respect to neurocognitive outcomes.[32] There is wide variability among studies in terms of patient characteristics, neurocognitive assessment methodologies, and reported outcomes, and many studies have been underpowered.[32–34]

There is limited but consistent evidence that postoperative hypoperfusion following carotid revascularization is associated with cognitive decline.[35–37] Furthermore, in patients with baseline impairment of blood flow in the middle cerebral artery (MCA), carotid revascularization is associated with improved cognitive test scores following the procedure.[32,38]

## Risk Factors for Postoperative Cognitive Dysfunction

Risk factors that are associated with an increased incidence of early cognitive decline include age older than 75 years, diabetes mellitus, apolipoprotein-ε4 polymorphism, absence of posterior communicating arteries, and several complement polymorphisms.[32,39–42]

Recent research has focused on modifiable factors that may reduce the incidence of early cognitive decline. Blood pressure management is one such variable. MAP maintained at <20% above baseline during carotid clamping is associated with greater risk for early cognitive decline. MAP maintained at >20% above baseline is associated with lower risk for early cognitive decline.[7]

## MONITORING FOR NEUROLOGICAL INJURY
### Neuromonitoring for Carotid Endarterectomy

Maintaining normal arterial perfusion pressure is critical to ensure adequate collateral CBF during cross-clamping of the carotid artery. There is, however, a high likelihood of significant stenosis within one or more major vessels that supply collateral blood flow in CEA patients. Intraoperative neuromonitoring, with the focus on preventing a stroke during carotid cross-clamping and unclamping, is the primary technique used to verify that CBF is adequate during the CEA procedure.

To assure that there is adequate cerebral perfusion during the critical time of carotid clamp placement, four neuromonitoring methods may be employed: (1) clinical intraoperative examination, (2) electrophysiological monitoring, (3) cortical cerebral perfusion measurement, and (4) transcranial oxygen saturation measurement. Based on neuromonitoring changes consistent with cerebral ischemia, the majority of surgeons selectively place a temporary shunt during carotid clamping. This is not standard practice; some surgeons place a shunt routinely and others never do.[8]

It is important to consider that physiological interventions (e.g., hypothermia) and pharmacological interventions (e.g., anesthetics including lidocaine, induction agents, or volatile agents) may cause neuromonitoring changes that can mimic ischemia during cross-clamping; these changes should not be misinterpreted.

### Intraoperative Clinical Examination

Intraoperative clinical examination is the gold standard for neuromonitoring during CEA. It requires that the patient be sufficiently awake and responsive during the procedure in order to evaluate mental status, and language, motor, and sensory functions. This requires that the surgical area be anesthetized using a regional technique (i.e., either superficial or deep cervical block), and that the patient accepts being aware during surgery and cooperating with neurological testing upon request. A major advantage to awake, intraoperative neurological testing is that there is no requirement for electrophysiological or CBF monitoring equipment and personnel with expertise in interpreting the monitoring data. The major disadvantage of this technique is the possibility of sudden airway compromise due to concurrent sedation, surgical complications, or acute neurological deterioration during the procedure.

### Electrophysiological Monitoring

Electrophysiological examination can be performed using intraoperative electroencephalography (EEG) and evoked potential monitoring. An advantage of intraoperative electrophysiological examinations over clinical examinations is that they can be performed on patients who are under general anesthesia. The EEG monitors spontaneous electric activity arising from the cerebral cortex. Evoked potential monitoring, such as somatosensory evoked potentials (SSEPs) and motor evoked potentials (MEPs), evaluates both subcortical and cortical regions.

Before Clamping        After Clamping   3 μV | 1 sec

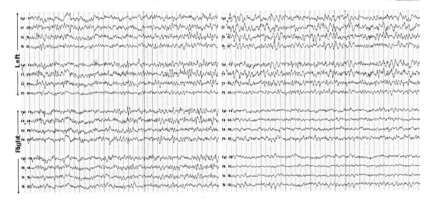

FIGURE 18.1 Spontaneous cortical activity before and after carotid artery clamping. Electroencephalogram amplitude decrease and slowing are produced by cerebral ischemia, but may also be produced by anesthetics and intravenous medications (propofol, etomidate, pentothal, lidocaine) and inhalational agents (isoflurane, halothane, sevoflurane, desflurane).

The EEG, however, is not responsive to decreases in CBF velocity unless it is reduced by more than 60% from baseline, probably due to the rich vascular supply to the brain (Figure 18.1).[43] Reductions of this magnitude also increase the likelihood of developing new neurological findings after surgery.[44] Interestingly, much lesser reductions (more than 28%) in intraoperative CBF velocity are associated with an increased likelihood of neurocognitive decline.[4]

Carotid artery clamping reduces blood flow but usually does not eliminate it.[45] With insufficient CBF, it may take a minute or more before EEG changes manifest, as compared to less than 10 seconds with the complete absence of CBF.[46] Depending on the adequacy of collateral flow, CBF reductions to less than 20 mL/100 g of brain tissue/minute may cause ipsilateral or bilateral decrease of fast-frequency EEG waves (>5 Hz) and a predominance of high-amplitude low-frequency waves (<4 Hz).[43,47–49]

SSEPs and MEPs can be added to EEG monitoring for patients under general anesthesia, but they have not been shown to be more predictive of ischemia during carotid clamping.

## Cerebral Perfusion Monitoring

Xenon-enhanced computed tomography (CT) scanning is a direct method of measuring CBF, but this technique is impractical for intraoperative use and only provides intermittent measurements. Therefore, TCD ultrasonography is used to continuously monitor CBF velocity in major cerebral arteries, as an indirect surrogate measure of CBF. Within the range of autoregulation, changes in cerebral perfusion pressure trigger compensatory changes in cerebrovascular resistance, resulting in a relatively constant blood flow. The TCD pulsatility index (PI) reflects change in cerebral vascular resistance, calculated as the systolic CBF velocity minus the diastolic CBF velocity, divided by the mean CBF velocity.[50] Normal values of PI are 0.6–1.1 (a unitless variable). Decreases in cerebrovascular resistance are reflected as a transient decrease in CBF velocity that partially recovers within several minutes (persistent declines in velocity are clinically significant).

Patient 1

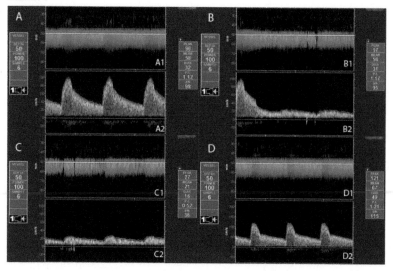

Patient 2

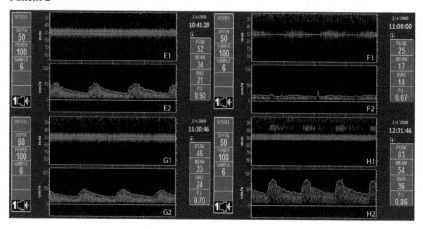

FIGURE 18.2 Transcranial Doppler (TCD) ultrasound tracings. Each tracing consists of two frames, 1 and 2. 1 is the Power M-mode tracing (analogous to the ultrasound mode) on the y-axis in mm and visualizes flow from 30 to 80 mm from the surface of the scalp. 2 is the Doppler velocity in cm/sec on the y-axis at a distance indicated by the yellow line in the Power M-mode. The x-axis is in seconds between the time markers. Patient 1: TCD tracings at four different time points relative to cross-clamping the carotid artery: (A) before, (B) immediately at, (C) during, and (D) after unclamping the carotid artery. The boxed numbers to the left of each tracing show the depth in mm, power, and sample volume. The boxed numbers to the right of each tracing show the peak, mean, diastolic velocities, pulsatility index, and the percentage change from baseline of the mean cerebral blood flow velocity. Patient 2: TCD tracings at four different time points relative to cross-clamping the carotid artery: (E) before, (F) immediately at, (G) after shunt insertion, and (H) after shunt removal and unclamping the carotid artery. The boxed numbers to the left of each tracing show the depth in mm, power, and sample volume. The boxed numbers on the right of each tracing show the peak, mean, diastolic velocities, and pulsatility index.

During CEA, changes in cerebral blood velocity occur immediately upon clamping the carotid artery and become apparent within seconds. In contrast, changes in the EEG that occur in response to clamping of the carotid artery develop more slowly over several minutes, depending on the degree of collateral blood flow. Decreases in CBF velocity reflect percentage decreases in CBF, assuming the diameter of the insonated vessel and cerebrovascular resistance remain constant (Figure 18.2).

## Transcranial Oxygen Saturation Measurement

Regional brain tissue oximetry using near infrared spectroscopy (NIRS) primarily measures the venous oxygen saturation of the cortex, which is dependent on the adequacy of oxygen delivery. Cerebral oximetry, however, has a poor positive predictive value for ischemia compared to intraoperative clinical monitoring and EEG monitoring.[51–52] Despite these findings, this technology is used increasingly due to its low cost, noninvasive nature, and ease of technical application.

## Neuromonitoring for Carotid Artery Stenting

In contrast to CEA, CAS requires no neuromonitoring devices because the procedure is performed with the patient awake under regional anesthesia. Clinical neuromonitoring in this setting, however, can still be useful because it allows for rapid detection of embolization or inadequate blood flow after stent placement. TCD ultrasound during CAS can be used to monitor for emboli (HITS) during stenting, and although monitoring for emboli does not prevent their occurrence, it can explain why a patient may have symptoms upon clinical testing or alert the clinical team to expect such changes.

## NEUROPROTECTION STRATEGIES
## Strategies Aimed at Preventing and Treating Cerebral Ischemia

### Carotid Endarterectomy

Patients who undergo CEA typically have diffuse vascular disease involving the heart, the peripheral vasculature, and the cerebral circulation.[53] When there is significant stenosis of one or more of the major vessels supplying blood flow to the brain (other than the carotid artery undergoing intervention), it is imperative to maintain normal or supranormal arterial blood pressure to ensure adequate blood flow to the brain.

Upon detecting reduced CBF by any monitoring technique, the surgical team should be notified and the arterial blood pressure should be increased. When significant changes occur in the EEG upon carotid artery clamping, most surgeons employ a shunt to prevent global hemispheric ischemia. A decline in CBF velocity by more than 60% is also used a criterion for shunt insertion by most clinicians.[54] Interestingly, shunt placement for lesser decrements in CBF velocity has been associated with better cognitive outcomes.[4]

An infusion of phenylephrine or other vasoconstrictive medications is commonly used to increase peripheral vascular resistance and systemic arterial pressure.[55] As arterial pressure is increased, the surgeon places a shunt connecting the vessel(s) below and above the surgical site. TCD monitoring can be used to ensure normalization of CBF with shunts in situ, reassuring the clinicians that the shunt is functioning as intended.[56–57]

Most new neurological deficits after CEA are not due to ischemia during cross-clamp, but rather due to emboli.[14] Emboli are not detected by the EEG (unless massive), but they are detected by TCD, especially during surgical manipulations such as dissection of the carotid artery and its bifurcation, and upon opening of the internal carotid artery clamp.[56] Most emboli are gaseous and not associated with adverse clinical events, but the presence of more than 10 particulate emboli is associated with cerebral complications, including carotid artery thrombosis, new lesions on magnetic resonance imaging (MRI), and development of neurological deficits.[58–59]

Steps that surgeons use to avoid emboli include gentle handling of the carotid artery prior to clamping, avoidance of repetitive clamping of the area with plaque involvement, and performing "backflow" prior to unclamping the vessel to flush particulate emboli from the cerebral circulation. "Backflow" consists of releasing each of the three clamps—common carotid artery, external carotid artery, and internal carotid artery—individually and sequentially to allow debris to enter the surgical site and be removed by suctioning.

## Carotid Artery Stenting

Cerebral protective devices (CPD) have been developed recently to prevent distal embolization of plaque debris and thrombus formation caused by manipulation of wires and stent deployment during CAS.[60] A review of nonrandomized studies of patients with symptomatic or asymptomatic carotid artery stenosis who underwent CAS reported that CAS performed with a CPD was associated with lower 30-day stroke rate than CAS without a CPD (0.8% vs. 4.8%).[61] Furthermore, the use of a CPD was associated with reduced incidence of clinically silent ischemic brain lesions on DW-MRI (33% vs. 45%).[62] The use of CPDs was mandated during the EVA-3S trial after an interim analysis of 73 CAS patients showed a four times greater risk of stroke in unprotected stenting compared to patients in whom a CPD was used.[63] In the full trial report, stroke rates were 25% and 7.9%, respectively.[64] In contrast, the SPACE trial and ICSS trials found that stroke risk did not differ between unprotected and protected stenting.[65]

The only randomized trials comparing CAS with versus without CPDs using DW-MRI lesions as the outcome measure found that the risk of new ischemic brain lesions was greater with use of CPDs.[66–67] This may seem counterintuitive, but in these studies the most commonly used CPDs were distal filter devices, and it is conceivable that crossing the stenotic region with the device prior to filter deployment may dislodge embolic material from the arterial wall.[66]

Proximal occlusion devices used during CAS produce retrograde blood flow across the stenosis during the time of intervention, which theoretically should lower the risk of distal embolism.[68] Use of flow reversal systems is associated with lower risk for clinical stroke and new cerebral ischemic lesions on DW-MRI, compared to distal filter devices. Not all patients, however, can tolerate flow reversal in the carotid artery undergoing intervention.[69–70] The current evidence is therefore inconclusive about whether use of CPDs during CAS is effective in preventing perioperative stroke, and about which type of CPD (if any) is most beneficial.

## Pharmacologic Neuroprotection

Statins, which are widely prescribed as cardiovascular risk reduction therapy, also exert cholesterol-independent effects and may improve acute stroke recovery. Retrospective studies have shown an association between ongoing statin therapy and improved outcome in patients presenting with ischemic stroke.[71-72] A large meta-analysis also showed that statin therapy begun prior to stroke onset was associated with improved outcome.[73] Statin use has been found to be associated with decreased risk of early cognitive decline in the asymptomatic CEA population.[74] The time course and mechanism of protection, however, are unclear.

Magnesium has shown promise for neuroprotection during CEA and cardiac bypass surgery.[75-76] The FAST-MAG trial, however, found that while pre-hospital initiation of magnesium sulfate therapy within 2 hours after the onset of stroke symptoms was safe, it did not improve disability outcomes at 90 days.[77]

Multiple pharmacologic agents have shown great promise as neuroprotectants in animal models of ischemic stroke. These treatment strategies are pertinent to CEA and CAS because these procedures may induce global and focal cerebral ischemia, whether for limited time intervals during cross-clamping or for prolonged intervals in the case of embolic stroke. To date, however, there are no clinical data supporting the role of any pharmacologic agent as a neuroprotective strategy for focal cerebral ischemia. A systematic review of all controlled acute ischemic stroke clinical treatment trials published in English to the year 2000 concluded that many trials have been handicapped in their ability to show agent efficacy because of inadequate sample sizes, inappropriate time windows for treatment and outcome assessment, or failure to target a specific stroke mechanism.[78]

## Hypothermia

It is well established that hypothermia is neuroprotective in experimental models of brain ischemia.[79] Hypothermia decreases cerebral metabolism, suppresses glutamate release, reduces neuroinflammatory responses, disrupts apoptotic pathways, reduces free radical generation, and minimizes edema formation.[80] Hypothermia has been associated with improved neurological outcome in patients surviving cardiac arrest, and it is the first neuroprotective strategy to be recommended by the American Heart Association in cardiac arrest patients who remain comatose after resuscitation.[81] No clinical trials to date have evaluated hypothermia as a form of neuroprotection during carotid revascularization. In the setting of potential focal cerebral ischemia during neurosurgical clipping of ruptured intracranial aneurysms, however, mild hypothermia has not been associated with improved outcomes.[82] Without conclusive evidence that hypothermia is beneficial in patients with focal cerebral ischemia, current recommendations are to maintain normothermia and to avoid hyperthermia in this patient population.[83]

## IMPLICATIONS FOR CLINICAL PRACTICE

Neuroprotective strategies for CEA focus on the prevention of ischemia by neuro-monitoring, and changes in management in response to neuromonitoring data such as shunt placement and alteration of blood pressure management. Neuroprotective strategies for CAS focus on avoiding embolization by using CPDs. These strategies should be used to optimize neurological and neurocognitive outcomes after CEA and CAS.

Given the strong associative data, it is reasonable to continue statin therapy in patients undergoing CAS or CEA who are at high risk of stroke or in those who are already on statin therapy.

## FUTURE DIRECTIONS

Future directions for reducing the perioperative risk of CAS will a focus on further development of CPDs to prevent distal embolization of plaque debris and thrombus caused by manipulation of intravascular wires and stent deployment.[60] CPDs that are well tolerated by patients and decrease embolization are likely to increase the safety of CAS. Perioperative medical management strategies for both CAS and CEA, such as statins, antiplatelet agents, hypothermia, and pharmacologic neuroprotection, also are promising areas for ongoing investigation. Investigations in neuroprotection for CEA and CAS should include assessment of cognitive decline, an adverse outcome that is more subtle than clinical stroke but occurs with greater frequency, given the limitations of power and sample size in studies that utilize clinical stroke as the sole outcome measure.

## REFERENCES

1. de Borst GJ, Moll FL, van de Pavoordt HD, Mauser HW, Kelder JC, Ackerstaf RG. Stroke from carotid endarterectomy: when and how to reduce perioperative stroke rate? *Eur J Vasc Endovasc Surg.* 2001;21(6):484–9.

2. Ferguson GG, Eliasziw M, Barr HW, et al. The North American Symptomatic Carotid Endarterectomy Trial: surgical results in 1415 patients. *Stroke.* 1999;30(9):1751–8.

3. Ederle J, Dobson J, Featherstone RL, et al.; International Carotid Stenting Study investigators. Carotid artery stenting compared with endarterectomy in patients with symptomatic carotid stenosis (International Carotid Stenting Study): an interim analysis of a randomised controlled trial. *Lancet.* 2010;375(9719):985–97.

4. Mergeche JL, Bruce SS, Sander Connolly E, Heyer EJ. Reduced middle cerebral artery velocity during cross-clamp predicts cognitive dysfunction after carotid endarterectomy. *J Clin Neurosci.* 2014;21(3):406–11.

5. Heyer EJ, Adams DC, Solomon RA, et al. Neuropsychometric changes in patients after carotid endarterectomy. *Stroke.* 1998;29(6):1110–5.

6. Heyer EJ, Sharma R, Rampersad A, et al. A controlled prospective study of neuropsychological dysfunction following carotid endarterectomy. *Arch Neurol.* 2002;59(2):217–22.

7. Heyer EJ, Mergeche JL, Anastasian ZH, Kim M, Mallon KA, Connolly ES. Arterial blood pressure management during carotid endarterectomy and early cognitive dysfunction. *Neurosurgery.* 2014;74(3):245–51; discussion 251–3.

8. Fode NC, Sundt TM, Robertson JT, Peerless SJ, Shields CB. Multicenter retrospective review of results and complications of carotid endarterectomy in 1981. *Stroke.* 1986; 17(3):370–5.

9. Brott TG, Halperin JL, Abbara S, et al. 2011 ASA/ACCF/AHA/AANN/AANS/ ACR/ASNR/CNS/SAIP/SCAI/SIR/SNIS/SVM/SVS guideline on the management of patients with extracranial carotid and vertebral artery disease. A report of the American College of Cardiology Foundation/American Heart Association Task Force on Practice Guidelines, and the American Stroke Association, American Association of Neuroscience

Nurses, American Association of Neurological Surgeons, American College of Radiology, American Society of Neuroradiology, Congress of Neurological Surgeons, Society of Atherosclerosis Imaging and Prevention, Society for Cardiovascular Angiography and Interventions, Society of Interventional Radiology, Society of NeuroInterventional Surgery, Society for Vascular Medicine, and Society for Vascular Surgery. *Circulation.* 2011;124(4):e54–130.

10. Cina CS, Clase CM, Haynes RB. Carotid endarterectomy for symptomatic carotid stenosis. *Cochrane Database Syst Rev.* 2000;(2):CD001081.

11. Barnett HJM, Taylor DW, Eliasziw M, et al.; Collaborators NASCET. Benefit of carotid endarterectomy in patients with symptomatic moderate or severe stenosis. *NEJM.* 1998;339(20):1415–25.

12. Liu ZJ, Fu WG, Guo ZY, Shen LG, Shi ZY, Li JH. Updated systematic review and meta-analysis of randomized clinical trials comparing carotid artery stenting and carotid endarterectomy in the treatment of carotid stenosis. *Ann Vasc Surg.* 2012;26(4):576–90.

13. Gupta PK, Ramanan B, Mactaggart JN, et al. Risk index for predicting perioperative stroke, myocardial infarction, or death risk in asymptomatic patients undergoing carotid endarterectomy. *J Vasc Surg.* 2013;57(2):318–26.

14. Krul JM, van Gijn J, Ackerstaff RG, Eikelboom BC, Theodorides T, Vermeulen FE. Site and pathogenesis of infarcts associated with carotid endarterectomy. *Stroke.* 1989; 20(3):324–8.

15. Doig D, Turner EL, Dobson J, et al.; ICSS Investigators. Risk factors for stroke, myocardial infarction, or death following carotid endarterectomy: results from the International Carotid Stenting Study. *Eur J Vasc Endovasc Surg.* 2015;50(6):688–94.

16. Rothwell PM, Slattery J, Warlow CP. Clinical and angiographic predictors of stroke and death from carotid endarterectomy: systematic review. *BMJ.* 1997;315(7122):1571–7.

17. Altinbas A, Algra A, Brown MM, et al.; International Carotid Stenting Study Investigators. International Carotid Stenting Study I: effects of carotid endarterectomy or stenting on hemodynamic complications in the International Carotid Stenting Study: a randomized comparison. *Int J Stroke.* 2014;9(3):284–90.

18. Wong JH, Findlay JM, Suarez-Almazor ME. Hemodynamic instability after carotid endarterectomy: risk factors and associations with operative complications. *Neurosurgery.* 1997;41(1):35–41; discussion 41–3.

19. Bond R, Narayan SK, Rothwell PM, Warlow CP; European Carotid Surgery Trialists' Collaborative Group. Clinical and radiographic risk factors for operative stroke and death in the European carotid surgery trial. *Eur J Vasc Endovasc Surg.* 2002;23(2):108–16.

20. Brown MM, Raine R. Should sex influence the choice between carotid stenting and carotid endarterectomy? *Lancet Neurol.* 2011;10(6):494–7.

21. Naylor AR, AbuRahma AF. Debate: whether carotid endarterectomy is safer than stenting in the hyperacute period after onset of symptoms. *J Vasc Surg.* 2015;61(6):1642–51.

22. Strömberg S, Gelin J, Osterberg T, Bergström GM, Karlström L, Osterberg K; Swedish Vascular Registry (Swedvasc) Steering Committee. Very urgent carotid endarterectomy confers increased procedural risk. *Stroke.* 2012;43(5):1331–5.

23. Rantner B, Schmidauer C, Knoflach M, Fraedrich G. Very urgent carotid endarterectomy does not increase the procedural risk. *Eur J Vasc Endovasc Surg.* 2015;49(2):129–36.

24. Sharpe R, Sayers RD, London NJ, et al. Procedural risk following carotid endarterectomy in the hyperacute period after onset of symptoms. *Eur J Vasc Endovasc Surg.* 2013;46(5):519–24.

25. Connolly ES, Jr, Winfree CJ, Rampersad A, et al. Serum S100B protein levels are corre-lated with subclinical neurocognitive declines after carotid endarterectomy. *Neurosurgery.* 2001;49(5):1076–82; discussion 1082–3.

26. Wilson DA, Mocco J, D'Ambrosio AL, et al. Post-carotid endarterectomy neurocognitive decline is associated with cerebral blood flow asymmetry on post-operative magnetic resonance perfusion brain scans. *Neurol Res.* 2008;30(3):302–6.

27. Crawley F, Stygall J, Lunn S, Harrison M, Brown MM, Newman S. Comparison of micro-embolism detected by transcranial Doppler and neuropsychological sequelae of carotid surgery and percutaneous transluminal angioplasty. *Stroke.* 2000;31(6):1329–34.

28. Gupta N, Corriere MA, Dodson TF, et al. The incidence of microemboli to the brain is less with endarterectomy than with percutaneous revascularization with distal filters or flow reversal. *J Vasc Surg.* 2011;53(2):316–22.

29. Martin KK, Wigginton JB, Babikian VL, Pochay VE, Crittenden MD, Rudolph JL. Intraoperative cerebral high-intensity transient signals and postoperative cognitive func-tion: a systematic review. *Am J Surg* 2009;197(1):55–63.

30. Zhou W, Hitchner E, Gillis K, et al. Prospective neurocognitive evaluation of patients undergoing carotid interventions. *J Vasc Surg* 2012;56(6):1571–8.

31. Schnaudigel S, Groschel K, Pilgram SM, Kastrup A. New brain lesions after carotid stenting versus carotid endarterectomy – a systematic review of the literature. *Stroke.* 2008;39(6):1911–9.

32. Plessers M, Van Herzeele I, Vermassen F, Vingerhoets G. Neurocognitive functioning after carotid revascularization: a systematic review. *Cerebrovasc Dis Extra.* 2014;4(2):132–48.

33. De Rango P, Caso V, Leys D, Paciaroni M, Lenti M, Cao P. The role of carotid artery stenting and carotid endarterectomy in cognitive performance a systematic review. *Stroke.* 2008;39(11):3116–27.

34. Berman L, Pietrzak RH, Mayes L. Neurocognitive changes after carotid revasculariza-tion: a review of the current literature. *J Psychosom Res.* 2007;63(6):599–612.

35. Chida K, Ogasawara K, Suga Y, et al. Postoperative cortical neural loss associated with cerebral hyperperfusion and cognitive impairment after carotid endarterectomy: [123]I-iomazenil SPECT study. *Stroke.* 2009;40(2):448–53.

36. Nanba T, Ogasawara K, Nishimoto H, et al. Postoperative cerebral white matter dam-age associated with cerebral hyperperfusion and cognitive impairment after carotid endarterectomy: a diffusion tensor magnetic resonance imaging study. *Cerebrovasc Dis.* 2012;34(5-6):358–67.

37. Hirooka R, Ogasawara K, Sasaki M, et al. Magnetic resonance imaging in patients with cerebral hyperperfusion and cognitive impairment after carotid endarterectomy. *J Neurosurg.* 2008;108(6):1178–83.

38. Lal BK, Younes M, Cruz G, Kapadia I, Jamil Z, Pappas PJ. Cognitive changes after sur-gery vs stenting for carotid artery stenosis. *J Vasc Surg.* 2011;54(3):691–8.

39. Mocco J, Wilson DA, Komotar RJ, et al. Predictors of neurocognitive decline after carotid endarterectomy. *Neurosurgery.* 2006;58(5):844–50; discussion 844–50.

40. Heyer EJ, Wilson DA, Sahlein DH, et al. APOE-epsilon4 predisposes to cogni-tive dysfunction following uncomplicated carotid endarterectomy. *Neurology.* 2005; 65(11):1759–63.

41. Heyer EJ, Kellner CP, Malone HR, et al. Complement polymorphisms and cognitive dysfunction after carotid endarterectomy. *J Neurosurg.* 2013;119(3):648–54.

42. Sussman ES, Kellner CP, Mergeche JL, et al. Radiographic absence of the posterior com-municating arteries and the prediction of cognitive dysfunction after carotid endarterec-tomy. *J Neurosurg.* 2014;121(3):593–8.

43. Sundt TM Jr, Sharbrough FW, Piepgras DG, Kearns TP, Messick J Jr, O'Fallon WM. Correlation of cerebral blood flow and electroencephalographic changes during carotid endarterectomy: with results of surgery and hemodynamics of cerebral ischemia. *Mayo Clinic Proceedings.* 1981;56(9):533–43.

44. Halsey JH Jr. Risks and benefits of shunting in carotid endarterectomy. The International Transcranial Doppler Collaborators. *Stroke.* 1992;23(11):1583–7.

45. Adams DC, Heyer EJ, Emerson RG, et al. Implantable cardioverter defibrillator: evaluation of clinical neurologic outcome and electroencephalographic changes during implantation. *J Thoracic Cardiovasc Surg.* 1995;109(3):565–73.

46. Adams D, Heyer E, Emerson R, Spotnitz H, Delphin E. Implantable cardioverter defibrillator: evaluation of neurologic outcome and EEG changes during implantation. *Anesthesiology.* 1993;79:A214.

47. Michenfelder JD, Sundt TM, Fode N, Sharbrough FW. Isoflurane when compared to enflurane and halothane decreases the frequency of cerebral ischemia during carotid endarterectomy. *Anesthesiology.* 1987;67(3):336–40.

48. Nuwer MR. Intraoperative electroencephalography. *J Clin Neurophysiol.* 1993;10(4): 437–44.

49. Sharbrough FW, Messick JM, Sundt TMJ. Correlation of continuous electroencephalograms with cerebral blood flow measurements during carotid endarterectomy. *Stroke.* 1973;4(4):674–83.

50. Aleksic M, Heckenkamp J, Gawenda M, Brunkwall J. Pulsatility index determination by flowmeter measurement: a new indicator for vascular resistance? *Eur Surg Res.* 2004;36(6):345–49.

51. Mauermann WJ, Crepeau AZ, Pulido JN, et al. Comparison of electroencephalography and cerebral oximetry to determine the need for in-line arterial shunting in patients undergoing carotid endarterectomy. *J Cardiothorac Vasc Anesth.* 2013;27(6):1253–9.

52. Stilo F, Spinelli F, Martelli E, et al. The sensibility and specificity of cerebral oximetry, measured by INVOS-4100, in patients undergoing carotid endarterectomy compared with awake testing. *Minerva Anestesiol.* 2012;78(10):1126–35.

53. Hertzer NR, O'Hara PJ, Mascha EJ, Krajewski LP, Sullivan TM, Beven EG. Early outcome assessment for 2228 consecutive carotid endarterectomy procedures: the Cleveland Clinic experience from 1989 to 1995. *J Vasc Surg.* 1997; 26(1):1–10.

54. Costin M, Rampersad A, Solomon RA, Connolly ES, Heyer EJ. Cerebral injury predicted by transcranial Doppler ultrasonography but not electroencephalography during carotid endarterectomy. *J Neurosurg Anesthesiol.* 2002;14(4):287–92.

55. Drummond JC, Oh YS, Cole DJ, Shapiro HM. Phenylephrine-induced hypertension reduces ischemia following middle cerebral artery occlusion in rats. *Stroke.* 1989;20(11):1538–44.

56. Smith JL, Evans DH, Gaunt ME, London NJ, Bell PR, Naylor AR. Experience with transcranial Doppler monitoring reduces the incidence of particulate embolization during carotid endarterectomy. *Br J Surg.* 1998;85(1):56–9.

57. Heyer E, Winfree C, Mack W, Connolly ES Jr. Transcranial Doppler monitoring during carotid endarterectomy: a technical case report. *J Neurosurgical Anesthesia.* 2000;12(3):233–39.

58. Gaunt ME, Martin PJ, Smith JL, et al. Clinical relevance of intraoperative embolization detected by transcranial Doppler ultrasonography during carotid endarterectomy: a prospective study of 100 patients. *Br J Surg.* 1994;81(10):1435–9.

59. Ackerstaff RG, Jansen C, Moll FL, Vermeulen FE, Hamerlijnck RP, Mauser HW. The significance of microemboli detection by means of transcranial Doppler ultrasonography monitoring in carotid endarterectomy. *J Vasc Surg.* 1995;21(6):963–9.

60. Theron JG, Payelle GG, Coskun O, Huet HF, Guimaraens L. Carotid artery stenosis: treatment with protected balloon angioplasty and stent placement. *Radiology.* 1996;201(3):627–36.

61. Kastrup A, Groschel K, Krapf H, Brehm BR, Dichgans J, Schulz JB. Early outcome of carotid angioplasty and stenting with and without cerebral protection devices: a systematic review of the literature. *Stroke.* 2003;34(3):813–9.

62. Schnaudigel S, Groschel K, Pilgram SM, Kastrup A. New brain lesions after carotid stenting versus carotid endarterectomy: a systematic review of the literature. *Stroke.* 2008;39(6):1911–9.

63. Mas JL, Chatellier G, Beyssen B; EVA-3S Investigators. Carotid angioplasty and stenting with and without cerebral protection: clinical alert from the Endarterectomy Versus Angioplasty in Patients With Symptomatic Severe Carotid Stenosis (EVA-3S) trial. *Stroke.* 2004;35(1):e18–20.

64. Mas JL, Chatellier G, Beyssen B, et al.; EVA-3S Investigators Endarterectomy versus stenting in patients with symptomatic severe carotid stenosis. *N Engl J Med.* 2006;355(16):1660–71.

65. Ringleb PA, Hennerici M, Hacke W. Stent-protected angioplasty of symptomatic carotid artery stenosis. The European point of view. *Int J Stroke.* 2006;1(2):94–6.

66. Barbato JE, Dillavou E, Horowitz MB, et al. A randomized trial of carotid artery stenting with and without cerebral protection. *J Vasc Surg.* 2008;47(4):760–5.

67. Macdonald S, Evans DH, Griffiths PD, et al. Filter-protected versus unprotected carotid artery stenting: a randomised trial. *Cerebrovasc Dis.* 2010;29(3):282–9.

68. Parodi JC, Ferreira LM, Sicard G, La Mura R, Fernandez S. Cerebral protection during carotid stenting using flow reversal. *J Vasc Surg.* 2005;41(3):416–22.

69. Clair DG, Hopkins LN, Mehta M, et al.; EMPiRE Clinical Study Investigators. Neuroprotection during carotid artery stenting using the GORE flow reversal system: 30-day outcomes in the EMPiRE Clinical Study. *Catheter Cardiovasc Interv.* 2011;77(3):420–9.

70. Nikas D, Reith W, Schmidt A, et al. Prospective, multicenter European study of the GORE flow reversal system for providing neuroprotection during carotid artery stenting. *Catheter Cardiovasc Interv.* 2012;80(7):1060–8.

71. Moonis M, Kane K, Schwiderski U, Sandage BW, Fisher M. HMG-CoA reductase inhibitors improve acute ischemic stroke outcome. *Stroke.* 2005;36(6):1298–300.

72. Elkind MS, Flint AC, Sciacca RR, Sacco RL. Lipid-lowering agent use at ischemic stroke onset is associated with decreased mortality. *Neurology.* 2005;65(2):253–8.

73. Ní Chróinín D, Åsplund K, Asberg S, et al. Statin therapy and outcome after ischemic stroke: systematic review and meta-analysis of observational studies and randomized trials. *Stroke.* 2013;44(2):448–56.

74. Heyer EJ, Mergeche JL, Bruce SS, et al. Statins reduce neurologic injury in asymptomatic carotid endarterectomy patients. *Stroke.* 2013;44(4):1150–2.

75. Mack WJ, Kellner CP, Sahlein DH, et al. Intraoperative magnesium infusion during carotid endarterectomy: a double-blind placebo-controlled trial. *J Neurosurg.* 2009;110(5):961–7.

76. Bhudia SK, Cosgrove DM, Naugle RI, et al. Magnesium as a neuroprotectant in cardiac surgery: a randomized clinical trial. *J Thorac Cardiovasc Surg.* 2006;131(4):853–61.

77. Saver JL, Starkman S, Eckstein M, et al.; FAST-MAG Investigators and Coordinators. Prehospital use of magnesium sulfate as neuroprotection in acute stroke. *N Engl J Med.* 2015;372(6):528–36.

78. Kidwell CS, Liebeskind DS, Starkman S, Saver JL. Trends in acute ischemic stroke trials through the 20th century. *Stroke.* 2001;32(6):1349–59.

79. Yenari MA, Han HS. Neuroprotective mechanisms of hypothermia in brain ischaemia. *Nat Rev Neurosci.* 2012;13(4):267–78.

80. Wu TC, Grotta JC. Hypothermia for acute ischaemic stroke. *Lancet Neurol.* 2013;12(3):275–84.

81. Nolan JP, Neumar RW, Adrie C, et al. Post-cardiac arrest syndrome: epidemiology, pathophysiology, treatment, and prognostication. A scientific statement from the International Liaison Committee on Resuscitation; the American Heart Association Emergency Cardiovascular Care Committee; the Council on Cardiovascular Surgery and Anesthesia; the Council on Cardiopulmonary, Perioperative, and Critical Care; the Council on Clinical Cardiology; the Council on Stroke. *Resuscitation.* 2008;79(3):350–79.

82. Todd MM, Hindman BJ, Clarke WR, Torner JC; Intraoperative Hypothermia for Aneurysm Surgery Trial (IHAST) Investigators. Mild intraoperative hypothermia during surgery for intracranial aneurysm. *N Engl J Med.* 2005;352(2):135–45.

83. Talke PO, Sharma D, Heyer EJ, Bergese SD, Blackham KA, Stevens RD. Society for Neuroscience in Anesthesiology and Critical Care Expert consensus statement: anesthetic management of endovascular treatment for acute ischemic stroke: endorsed by the Society of NeuroInterventional Surgery and the Neurocritical Care Society. *J Neurosurg Anesthesiol.* 2014;26(2):95–108.

# 19 Neuroprotection for Vascular and Endovascular Neurosurgery

Travis R. Ladner, Nishant Ganesh Kumar,

Lucy He, and J Mocco

## INTRODUCTION

The complexity of neurovascular disease presents a challenge to the surgical and anesthesia teams managing patients with such conditions. With open or endovascular techniques, abrupt changes in hemodynamic status and intracranial pressure (ICP) are an ever-present concern perioperatively. Moreover, vascular procedures inherently involve manipulating critical vascular and neural structures, including friable structures that may have recently ruptured, furthering risk of neurological damage. Clinical experience over the past several decades has generated several effective strategies to reduce neurological complications of neurovascular procedures. This chapter reviews common complications of cerebrovascular and endovascular operations and their risk factors, and summarizes clinical principles, strategies, and considerations for maximizing neuroprotection in the treatment of neurovascular disease.

## MECHANISMS OF AND RISKS FOR NEUROLOGICAL INJURY IN NEUROVASCULAR SURGERY

Neurological complications of neurovascular surgery can be classified broadly into primary (i.e., occurring in the operating room [OR]) and secondary (i.e., occurring in the intensive care unit [ICU]) injury. As a consequence of primary injury, pathological processes can be set into motion that present in a delayed clinical manner. Examples of primary injury include edema, hemorrhage, and ischemia. Secondary injuries include delayed vasospasm/cerebral ischemia, hydrocephalus, and seizures.

### General Concerns for Injury During Open Procedures

Brain edema during craniotomy may cause ischemia and also impede the surgeon's access to and visualization of vital structures. Retraction during the case can further increase ischemia and/or impede venous outflow, increasing edema. As a result, many physicians have begun to avoid the use of retractors completely.[1] Direct injury to cranial nerves during aneurysm clipping is another potential complication.

Intraoperative hemorrhage, although infrequent (up to 20% in some series, but usually much less) is a potential risk that the team should be prepared to address.[2] Ruptured aneurysms are at an increased risk of re-rupture within 24 hours after the initial rupture, especially within the first 2 hours.[3] Surgical dissection of the aneurysm and clip placement are the most frequent causes of intraoperative rupture.[2] As a result, it is crucial to have a stringent practice of maintaining access to proximal vasculature for possible temporary occlusion during clipping or in the face of rupture. Intraoperative bleeding may require prolonged proximal vessel temporary clipping time while bleeding is controlled, or even sacrifice of the proximal vessel with resultant ischemia or infarction. Delayed edema can also result from ischemia as a result of the reduced perfusion from the sacrificed segment. Arteriovenous malformations (AVMs) always have the potential for abrupt, massive blood loss from arterial feeders during resection, even with preoperative embolization. Increased ICP can further increase secondary ischemia and may result in brain herniation through the opened cranium. Resection of normal cortex may be required to identify sources of bleeding or manage intractable cerebral swelling. In the acute management of visually limiting bleeding within the operative field, induced hypotension may be required.[4] Extensive or prolonged hypotension during active blood loss, however, may exacerbate ischemia, especially in older patients.

Direct ischemic complications may also occur during surgery. Vessel spasm during vessel manipulation and/or after aneurysmal subarachnoid hemorrhage (SAH) can be flow limiting. While this is often visualized directly by the operating surgeon and treated with papaverine or sodium nitroprusside, use of micro-Doppler ultrasonography or intraoperative indocyanine green (ICG) angiography can further help confirm vessel patency and flow.[5-7] During aneurysm clipping, temporary occlusion of the parent artery provides hemostatic control and can lower hemorrhage risk by softening the aneurysm during dissection. Prolonged temporary clip time, however, increases the stroke risk. One group reported a 9.4-fold increase for total temporary clip times longer than 20 minutes.[8] During final clip application, small perforating arteries may also be compromised. Vascular steal during AVM resection may also cause regional ischemia.[9] During extracranial-intracranial bypass operations in cases of direct bypass, ischemia may occur during temporary arterial occlusion. In cases of stenotic diseases, such as moyamoya, flow-limiting vascular steal in anesthetized patients may cause hypotensive cerebral ischemia.[10]

## General Concerns for Injury During Endovascular Procedures

Hemorrhage, edema, and ischemia are always of concern during endovascular procedures. Arterial injury during all stages of interventional procedures may cause vessel dissection or even perforation. As a result, care must be taken to limit the force and nature of endovascular manipulations. In the case of AVM embolization, an overzealous approach may lead to impediment of venous outflow, precipitating hemorrhage or edema.[11] Permanent neurological complications were observed in 4.2% of AVM embolization procedures in one series.[12] Delayed intraparenchymal hemorrhage after flow diversion of aneurysms using the Pipeline Embolization Device is a feared complication of unknown etiology that has been reported in 2.5% of cases.[13]

Ischemia may result from vessel spasm during catheter manipulation or distal embolization of dislodged plaques in cases of atherosclerosis. Coil embolization of aneurysms may result in coil mass herniation into the parent vessel or distal coil migration, with damage to the endothelium that precipitates acute or delayed thrombosis and ischemic stroke, as has been observed in up to 2.5% of cases.[14] Inadvertent migration of liquid embolic agents, such as Onyx or N-butyl cyanoacrylate (n-BCA), can also lead to ischemia via nontarget embolization and has been reported in 5.6% of cases.[15] In-stent stenosis due to intimal damage and remodeling following stenting may also cause delayed cerebral ischemia (DCI), notably occurring in 29.7% of cases in the Wingspan intracranial stent registry.[16]

## Secondary Neurologic Injury

In addition to these primary brain injuries, delayed secondary brain injury following vascular and endovascular surgery includes cerebral edema, infection, seizures, hematoma, hydrocephalus, vasospasm, elevated ICP, ischemia, and metabolic complications. Secondary brain injury can exert its effects over a period of minutes to hours, as occurs with arterial ischemia, or over a period of days, as occurs with inflammation, venous ischemia, and edema formation.

One classic example is the delayed sequela of aneurysmal SAH, which may cause vasospasm and DCI secondary to an inflammatory cascade triggered by extravasated blood in the cerebrospinal fluid (CSF).[17] Clinical decline with concurrent radiographic vasospasm occurs in approximately 20–30% of aneurysmal SAH patients, although in some poor-grade patients infarction from DCI can develop in the absence of clinically obvious neurological deterioration. Hydrocephalus is another delayed complication of hemorrhagic events, resulting from disruption to CSF flow from intraventricular hemorrhage and/or interruption of CSF absorption by arachnoid granulations; it occurs in approximately 20% of SAH cases.[18–19] Seizures may result from parenchymal irritation from extravascular blood, a phenomenon reported in 15–18% of cases acutely, with approximately 3% developing late epilepsy.[20]

## Risk Factors for Neurological Injury in Neurovascular Surgery

Medical comorbidities conferring increased risk for stroke in the intraoperative and perioperative period are well described and include pre-existing atherosclerosis, hypertension, and cardiac arrhythmia (e.g., atrial fibrillation).[21] In open clipping of unruptured aneurysms, increasing patient age is a predictor of poorer neurological outcomes, especially in patients over the age of 60 years.[22] Aneurysms that are large, complex, and/or in the posterior circulation are associated with an increased risk of perioperative stroke and worse neurological outcomes.[22] Clipping of ruptured aneurysms in the posterior circulation, particularly the basilar and posterior inferior cerebellar arteries, is also associated with poor outcomes.[23]

In SAH, the probability of cerebral vasospasm increases with the amount of subarachnoid blood observed on head computed tomography (CT), particularly with thick clot completely filling at least one cistern or fissure or with bilateral intraventricular hemorrhage. The combination of these two CT features on admission implies the highest risk of DCI, as codified in the modified Fisher Scale. Patients with poor neurological status (i.e., Hunt-Hess grade 3 or 4 indicating stupor or coma) on presentation also tend to have worse neurologic outcomes, with an increased risk of DCI with increasing grade.[24] Polymorphisms of the endothelial nitric oxide synthase (eNOS), plasminogen activator inhibitor-1 (PAI-1), apolipoprotein E (ApoE), ryanodine receptor 1 (RyR1), and cystathionine-β synthase (CBS) genes have also been implicated in vasospasm and/or DCI risk.[17]

Early seizures after SAH are associated with younger age, poor clinical grade, thick hemorrhage, acute hydrocephalus, and rebleeding.[20] Presence of intraventricular blood is a risk factor for acute hydrocephalus.[25] Delayed shunt-dependent hydrocephalus, which occurs in approximately 40% of patients, has been associated with increasing age, female sex, poor Hunt-Hess grade, thick SAH, intraventricular hemorrhage, hydrocephalus on admission, ruptured aneurysm within the distal posterior circulation, clinical vasospasm, and endovascular treatment.[19]

In the case of AVMs, the Spetzler-Martin grading system was created to risk-stratify patients undergoing open AVM resection.[9] Risk factors in AVM surgery include large size, critical functional areas within adjacent brain tissue, and presence of deep venous drainage. The Spetzler-Martin grading system assigns a score of I–V based on these factors, with more frequent peri- and postoperative complications in higher grade AVMs. The rates of major deficits for each of grades I–V are 0%, 0%, 4%, 7%, and 12%, respectively.[9]

## MONITORING FOR NEUROLOGICAL INJURY

It is critical to monitor for primary injuries during a neurovascular operation as well as for secondary injuries postoperatively. These include intracranial processes such as cerebral edema, hematoma, metabolic dysfunction, and elevated intracranial hypertension, as well as extracranial processes such as hypotension, hypercapnia, acid–base disorders, and hypothermia.[26] Important aspects of monitoring for secondary injury include recording hemodynamic and neurophysiologic parameters using both invasive and noninvasive means.

### Balloon Test Occlusion

Preoperatively, balloon test occlusion (BTO) can be performed via proximal inflation of a balloon in the territory of interest to determine the functional sufficiency of collateral flow and clinical tolerance of temporary and possible permanent occlusion. This is performed in awake patients, identifying neurological status following occlusion and a hypotensive challenge, with imaging adjuncts such as xenon-enhanced CT to assess blood flow or electroencephalography (EEG) to assess neural activity.[27-28] In cases of complex aneurysms requiring complete parent vessel sacrifice, BTO is a useful adjunct to confirm clinical tolerability.[27,29] The procedure itself is relatively safe. Mathis et al. reported a permanent neurological complication rate of 0.4% in a series of 500 patients undergoing BTO.[29] In general, postoperative stroke rates for clinically tolerated BTO studies range from about 5% to 20%.[30] For internal carotid artery (ICA) sacrifice, Linskey et al. found a lower infarct frequency using a preoperative BTO/xenon CT protocol (10%), compared to literature-derived controls (26%).[27] Similarly, a protocol combining BTO with hypotension showed a stroke rate of 5.2% with ICA sacrifice.[30] Vessel sacrifice may be performed endovascularly or via open trapping, and while the decision for the type of operation is dependent on patient clinical and anatomic considerations, BTO remains a key procedure in preoperative planning for both operative modalities.

## Microvascular Doppler Ultrasonography

Microvascular Doppler ultrasonography via direct probe recording can be used intraoperatively to measure the cerebral blood flow (CBF) of the microcirculation of the target vessel, both quantitatively and qualitatively. This allows for a relatively inexpensive, real-time assessment of regional CBF changes as the case progresses, and has been described in AVM resection as well as aneurysm clipping.[6,31] This can assist the anesthesiologist in understanding ongoing hemodynamic parameters in the brain and can direct the surgeon to intervene (e.g., in cases needing repositioning of an aneurysm clip). According to the literature, such a technique has been used to guide the successful repositioning of 18–31% of aneurysm clips.[6,32-33] Stendel et al. reported that the technique resulted in clip repositioning of middle cerebral artery (MCA) aneurysms more than twice as often as anterior cerebral artery (ACA) aneurysms.[33] Moreover, repositioning occurred more frequently in ruptured cases than in unruptured cases. Doppler may be a rapid intraoperative adjunct with desirable sensitivity and specificity. Bailes et al. compared ultrasound versus intraoperative angiography in 35 patients and found complete concordance in all cases.[32] While Doppler alone cannot demonstrate a residual aneurysm neck, it may be able to assess the degree of flow preservation within a visually confirmed neck. Other intraoperative adjuncts may be of assistance in this situation.

## Indocyanine Green Angiography

Intraoperative microscopic videoangiography with indocyanine green (ICG) dye is routinely used to visualize vascular flow during open neurovascular surgery. The dye is injected as an intravenous bolus and allows for assessment of blood flow in perforating arteries and distal segments following clip placement or AVM resection. Moreover, ICG can aid the surgeon in identifying any residual flow into a clipped aneurysm. Use of ICG therefore informs the need for clip repositioning to ensure perforator patency and maximal aneurysm occlusion. There is an imperfect correlation, however, between ICG videoangiography and intraoperative digital subtraction angiography. In a series reported by Washington et al., there was no agreement between the two methods in 24.5% of cases.[7] In 14.3% of cases, ICG videoangiography did not suggest need for clip repositioning, whereas digital subtraction angiography did. Other evaluations, however, have reported higher rates of agreement in 90% of aneurysm cases, with discrepancies being of little clinical or surgical consequence.[34]

Intraoperative angiography is time- and resource-intensive and not practical in all centers; therefore, some have advocated for multimodal monitoring. In a comparison of ICG with microvascular Doppler, Fischer et al. found that both techniques were similarly useful during surgery, although they noted several complementary advantages and disadvantages for each.[35] ICG better demonstrated perfusion in small perforators and visualization of the aneurysm neck remnant, but it was less reliable in deep surgical fields and in cases where visualization was limited by blood clots, intramural thrombi, or calcifications. With these combined modalities, branch occlusions occurred in 4% of cases, and neck remnants were observed in 6%.

## Intraoperative Neurophysiologic Monitoring

EEG is used to monitor for ischemia and is essential to confirm burst suppression during temporary clipping for aneurysm surgery. It may also identify injury from direct vessel compromise, vasospasm, retractor placement, or clip placement.

Somatosensory evoked potentials (SSEP) are used to monitor for injury to somatosensory cortex and sensory fibers along the dorsal column-medial lemniscus pathway. As such, SSEP monitoring for aneurysms of the MCA is very accurate and has been well described.[36] In a series of 131 operations, Penchet et al. noted significant monitoring changes in 26% of patients, most commonly occurring during temporary clipping and accounting for 74% of such monitoring changes.[37] In all cases with SSEP changes that could not be reversed, a postoperative stroke occurred. The false-negative rate was 4.6%, wherein patients without a monitoring change or a reversal of change still developed a stroke. In the resection of vascular malformations, Chang et al. found comparable test characteristics for SSEP monitoring.[38]

Motor evoked potentials (MEPs) allow monitoring of the pyramidal tracts because motor deficits may occur in absence of SSEP changes.[36] MEPs may be elicited via direct cortical stimulation with a strip electrode or placement of transcranial electrodes. Strip electrode placement has been associated with a 2% risk of clinically insignificant subdural bleeding.[39] Szelényi et al. demonstrated that MEPs are safe and effective at predicting postoperative outcome during aneurysm surgery.[40] In one nonrandomized prospective study of MEP monitoring versus controls, Yue et al. found a reduced incidence of new motor deficits in the monitored group (9% vs. 27%).[41] For AVMs in language or motor areas, awake craniotomy with electrocortical stimulation mapping has also been performed with success.[42]

Bispectral index (BIS) monitoring is becoming more commonly used in the OR to assess anesthesia awareness, although the reliability of this modality is not completely proved.[43] It is based on an empirically derived proprietary formula combining several weighted EEG parameters. BIS typically ranges from 0 (EEG silence) to 100 (fully awake). BIS during embolization of ruptured aneurysms in good-grade SAH patients has shown a very favorable correlation with the eyelash reflex (area under the curve = 0.932).[44] In craniotomy for supratentorial tumors, some BIS-guided protocols may result in lower maintenance anesthetic concentration and reduce anesthesia recovery time.[45]

## Continuous EEG

The Neurocritical Care Society currently recommends continuous EEG monitoring in poor-grade SAH patients who fail to improve or have unexplained neurological deterioration.[46] EEG monitoring is particularly useful for detecting subclinical seizures and characterizing seizures, especially in poor-grade SAH patients in whom clinical exam is challenging.[47]

EEG changes occur when CBF dips below approximately 30 mL/100 g/min, and therefore continuous EEG may also detect ischemia in patients at risk for DCI due to vasospasm.[48] One hypothesis is that perturbation of ion homeostasis in the cellular microenvironment of SAH generates a depolarization event that incites a self-propagating depolarization front.[49] Cortical spreading depolarization leads to excitotoxicity as well as a decrease in regional CBF, thereby initiating cerebral ischemia and resultant EEG changes.

Continuous EEG is accurate in predicting DCI/vasospasm after SAH, particularly in assessing the α-to-δ power ratio or the α-to-total power ratio.[48] The presence of periodic lateralized epileptiform discharges and absence of sleep architecture is prognostic for poor 3-month outcome in patients with poor-grade SAH.[50] Continuous EEG may identify the need for interventions, such as antiepileptic medication or further diagnostic imaging.[47] It is also important in diagnosing nonconvulsive status epilepticus, which occurs in approximately 3% of SAH patients and is difficult to treat.[51]

## Transcranial Doppler

Transcranial Doppler (TCD) ultrasonography is a noninvasive monitoring modality that is useful for detecting vasospasm after SAH and identifying patients who need targeted interventions.[52] The quality of TCD assessment, however, is dependent on the operator and the adequacy of acoustic windows. A mean flow velocity greater than 120 cm/sec has generally been used to define vasospasm. TCD flow studies accurately identify MCA vasospasm; however, prediction of vasospasm within the ACA, posterior circulation, and distal cerebral vasculature remains poor.[53] A meta-analysis of 26 studies comparing TCD to angiography found a positive predictive value of 97% and a negative predictive value of 78% for TCD assessment of the MCA territory.[54] Thus, a positive TCD can accurately predict angiographic MCA vasospasm, but a negative TCD does not rule it out. A separate meta-analysis of 17 studies comparing TCD to DCI (defined as clinical or angiographic vasospasm) found a positive predictive value of 57% and a negative predictive value of 92%.[55] Despite these findings, there is limited evidence that TCD monitoring improves clinically relevant outcomes, although its use is often encouraged.[56] TCD therefore remains an adjunct to other monitoring modalities in the assessment of neurological status and cannot be used in isolation.

## Postprocedure Magnetic Resonance Imaging

Magnetic resonance imaging (MRI) assessment of ischemic injury can be accomplished using diffusion weighted imaging (DWI) sequences after neurovascular surgery. Some centers have reported new ischemic lesions in up to 24% of unruptured aneurysms treated endovascularly; these lesions may not be clinically apparent and may reflect small emboli.[57] MRI after stroke is useful to assess the extent of infarction and to aid in prognostication and risk stratification for ICP management, including hyperosmolar therapy or decompressive hemicraniectomy.[58] In particular, an infarct larger than approximately 80 mL on DWI within 6 hours of onset is predictive of poor clinical outcomes.[59] MRI has not been found to predict subsequent swelling, brainstem shift, or secondary damage to other structures.[58] For AVMs with plans for radiosurgery, pre- or postembolization MRI with specific thin-cut sequences can be merged for radiation planning.[60]

In the event of large territory ischemic injury or large mass effect from hemorrhagic injury, ICP management is prudent. In SAH, the risk for high ICP (>20 mm Hg) peaks on day 3 and typically declines after day 7.[61] External ventricular drains (EVDs) and ICP probes are most commonly placed in patients with poorer neurological status. Placement of EVDs may be preferable to ICP monitors, given the potential for therapeutic CSF diversion. ICP monitoring allows for stratification for ICP-lowering interventions, such as sedation, cerebral perfusion pressure optimization, hyperosmolar therapy, hyperventilation, hypothermia, and hemicraniectomy. One randomized trial comparing two ICP goal-directed management strategies (i.e., mean ICP <20 mm Hg vs. mean ICP wave amplitude [MWA] <5 mm Hg) after SAH showed better overall outcomes at 1 year in the MWA group (31% vs. 10% favorable outcome).[62] The authors attributed this to a 50% increase in total CSF drainage during the first week with the MWA strategy. While ICP is commonly monitored, it is also important to consider the entire clinical situation of the individual patient.

## NEUROPROTECTION STRATEGIES
### Physiologic Interventions for Open Neurovascular Surgery

#### Aneurysms

Temporary occlusion of the parent artery is a common technique during aneurysm clipping as it provides proximal hemostatic control and can lower hemorrhage risk by softening the aneurysm during dissection. The primary limitation of this technique is stroke risk. Ogilvy et al. prospectively observed that temporary clipping longer than 20 minutes and intraoperative aneurysm rupture were significant predictors of subsequent infarct.[8]

Because of the risk of vasospasm during surgery, as well as the use of temporary clipping, normotension or mild hypertension is preferred.[63] In cases of aneurysmal SAH, it is useful to know the interval since rupture since this informs vasospasm risk, which is greatest at 7 days and tapers off over about 14 days post-bleed.[18] Patients may have exaggerated hemodynamic responses to inhalational anesthetics when on nimodipine or nicardipine. One study found that nicardipine-induced hypotension was more profound with sevoflurane, but more persistent with isoflurane.[64] Hypotension should be minimized intraoperatively. Doing so may enhance collateral flow during temporary clipping, but this must be balanced against the risk of causing rupture of an unsecured aneurysm at elevated pressures. Certainly, abrupt changes in mean arterial pressure (MAP) should be avoided.

Avoidance of intraoperative hyperglycemia may improve neurological outcomes in SAH patients. In the Intraoperative Hypothermia for Aneurysm Surgery Trial (IHAST), post hoc analyses revealed that patients with elevated intraoperative blood glucose concentration were more likely to have cognitive (at >129 mg/dL) and neurological (at >152 mg/dL) deficits 3 months postoperatively.[65] While there is no high-level evidence for glucose control during open aneurysm repair, hyperglycemia is associated with increased inflammation and poor outcomes in many disease states, and it may exacerbate the extent of any ischemic insult encountered during surgery.[66]

Other physiologic interventions include adjustment of ventilation to ensure normocarbia in order to avoid cerebrovascular vasoconstriction in areas at risk for vasospasm.[63] Brain relaxation, through the use of mannitol and propofol when tolerated, is recommended to increase brain compliance and possibly reduce the need for brain retraction and the risk of retraction-associated injury.[67] Some have successfully eliminated the need for static retraction in open vascular and skull base surgery by emphasizing gravity-based retraction and use of a dynamic handheld sucker retraction technique.[1] At the end of the case, extubation should be attempted early, once the patient is ready with regard to neurologic, temperature, and cardiopulmonary status.

Hypothermia has a long history of use in reducing metabolic rate to protect against ischemia in various organ systems. A Cochrane review of three randomized trials determined that there may be a neurological benefit for mild hypothermia (18% increase in likelihood of a good outcome) in good-grade SAH (i.e., Hunt-Hess I–III) patients undergoing ruptured aneurysm clipping.[68] This finding may be related to more severe metabolic deregulation in poor-grade patients. For all levels of hemorrhage severity, however, there was no evidence that intraoperative mild hypothermia was harmful. Despite these promising results, clinicians are cautioned that there is a hypothetical risk of coagulopathy and other potentially detrimental results with hypothermia.

Cardiac arrest by either hypothermia or chemical means has been employed in aneurysm surgery as early as the 1950s.[69] The current practice is that complete hypothermic cardiac arrest should be limited in its application to cases of giant or posterior circulation aneurysms that are not amenable to conventional techniques, including endovascular repair.[70] Four key predictors of success are the depth of hypothermia, duration of total circulatory arrest, barbiturate use, and hemostasis.[71] More recently, pharmacological arrest with adenosine alone has been tried successfully and may be particularly useful when operating in a narrow field with limited exposure and impeded clip placement.[72] This is rarely practiced, however, as many of these cases are now treated endovascularly using flow diversion.

## Arteriovenous Malformations

Management considerations for AVMs are similar to those for aneurysm surgery, including anesthetic agents that promote brain relaxation, facilitate blood pressure control, and expedite emergence.[4] Homeostasis during surgery is maintained with euvolemia, normotension, isotonicity, normoglycemia, and normocapnia.

With AVMs, it is important to be cognizant of the potential for abrupt, massive blood loss. Therefore, it is paramount to ensure that blood products are available and intravenous access for potentially rapid transfusion is adequate. Knowledge of the extent of any preoperative embolization and the size of the AVM can help anticipate the likelihood and severity of intraoperative blood loss.

We recommend use of hemodynamic monitoring for MAP. A reasonable hemodynamic goal is mild hypotension to normotension in the absence of other comorbidities. Induced hypotension, especially for large AVMs with deep arterial feeders, may improve surgical hemostasis by limiting brisk bleeding from small feeding vessels.[4] Preoperatively, it is also recommended to identify whether a coexisting intracranial aneurysm is present on a feeding artery because AVMs are frequently associated with aneurysms.[73] Cerebral vasodilating agents should be avoided when possible.

The most frequent contemporary indication for extracranial-intracranial (EC-IC) bypass is moyamoya disease. A less common indication is atherosclerotic large vessel occlusive disease. These operations include direct bypass by anastomosis of the superficial temporal artery (STA) to the MCA, or indirect bypass (encephalo-duro-arterio-synangiosis [EDAS]) wherein a scalp artery, such as the STA, is overlaid on the cortex to promote neovascularization.

The anesthetic goal during surgery is to maintain adequate cerebral perfusion and hemodynamic stability.[74] Normocarbia and normothermia should be maintained perioperatively. Hypocapnia may lead to cerebral ischemia in regions already affected by steno-occlusive disease, in part due to hypercarbia-induced vascular steal to unaffected territories.[75] Patients should be normotensive or slightly hypertensive during surgery, with increase in MAP during temporary arterial occlusion performed during direct bypass.[74] Hypertension, however, may increase the risk of bleeding at the site of anastomosis. Therefore, normotension or mild induced hypertension to a blood pressure 10% to 20% above the preoperative baseline is recommended.[74]

The greatest risk to the patient is cerebral ischemia, especially during induction and temporary arterial occlusion.[10] However, in standard direct bypass, the risk of intraoperative ischemia is low because the occlusion time is typically brief, and, in indirect bypass, there is no temporary occlusion. Hypotension may increase the risk of graft thrombosis and failure.[76] Any episodes of hypotension should be aggressively corrected with vasopressors. Consideration should be given for preoperative admission for IV fluid hydration overnight for volume regulation.[77] Prolonged fasting leading to dehydration, in combination with any episodes of hypotension, could lead to cardiovascular collapse.

## Pharmacologic Interventions for Open Neurovascular Surgery

In addition to maintaining adequate cerebral perfusion pressure during surgery, reduction of metabolic rate is an important strategy. There are limited clinical trial data for anesthetic-induced neuroprotection in vascular and endovascular neurosurgery, and often decisions are made based on the clinical scenario. There are no randomized trials for neuroprotective agents during temporary clipping for aneurysm surgery, but post hoc analysis of the IHAST data did not find that supplemental protective drugs (thiopental or etomidate) had any association with neurological outcome.[78]

There are, however, many supportive preclinical studies for neuroprotection in general. The pathophysiology of cerebral ischemia and reperfusion is mainly driven by excess adenosine triphosphate (ATP) consumption, glutamatergic excitotoxicity, ionic concentration imbalance, and free radical formation.[79] Laboratory investigations demonstrate that conventional anesthetics (both inhalational and intravenous) offer protection against ischemia.[79-81] Inhalational anesthetics can improve outcomes from both focal and global ischemia by many mechanisms, including suppression of energy requirements, inhibition of glutamatergic signaling, and reduction in inflammation/oxidation. Propofol has anti-inflammatory and antiapoptotic properties, but it also appears to greatly suppress the cerebral metabolic rate.[79,82] A summary of proposed mechanisms of neuroprotection for these agents is presented in Table 19.1.

**Table 19.1** Mechanisms of Neuroprotection for Inhalational and Propofol Anesthetics

| Mechanism of Neuroprotection | Inhalational | Propofol |
|---|---|---|
| Inhibition of glutamate release and signaling | Yes | Yes |
| Stimulation of GABA$_A$ receptors | Yes | Yes |
| Inhibition of the peripheral sympathetic response to ischemia | Yes | No |
| Prevention of apoptosis | Yes | Yes |
| Antioxidative effect | Yes | Yes |
| Direct scavenger of free radicals and decreasing lipid peroxidation | No | Yes |
| Preconditioning | Yes | No |
| Anti-inflammatory | Yes | Yes |

Adapted from Jovic M, Unic-Stojanovic D, Isenovic E, et al. Anesthetics and cerebral protection in patients undergoing carotid endarterectomy. *J Cardiothorac Vasc Anesth*. 2015;29(1):178–84 (Table 3).

## Barbiturates

Barbiturates such as thiopental have a well-established efficacy in establishing cerebral protection during experimental focal ischemia, likely reducing the metabolic rate to accommodate for planned reduction in blood flow. Very high doses of barbiturates are often required to achieve maximal burst suppression, but large doses may be associated with hemodynamic instability and will prevent early neurological examination postoperatively.[43] Thiopental is typically induced in relatively small doses immediately prior to temporary clipping. During temporary clipping, burst suppression is induced and confirmed via monitoring to help minimize the risk of ischemic injury. Thiopental has classically been well-tolerated during burst suppression for aneurysm clipping.[71]

## Propofol

Propofol increases γ-aminobutyric acid (GABA)-mediated inhibitory tone in the central nervous system.[83] Ravussin and de Tribolet described the use of propofol for induction and maintenance, and also for EEG burst suppression, during aneurysm clipping.[67] In a study of patients undergoing brain tumor resection, this group found similar decreases in ICP with propofol versus thiopental, but with more stable hemodynamic parameters and faster recovery in the propofol group.[84] In aneurysm surgery just before temporary clipping, burst suppression was achieved by increasing the propofol infusion rate to 500 µg/kg/min, while increasing MAP to 100 mm Hg with volume loading and dopamine to augment collateral flow. No deterioration in patients undergoing temporary clipping was observed with this protocol.

## Etomidate

Batjer et al. have had success with the use of etomidate for suppression during temporary clipping.[85] Etomidate suppresses electrical activity in a dose-dependent manner, progressing through burst suppression to complete electrical silence. In the OR, general anesthesia was induced via thiopental, sufentanil, and vecuronium bromide. Then, etomidate dosage was titrated to burst suppression prior to temporary clipping, requiring a dose of 0.4–0.5 mg/kg. The authors did not report any complications directly related to temporary clipping; a good neurological outcome occurred in 71% of patients.

## Inhalational Anesthetics

There is no clear benefit for inhaled versus intravenous anesthetic agents for vascular neurosurgery. One nonrandomized study in aneurysmal SAH reported reduced operative time and length of stay with intravenous compared to inhalational anesthesia, with no other effects on clinical outcomes.[86] The choice of anesthetic technique should be based on the clinical context. With elevated ICP, propofol-based techniques may be preferred over inhalational agents. In general, inhalational agents can increase CBF, cerebral blood volume (CBV), and ICP.[87] They can also uncouple CBF and metabolic demand ($CMRO_2$), and generate postanesthetic hyperemia.[87-88] Of the currently available inhalational anesthetics, sevoflurane has the lowest risk for increasing CBF and ICP, and is associated with a relatively quick recovery period.[87]

In steno-occlusive disease, such as moyamoya, there is no definitive evidence for superiority of one anesthetic agent over another. A study of 216 moyamoya patients who underwent surgery showed no difference in outcomes when comparing inhaled versus intravenous anesthetics; greater disease severity and choice of indirect bypass were the strongest predictors of worse neurological outcomes.[89] The principal hemodynamic goal in revascularization surgery for moyamoya is avoidance of hypoperfusion; therefore, use of inhaled agents is reasonable. Permissive hypertension during the procedure and close monitoring during induction is also key.[74] Neuromonitoring is a useful adjunct to augmenting hemodynamic status.

## Neuroprotection for Endovascular Neurosurgery

The primary anesthetic goal for endovascular cases is an immobile, hemodynamically stable patient. There is no clearly superior anesthetic agent or technique for neuroprotection in endovascular neurosurgery.[90] For embolizations, general anesthesia offers the advantage of ensuring complete patient immobility. This improves the quality of fluoroscopic imaging and may facilitate greater procedural safety. General anesthesia also offers patient comfort and easier control of respiratory and hemodynamic status. It does limit intraoperative neurological testing, but neuromonitoring adjuncts may reduce this concern.[91] Induction of anesthesia is typically rapid with the use of conventional agents (propofol, desflurane, and sevoflurane). General anesthesia also allows for more rapid management of complications.

In cases of acutely ruptured aneurysms, tight control of ICP and circulatory hemodynamics is important. As in aneurysm clipping, this may include the use of mannitol, mild hyperventilation, and head elevation to improve venous outflow.[56,63] Tight blood pressure control is critical. For patients undergoing embolization of high-flow lesions such as AVMs, avoiding abrupt changes in blood pressure can help minimize hemorrhage risk. This is especially critical during the act of embolization, which can cause sudden changes in vessel pressures.[12] In cases of SAH at risk for vasospasm, controlled hypertension may be useful.[63]

Electrophysiologic monitoring is not always indicated but can be useful in more complex cases, such as giant or wide-necked aneurysms, aneurysms with necks adjacent to critical vessels, high ICP, large SAH, or other medically complex scenarios.[92] In one series of aneurysm coiling procedures with concurrent neuromonitoring (EEG, SSEP, or brainstem auditory evoked potentials), monitoring changes were observed in 26% of cases, leading to alterations in management in 14% of cases.[91] Neuromonitoring is also useful in patients who are obtunded (e.g., due to SAH) or under general anesthesia.

Direct thromboembolic complications can occur during embolization procedures and can occur postoperatively in a delayed fashion. Dual antiplatelet therapy may reduce this risk.[93] Delayed hemorrhagic complications can occur, especially after the treatment of high-flow shunting states such as dural arteriovenous fistula or AVMs.[94] Therefore, close neurological monitoring and blood pressure control are critical during and immediately after the procedure.

## Aneurysmal Subarachnoid Hemorrhage

The drug with the best supporting evidence for effective neuroprotection against vasospasm and DCI after SAH is oral nimodipine, although the mechanism of action is not completely clear. An early randomized controlled trial of nimodipine demonstrated an absolute risk reduction of neurological decline by 11.5%. Nimodipine administration, however, is limited by systemic hypotension.[95] A randomized controlled trial titled Nimodipine Microparticles to Enhance Recovery While Reducing Toxicity After Subarachnoid Hemorrhage (NEWTON) is comparing an intrathecal slow-release formulation to standard enteral nimodipine in an effort to limit systemic hypotension.[96] Rescue therapies for symptomatic, angiographic vasospasm following aneurysmal SAH include local intra-arterial verapamil and angioplasty.[97]

Seizure prophylaxis with the antiepileptics levetiracetam or phenytoin should also be considered to prevent secondary ischemic injury and possibly to reduce the risk of aneurysmal rerupture.[98] While there is high-level evidence for seizure prophylaxis in traumatic brain injury, none exists for aneurysmal SAH. In contrast, there is some evidence that prophylactic antiepileptic drug use (particularly phenytoin) may be deleterious in this population.[99] The decision for seizure prophylaxis must be judicious and take into account the extent of cortical damage as well as known seizure risk factors, including age, poor clinical grade, thick hemorrhage, acute hydrocephalus, and rebleeding.[20] Most centers limit prophylactic use of antiepileptic drugs during the ICU phase of the illness to poor-grade patients, although the Neurocritical Care Society SAH guidelines recommend against prophylactic use of these agents altogether.[46]

## IMPLICATIONS FOR CLINICAL PRACTICE

As detailed earlier, high-level evidence does not exist for many of the neuroprotection practices routinely employed in vascular and endovascular neurosurgery. The guidelines we do have are often derived from expert consensus and review of observational, noncontrolled, and/or nonrandomized studies. Despite this, there are many safe techniques that are frequently used, as described here.

## Neuromonitoring

Intraoperative neuromonitoring is recommended during surgery for aneurysm, AVM, and steno-occlusive disease. EEG is important during temporary clipping and, along with SSEP/MEP, can reveal ischemia at a very early stage before it becomes irreversible.[40] Electrophysiologic monitoring can also be useful in endovascular procedures when general anesthesia is used in patients who are obtunded and in SAH.[91] For AVMs adjacent to eloquent cortex (i.e., areas where damage produces major focal neurological deficits affecting motor, sensory or language function), monitoring is imperative and may be combined with advanced modalities, such as preoperative functional MRI, Wada testing (intracarotid sodium amobarbital procedure), and cortical stimulation mapping to maximize safe resection.[42] ICG and microvascular Doppler ultrasonography are important complementary modalities for open vascular surgery to minimize iatrogenic injury.[32] In SAH, postoperative monitoring with continuous EEG, TCD, and ICP monitoring helps assess neurophysiologic status and the need for further interventions.

## Anesthesia

It is important to recognize procedures and situations where permissive hypertension is desirable to reduce the risk of perioperative stroke (i.e., steno-occlusive disease), as opposed to conditions in which hemorrhagic complications are more likely and relative mild intraoperative hypotension is desirable (i.e., AVM or aneurysm). Depending on the case, the anesthesiologist should tailor the choice of anesthetic and hemodynamic goals to the setting. Agents that increase CBF (i.e., inhalational agents) should be used with caution in the setting of increased ICP. Abrupt changes in hemodynamic and ICP status must be avoided to reduce risk of hemorrhagic and ischemic complications. In endovascular neurosurgery, there is no clearly superior anesthetic agent for neuroprotection. The primary goal for interventional cases is to select an agent that maximizes safety by reducing patient mobility and improving fluoroscopic imaging quality.

## Intracranial Pressure Management

Maintenance of an appropriate ICP is crucial to ensure adequate cerebral perfusion intra- and postprocedurally. Goal-directed ICP monitoring in the intensive care unit may inform the need for CSF drainage and improve long-term outcomes.[62] For open craniotomies, CSF diversion with an EVD is often helpful from the standpoint of brain relaxation. For endovascular procedures, ICP monitoring is useful for rapidly identifying hemorrhagic complications during embolization of ruptured AVM or aneurysm (i.e., between angiographic runs and before the complication would otherwise be visualized).[11] Most importantly, ICP monitoring is useful to identify patients at risk for secondary ischemic injury, and to guide medical management and direct potential surgical decompression in cases of refractory intracranial hypertension.[62]

# FUTURE DIRECTIONS

Perhaps the quickest growing segment of neurovascular intervention is the treatment of acute ischemic stroke. While acute ischemic stroke was not a focus of this chapter, as systems of care and endovascular options for acute ischemic stroke evolve, it will be important to identify the most appropriate neuroprotective anesthetic protocols for these patients. Currently, there is no high-level evidence for general anesthesia versus monitored anesthesia care (MAC) for intra-arterial therapy. General anesthesia with intubation prevents excessive patient motion and improves image quality; however, retrospective studies indicate worse outcomes with general anesthesia.[100] Until there is better evidence to guide decision-making, the choice of anesthesia type should be tailored to patient parameters: general anesthesia for patients with significant neurological or airway compromise; MAC for patients with less severe deficits and/or those who are less hemodynamically stable.

The complexity of neurovascular disease presents a challenge to the surgical and anesthesia teams managing such patients. Monitoring of neurological status, hemodynamic parameters, and ICP are important adjuncts. Targeted physiologic and pharmacological interventions hold the promise of preventing perioperative injury, but strong evidence that these strategies are effective is still lacking. Conventional anesthetic agents used in vascular and endovascular neurosurgery appear to provide some protection against ischemia by various mechanisms elucidated in the laboratory. Further translational work to develop and investigate neuroprotective agents is warranted.

# REFERENCES

1. Spetzler RF, Sanai N. The quiet revolution: retractorless surgery for complex vascular and skull base lesions. *J Neurosurg.* 2012;116(2):291–300.

2. Batjer H, Samson D. Intraoperative aneurysmal rupture: incidence, outcome, and suggestions for surgical management. *Neurosurgery.* 1986;18(6):701–7.

3. Ohkuma H, Tsurutani H, Suzuki S. Incidence and significance of early aneurysmal rebleeding before neurosurgical or neurological management. *Stroke.* 2001;32(5):1176–80.

4. Ogilvy CS, Stieg PE, Awad I, et al. Recommendations for the management of intracranial arteriovenous malformations: a statement for healthcare professionals from a special writing group of the Stroke Council, American Stroke Association. *Circulation.* 2001;103(21):2644–57.

5. Zygourakis CC, Vasudeva V, Lai PMR, Kim AH, Wang H, Du R. Transient pupillary dilation following local papaverine application in intracranial aneurysm surgery. *J Clin Neurosci.* 2015;22(4):676–9.

6. Marchese E, Albanese A, Denaro L, Vignati A, Fernandez E, Maira G. Intraoperative microvascular Doppler in intracranial aneurysm surgery. *Surg Neurol.* 2005;63(4): 336–42; discussion 342.

7. Washington CW, Zipfel GJ, Chicoine MR, et al. Comparing indocyanine green videoangiography to the gold standard of intraoperative digital subtraction angiography used in aneurysm surgery. *J Neurosurg.* 2013;118(2):420–7.

8. Ogilvy CS, Carter BS, Kaplan S, Rich C, Crowell RM. Temporary vessel occlusion for aneurysm surgery: risk factors for stroke in patients protected by induced hypothermia and hypertension and intravenous mannitol administration. *J Neurosurg.* 1996;84(5):785–91.

9. Spetzler RF, Martin NA. A proposed grading system for arteriovenous malformations. *J Neurosurg.* 1986;65(4):476–83.

10. Sato K, Shirane R, Yoshimoto T. Perioperative factors related to the development of ischemic complications in patients with moyamoya disease. *Childs Nerv Syst.* 1997;13(2):68–72.

11. Cronqvist M, Wirestam R, Ramgren B, et al. Endovascular treatment of intracerebral arteriovenous malformations: procedural safety, complications, and results evaluated by MR imaging, including diffusion and perfusion imaging. *AJNR Am J Neuroradiol.* 2006;27(1):162–76.

12. Jayaraman MV, Marcellus ML, Hamilton S, et al. Neurologic complications of arteriovenous malformation embolization using liquid embolic agents. *AJNR Am J Neuroradiol.* 2008;29(2):242–6.

13. Brinjikji W, Lanzino G, Cloft HJ, Siddiqui AH, Kallmes DF. Risk factors for hemorrhagic complications following pipeline embolization device treatment of intracranial aneurysms: results from the International Retrospective Study of the Pipeline Embolization Device. *AJNR Am J Neuroradiol.* 2015;36(12):2308–13.

14. Henkes H, Fischer S, Weber W, et al. Endovascular coil occlusion of 1811 intracranial aneurysms: early angiographic and clinical results. *Neurosurgery.* 2004;54(2):268–80; discussion 280–5.

15. Thiex R, Williams A, Smith E, Scott RM, Orbach DB. The use of Onyx for embolization of central nervous system arteriovenous lesions in pediatric patients. *AJNR Am J Neuroradiol.* 2010;31(1):112–20.

16. Levy EI, Turk AS, Albuquerque FC, et al. Wingspan in-stent restenosis and thrombosis: incidence, clinical presentation, and management. *Neurosurgery.* 2007;61(3): 644–50; discussion 650–1.

17. Ladner TR, Zuckerman SL, Mocco J. Genetics of cerebral vasospasm. *Neurol Res Int.* 2013;2013:291895.

18. Dorsch N. A clinical review of cerebral vasospasm and delayed ischaemia following aneurysm rupture. *Acta Neurochir Suppl.* 2011;110(Pt 1):5–6.

19. Dorai Z, Hynan LS, Kopitnik TA, Samson D. Factors related to hydrocephalus after aneurysmal subarachnoid hemorrhage. *Neurosurgery.* 2003;52(4):763–9; discussion 769–71.

20. Choi KS, Chun HJ, Yi HJ, Ko Y, Kim YS, Kim JM. Seizures and epilepsy following aneurysmal subarachnoid hemorrhage: incidence and risk factors. *J Korean Neurosurg Soc.* 2009;46(2):93–8.

21. Kam PC, Calcroft RM. Peri-operative stroke in general surgical patients. *Anaesthesia.* 1997;52(9):879–83.

22. Khanna RK, Malik GM, Qureshi N. Predicting outcome following surgical treatment of unruptured intracranial aneurysms: a proposed grading system. *J Neurosurg.* 1996;84(1):49–54.

23. Spetzler RF, McDougall CG, Zabramski JM, et al. The Barrow Ruptured Aneurysm Trial: 6-year results. *J Neurosurg.* 2015; 123(3):609–17.

24. Hunt WE, Hess RM. Surgical risk as related to time of intervention in the repair of intracranial aneurysms. *J Neurosurg.* 1968;28(1):14–20.

25. Van Gijn J, Hijdra A, Wijdicks EF, Vermeulen M, van Crevel H. Acute hydrocephalus after aneurysmal subarachnoid hemorrhage. *J Neurosurg.* 1985;63(3):355–62.

26. Haddad SH, Arabi YM. Critical care management of severe traumatic brain injury in adults. *Scand J Trauma Resusc Emerg Med.* 2012;20:12.

27. Linskey ME, Jungreis CA, Yonas H, et al. Stroke risk after abrupt internal carotid artery sacrifice: accuracy of preoperative assessment with balloon test occlusion and stable xenon-enhanced CT. *AJNR Am J Neuroradiol.* 1994;15(5):829–43.

28. Morioka T, Matsushima T, Fujii K, Fukui M, Hasuo K, Hisashi K. Balloon test occlusion of the internal carotid artery with monitoring of compressed spectral arrays (CSAs) of electroencephalogram. *Acta Neurochir (Wien).* 1989;101(1-2):29–34.

29. Mathis JM, Barr JD, Jungreis CA, et al. Temporary balloon test occlusion of the internal carotid artery: experience in 500 cases. *AJNR Am J Neuroradiol.* 1995;16(4):749–54.

30. Standard SC, Ahuja A, Guterman LR, et al. Balloon test occlusion of the internal carotid artery with hypotensive challenge. *AJNR Am J Neuroradiol.* 1995;16(7):1453–8.

31. Rosenblum BR, Bonner RF, Oldfield EH. Intraoperative measurement of cortical blood flow adjacent to cerebral AVM using laser Doppler velocimetry. *J Neurosurg.* 1987;66(3):396–9.

32. Bailes JE, Tantuwaya LS, Fukushima T, Schurman GW, Davis D. Intraoperative microvascular Doppler sonography in aneurysm surgery. *Neurosurgery.* 1997;40(5):965–70; discussion 970–2.

33. Stendel R, Pietila T, Al Hassan AA, Schilling A, Brock M. Intraoperative microvascular Doppler ultrasonography in cerebral aneurysm surgery. *J Neurol Neurosurg Psychiatry.* 2000;68(1):29–35.

34. Raabe A, Nakaji P, Beck J, et al. Prospective evaluation of surgical microscope—integrated intraoperative near-infrared indocyanine green videoangiography during aneurysm surgery. *J Neurosurg.* 2005;103(6):982–9.

35. Fischer G, Stadie A, Oertel JMK. Near-infrared indocyanine green videoangiography versus microvascular Doppler sonography in aneurysm surgery. *Acta Neurochir (Wien).* 2010;152(9):1519–25.

36. Friedman WA, Chadwick GM, Verhoeven FJ, Mahla M, Day AL. Monitoring of somatosensory evoked potentials during surgery for middle cerebral artery aneurysms. *Neurosurgery.* 1991;29(1):83–8.

37. Penchet G, Arné P, Cuny E, Monteil P, Loiseau H, Castel JP. Use of intraoperative monitoring of somatosensory evoked potentials to prevent ischaemic stroke after surgical exclusion of middle cerebral artery aneurysms. *Acta Neurochir (Wien).* 2007;149(4):357–64.

38. Chang SD, Lopez JR, Steinberg GK. The usefulness of electrophysiological monitoring during resection of central nervous system vascular malformations. *J Stroke Cerebrovasc Dis.* 1999;8(6):412–22.

39. Szelényi A, Kothbauer K, de Camargo AB, Langer D, Flamm ES, Deletis V. Motor evoked potential monitoring during cerebral aneurysm surgery: technical aspects and comparison of transcranial and direct cortical stimulation. *Neurosurg.* 2005;57(4 Suppl):331–8.

40. Szelényi A, Langer D, Kothbauer K, de Camargo AB, Flamm ES, Deletis V. Monitoring of muscle motor evoked potentials during cerebral aneurysm surgery: intraoperative changes and postoperative outcome. *J Neurosurg.* 2006;105(5):675–81.

41. Yue Q, Zhu W, Gu Y, et al. Motor evoked potential monitoring during surgery of middle cerebral artery aneurysms: a cohort study. *World Neurosurg.* 2014;82(6):1091–9.

42. Gabarrós A, Young WL, McDermott MW, Lawton MT. Language and motor mapping during resection of brain arteriovenous malformations: indications, feasibility, and utility. *Neurosurgery.* 2011;68(3):744–52.

43. Yoon JR, Kim YS, Kim TK. Thiopental-induced burst suppression measured by the bispectral index is extended during propofol administration compared with sevoflurane. *J Neurosurg Anesthesiol.* 2012;24(2):146–51.

44. Duncan D, Kelly KP, Andrews PJD. A comparison of bispectral index and entropy monitoring, in patients undergoing embolization of cerebral artery aneurysms after subarachnoid haemorrhage. *Br J Anaesth.* 2006;96(5):590–6.

45. Boztuğ N, Bigat Z, Akyuz M, Demir S, Ertok E. Does using the bispectral index (BIS) during craniotomy affect the quality of recovery? *J Neurosurg Anesthesiol.* 2006 Jan;18(1):1–4.

46. Diringer MN, Bleck TP, Claude Hemphill J 3rd, et al.; Neurocritical Care Society. Critical care management of patients following aneurysmal subarachnoid hemorrhage: recommendations from the Neurocritical Care Society's Multidisciplinary Consensus Conference. *Neurocrit Care.* 2011;15(2):211–40.

47. Claassen J, Mayer SA, Hirsch LJ. Continuous EEG monitoring in patients with subarachnoid hemorrhage. *J Clin Neurophysiol.* 2005;22(2):92–8.

48. Claassen J, Hirsch LJ, Kreiter KT, et al. Quantitative continuous EEG for detecting delayed cerebral ischemia in patients with poor-grade subarachnoid hemorrhage. *Clin Neurophysiol.* 2004;115(12):2699–710.

49. Sánchez-Porras R, Zheng Z, Santos E, Schöll M, Unterberg AW, Sakowitz OW. The role of spreading depolarization in subarachnoid hemorrhage. *Eur J Neurol.* 2013;20(8):1121–7.

50. Claassen J, Hirsch LJ, Frontera JA, et al. Prognostic significance of continuous EEG monitoring in patients with poor-grade subarachnoid hemorrhage. *Neurocrit Care.* 2006;4(2):103–12.

51. Little AS, Kerrigan JF, McDougall CG, et al. Nonconvulsive status epilepticus in patients suffering spontaneous subarachnoid hemorrhage. *J Neurosurg.* 2007;106(5):805–11.

52. Kenney K, Amyot F, Haber M, et al. Cerebral vascular injury in traumatic brain injury. *Exp Neurol.* 2016;275 Pt 3:353–66.

53. Frontera JA, Fernandez A, Schmidt JM, et al. Defining vasospasm after subarachnoid hemorrhage: what is the most clinically relevant definition? *Stroke.* 2009;40(6):1963–8.

54. Lysakowski C, Walder B, Costanza MC, Tramèr MR. Transcranial Doppler versus angiography in patients with vasospasm due to a ruptured cerebral aneurysm: a systematic review. *Stroke.* 2001;32(10):2292–8.

55. Kumar G, Shahripour RB, Harrigan MR. Vasospasm on transcranial Doppler is predictive of delayed cerebral ischemia in aneurysmal subarachnoid hemorrhage: a systematic review and meta-analysis. *J Neurosurg.* 2015;124(5):1257–64.

56. Bederson JB, Connolly ES, Batjer HH, et al.; American Heart Association. Guidelines for the management of aneurysmal subarachnoid hemorrhage. A statement for healthcare professionals from a special writing group of the Stroke Council, American Heart Association. *Stroke.* 2009;40(3):994–1025.

57. Cronqvist M, Wirestam R, Ramgren B, et al. Diffusion and perfusion MRI in patients with ruptured and unruptured intracranial aneurysms treated by endovascular coiling: complications, procedural results, MR findings and clinical outcome. *Neuroradiology.* 2005;47(11):855–73.

58. Wijdicks EFM, Sheth KN, Carter BS, et al.; American Heart Association Stroke Council. Recommendations for the management of cerebral and cerebellar infarction with swelling: a statement for healthcare professionals from the American Heart Association/American Stroke Association. *Stroke J Cereb Circ.* 2014;45(4):1222–38.

59. Thomalla G, Hartmann F, Juettler E, et al. Prediction of malignant middle cerebral artery infarction by magnetic resonance imaging within 6 hours of symptom onset: a prospective multicenter observational study. *Ann Neurol.* 2010;68(4):435–45.

60. Bednarz G, Downes M, Werner-Wasik M, Rosenwasser RH. Combining stereotactic angiography and 3D time-of-flight magnetic resonance angiography in treatment planning for arteriovenous malformation radiosurgery. *Int J Radiat Oncol.* 2000;46(5):1149–54.

61. Zoerle T, Lombardo A, Colombo A, et al. Intracranial pressure after subarachnoid hemorrhage. *Crit Care Med.* 2015;43(1):168–76.

62. Eide PK, Bentsen G, Sorteberg AG, Marthinsen PB, Stubhaug A, Sorteberg W. A randomized and blinded single-center trial comparing the effect of intracranial pressure and intracranial pressure wave amplitude-guided intensive care management on early clinical state and 12-month outcome in patients with aneurysmal subarachnoid hemorrhage. *Neurosurgery.* 2011;69(5):1105–15.

63. Connolly ES, Rabinstein AA, Carhuapoma JR, et al.; American Heart Association Stroke Council; Council on Cardiovascular Radiology and Intervention; Council on Cardiovascular Nursing; Council on Cardiovascular Surgery and Anesthesia; Council on Clinical Cardiology. Guidelines for the management of aneurysmal subarachnoid hemorrhage: a guideline for healthcare professionals from the American Heart Association/American Stroke Association. *Stroke J Cereb Circ.* 2012;43(6):1711–37.

64. Nishiyama T, Matsukawa T, Hanaoka K, Conway CM. Interactions between nicardipine and enflurane, isoflurane, and sevoflurane. *Can J Anaesth.* 1997;44(10):1071–6.

65. Pasternak JJ, McGregor DG, Schroeder DR, et al. Hyperglycemia in patients undergoing cerebral aneurysm surgery: its association with long-term gross neurologic and neuropsychological function. *Mayo Clin Proc.* 2008;83(4):406–17.

66. Kruyt ND, Biessels GJ, de Haan RJ, et al. Hyperglycemia and clinical outcome in aneurysmal subarachnoid hemorrhage: a meta-analysis. *Stroke J Cereb Circ.* 2009;40(6):e424–30.

67. Ravussin P, de Tribolet N. Total intravenous anesthesia with propofol for burst suppression in cerebral aneurysm surgery: preliminary report of 42 patients. *Neurosurgery.* 1993;32(2):236–40; discussion 240.

68. Li LR, You C, Chaudhary B. Intraoperative mild hypothermia for postoperative neurological deficits in intracranial aneurysm patients. *Cochrane Database Syst Rev.* 2012;2:CD008445.

69. Wright JM, Huang CL, Sharma R, et al. Cardiac standstill and circulatory flow arrest in surgical treatment of intracranial aneurysms: a historical review. *Neurosurg Focus.* 2014;36(4):E10.

70. Lawton MT, Raudzens PA, Zabramski JM, Spetzler RF. Hypothermic circulatory arrest in neurovascular surgery: evolving indications and predictors of patient outcome. *Neurosurgery.* 1998;43(1):10–20; discussion 20–1.

71. Spetzler RF, Hadley MN, Rigamonti D, et al. Aneurysms of the basilar artery treated with circulatory arrest, hypothermia, and barbiturate cerebral protection. *J Neurosurg.* 1988;68(6):868–79.

72. Bendok BR, Gupta DK, Rahme RJ, et al. Adenosine for temporary flow arrest during intracranial aneurysm surgery: a single-center retrospective review. *Neurosurgery.* 2011;69(4):815–20; discussion 820–1.

73. Batjer H, Suss RA, Samson D. Intracranial arteriovenous malformations associated with aneurysms. *Neurosurgery.* 1986;18(1):29–35.

74. Chui J, Manninen P, Sacho RH, Venkatraghavan L. Anesthetic management of patients undergoing intracranial bypass procedures. *Anesth Analg.* 2015;120(1):193–203.

75. Arteaga DF, Strother MK, Faraco CC, et al. The vascular steal phenomenon is an incomplete contributor to negative cerebrovascular reactivity in patients with symptomatic intracranial stenosis. *J Cereb Blood Flow Metab.* 2014;34(9):1453–62.

76. Jafar JJ, Russell SM, Woo HH. Treatment of giant intracranial aneurysms with saphenous vein extracranial-to-intracranial bypass grafting: indications, operative technique, and results in 29 patients. *Neurosurgery.* 2002;51(1):138–44; discussion 144–6.

77. Ladner TR, Mahdi J, Attia A, et al. A multispecialty pediatric neurovascular conference: a model for interdisciplinary management of complex disease. *Pediatr Neurol.* 2015;52(2):165–73.

78. Hindman BJ, Bayman EO, Pfisterer WK, Torner JC, Todd MM; IHAST Investigators. No association between intraoperative hypothermia or supplemental protective drug and neurologic outcomes in patients undergoing temporary clipping during cerebral aneurysm surgery: findings from the Intraoperative Hypothermia for Aneurysm Surgery Trial. *Anesthesiology.* 2010;112(1):86–101.

79. Jovic M, Unic-Stojanovic D, Isenovic E, et al. Anesthetics and cerebral protection in patients undergoing carotid endarterectomy. *J Cardiothorac Vasc Anesth.* 2015;29(1):178–84.

80. Nunes RR, Duval Neto GF, Garcia de Alencar JC, et al. Anesthetics, cerebral protection and preconditioning. *Braz J Anesthesiol Elsevier.* 2013;63(1):119–28.

81. Wei H, Inan S. Dual effects of neuroprotection and neurotoxicity by general anesthetics: role of intracellular calcium homeostasis. *Prog Neuropsychopharmacol Biol Psychiatry.* 2013;47:156–61.

82. Unic-Stojanovic D, Babic S, Neskovic V. General versus regional anesthesia for carotid endarterectomy. *J Cardiothorac Vasc Anesth.* 2013;27(6):1379–83.

83. Peduto VA, Concas A, Santoro G, Biggio G, Gessa GL. Biochemical and electrophysiologic evidence that propofol enhances GABAergic transmission in the rat brain. *Anesthesiology.* 1991;75(6):1000–9.

84. Ravussin P, Tempelhoff R, Modica PA, Bayer-Berger MM. Propofol vs. thiopental-isoflurane for neurosurgical anesthesia: comparison of hemodynamics, CSF pressure, and recovery. *J Neurosurg Anesthesiol.* 1991;3(2):85–95.

85. Batjer HH, Frankfurt AI, Purdy PD, Smith SS, Samson DS. Use of etomidate, temporary arterial occlusion, and intraoperative angiography in surgical treatment of large and giant cerebral aneurysms. *J Neurosurg.* 1988;68(2):234–40.

86. Sato K, Karibe H, Yoshimoto T. Advantage of intravenous anaesthesia for acute stage surgery of aneurysmal subarachnoid haemorrhage. *Acta Neurochir (Wien).* 1999;141(2):161–3; discussion 163–4.

87. Goren S, Kahveci N, Alkan T, Goren B, Korfali E. The effects of sevoflurane and isoflurane on intracranial pressure and cerebral perfusion pressure after diffuse brain injury in rats. *J Neurosurg Anesth.* 2001;13(2):113–9.

88. Holmstrom A, Akeson J. Desflurane increases intracranial pressure more and sevoflurane less than isoflurane in pigs subjected to intracranial hypertension. *J Neurosurg Anesth.* 2004;16(2):136–43.

89. Sakamoto T, Kawaguchi M, Kurehara K, Kitaguchi K, Furuya H, Karasawa J. Risk factors for neurologic deterioration after revascularization surgery in patients with moyamoya disease. *Anesth Analg.* 1997;85(5):1060–5.

90. De Sloovere VT. Anesthesia for embolization of cerebral aneurysms. *Curr Opin Anaesthesiol.* 2014;27(4):431–6.

91. Liu AY, Lopez JR, Do HM, Steinberg GK, Cockroft K, Marks MP. Neurophysiological monitoring in the endovascular therapy of aneurysms. *AJNR Am J Neuroradiol.* 2003;24(8):1520–7.

92. Nadjat-Haiem C, Ziv K, Osborn I. Anesthesia for carotid and cerebrovascular procedures in interventional neuroradiology. *Int Anesthesiol Clin.* 2009;47(2):29–43.

93. McKevitt FM, Randall MS, Cleveland TJ, Gaines PA, Tan KT, Venables GS. The benefits of combined anti-platelet treatment in carotid artery stenting. *Eur J Vasc Endovasc Surg.* 2005;29(5):522–7.

94. Ledezma CJ, Hoh BL, Carter BS, Pryor JC, Putman CM, Ogilvy CS. Complications of cerebral arteriovenous malformation embolization: multivariate analysis of predictive factors. *Neurosurgery.* 2006;58(4):602–11.

95. Allen GS, Ahn HS, Preziosi TJ, et al. Cerebral arterial spasm--a controlled trial of nimodipine in patients with subarachnoid hemorrhage. *N Engl J Med.* 1983;308(11):619–24.

96. Hänggi D, Etminan N, Macdonald RL, et al. NEWTON: nimodipine microparticles to enhance recovery while reducing toxicity after subarachnoid hemorrhage. *Neurocrit Care.* 2015;23(2):274–84.

97. Lehmann E, Sagher O. Novel treatments for cerebral vasospasm following aneurysmal subarachnoid hemorrhage. *Acta Neurochir Suppl.* 2008;105:225–8.

98. Szaflarski JP, Sangha KS, Lindsell CJ, Shutter LA. Prospective, randomized, single-blinded comparative trial of intravenous levetiracetam versus phenytoin for seizure prophylaxis. *Neurocrit Care.* 2010;12(2):165–72.

99. Naidech AM, Kreiter KT, Janjua N, et al. Phenytoin exposure is associated with functional and cognitive disability after subarachnoid hemorrhage. *Stroke.* 2005;36(3):583–7.

100. John S, Thebo U, Gomes J, et al. Intra-arterial therapy for acute ischemic stroke under general anesthesia versus monitored anesthesia care. *Cerebrovasc Dis Basel Switz.* 2014;38(4):262–7.

# 20 Neuroprotection for Spine Surgery

Jess W. Brallier and Jonathan S. Gal

## INTRODUCTION

The 2012 Global Burden of Disease Study estimated that musculoskeletal conditions, such as arthritis and back pain, affect more than 1.7 billion people worldwide and are the second greatest cause of disability.[1] As the prevalence of spine pathology has increased, so has the frequency of surgery. The number of spinal fusion procedures has more than doubled between 1998 and 2011.[2]

In most instances, spine surgery is only considered after more conservative treatment options have failed. Primary conditions that often require surgical intervention include degenerative disk disease, spinal stenosis, isthmic spondylolisthesis, kyphosis, fractures, deformities, and tumors. Some procedures, such as laminectomy, foraminotomy, and discectomy, are relatively minor, while others, such as intervertebral fusions, disk replacements, deformity corrections, and spinal cord detetherings, are more complex.

Perioperative neurologic injury related to spine surgery may result in pain, weakness, paralysis, sexual dysfunction, or loss of bowel or bladder continence. Fortunately, these are infrequent complications. A 2009 retrospective study of 11,817 adult spine surgery patients found an overall incidence of major neurologic deficit presenting in the immediate postoperative period to be 0.178%. The incidence was 0.293% after cervical spine surgery, 0.488% after thoracic spine surgery, and 0.074% after lumbar/sacral spine surgery.[3] Although the overall incidence of such complications is relatively low, such injury can lead to substantial physical, emotional, and economic burden.

In addition to the standard precautions and monitoring modalities applied to every type of operation, the use of neuroprotective strategies during spine surgery is critical to minimizing the incidence of potentially life-altering complications. Multimodal intraoperative monitoring of neuronal elements (i.e., spinal cord and nerve roots) combined with physiologic optimization form the basis of these strategies.

## MECHANISMS OF NEUROLOGIC INJURY

An understanding of the causes and mechanisms of perioperative neurologic injury is an important cornerstone to its prevention. Intraoperatively, neurologic injury can result from direct surgical trauma to neuronal elements (i.e., the spinal cord and nerve roots) or hypoperfusion secondary to either compression of vascular structures or inadequate blood pressure. Postoperatively, injury may result from sustained hypotension, dislodgement of surgical instrumentation, or compression secondary to a hematoma. Physiologic abnormalities, such as hypotension, anemia, hypothermia, hypocapnia, and electrolyte imbalance, can induce injury or exacerbate a pre-existing insult. The 2009 retrospective study of 11,817 adult spine surgery patients found that of the 21 patients who suffered an immediate postoperative paraplegic or quadriplegic neurologic deficit, the etiology of injury, determined by either reoperation and/or imaging study, was epidural hematoma in 8 patients, inadequate decompression in 5 patients, presumed vascular compromise in 4 patients, graft/cage dislodgement in 2 patients, and presumed surgical trauma in 2 patients.[3] Of note, more than half of the deficits occurred when instrumentation was used.

The potential for neurologic injury is greatest in individuals with a spinal deformity, such as scoliosis. Not only are such operations more complex, they invariably involve instrumentation. A retrospective study of pediatric and adult patients with spinal deformity and fusion procedures found an overall incidence of intraoperative neurologic deficit to be 1.1%.[4] Surgical maneuvers associated with intraoperative neurologic deficit included curve overcorrection, spinal cord and/or cauda equina stretching, and pedicle screw impingement or breach. Physiologic factors associated with intraoperative neurologic deficit included hypotension, excessive bleeding, and choice of anesthetic agents.

Regardless of the etiology, clinical prognosis tends to depend on whether complete or incomplete injury has occurred. Incomplete spinal cord injury (SCI; e.g., spinal cord torsion due to temporary curve overcorrection) has a better prognosis than complete injury (e.g., spinal cord transection due to pedicle screw breach), with recovery from a complete injury being nearly full in one-third of patients, partial in another third, and absent in the remaining third.[5]

## RISK FACTORS FOR NEUROLOGIC INJURY
### Intraoperative Factors

The risk of perioperative neurologic injury varies directly with both the complexity of the spine pathology and the operation. Patients presenting with severe kyphosis, congenital scoliosis, and high-magnitude curves, as well as patients with pre-existing neurologic deficits, are at increased risk for neurologic injury. The surgical procedures used to treat such conditions are technically more complex, often involving significant spinal osteotomy and instrumentation (e.g., skeletal traction and insertion of Harrington rods, sublaminar wires, and pedicle screws), which increases the risk of neurologic injury.[6-9] In addition to increasing the technical complexity of the operation, spinal instrumentation increases surgical times and bleeding, thereby increasing the risk of hypoperfusion and ischemia. The risk of neurologic injury is further increased when a combined anterior/posterior technique is used than with either approach alone.[6]

Operative location also factors into neurologic risk stratification. The thoracic spine is particularly vulnerable to ischemia due to its poor collateralization and resultant arterial watershed areas, making it potentially vulnerable to intraoperative mechanical trauma.[3,10] As noted earlier, a retrospective study demonstrated that new-onset major neurologic deficit was highest in patients undergoing thoracic spine surgery.[3]

## Preoperative Factors

Neurologic risk is also increased in the setting of perioperative anticoagulation. Many patients presenting for spine operations have chronic medical problems managed with one or more drugs known to contribute to intraoperative bleeding, and these patients are at increased risk of spinal or epidural hematoma. While much controversy exists about the ideal time for preoperative cessation of these medications, most practitioners agree that anticoagulation should be interrupted for all but the most minor of spine operations.[11-12]

For patients taking nonsteroidal anti-inflammatory drugs (NSAIDs) as part of a pain management strategy, these medications should be temporarily discontinued or substituted with an analgesic that is not associated with bleeding (i.e., acetaminophen). For patients taking aspirin and/or clopidogrel for primary or secondary prevention of stroke or myocardial infarction, the guidelines for discontinuation are more complicated. In all but the most straightforward of clinical scenarios, the risks of continuing such medications perioperatively (i.e., intraoperative bleeding and postoperative hematoma) must be carefully weighed against the risks of their discontinuation (e.g., myocardial infarction due to coronary stent stenosis or perioperative stroke).[13-15] A multidisciplinary discussion regarding the associated risks and benefits of interrupting such therapy should occur with the patient and involve input from the primary care physician, cardiologist, surgeon, and anesthesiologist.

## MONITORING FOR NEUROLOGIC INJURY

Optimal management for prevention of perioperative neurologic injury begins with early detection. Intraoperative neuromonitoring of the spinal cord pathways and nerve roots has gained considerable momentum in the past three decades and is now used routinely to monitor for surgical trespass and hypoperfusion during spine surgery. Such monitoring allows for early detection of neural compromise and subsequent correction prior to the onset of irreversible injury.

### The Stagnara Wake-Up Test

In 1973, Stagnara and Vauzelle became pioneers in the field of intraoperative neuromonitoring with the publication of *Functional Monitoring of Spinal Cord Activity During Spinal Surgery*.[16] They described a method for monitoring the integrity of the motor tracts of the spinal cord during open operation by lightening the plane of anesthesia in order to permit spontaneous movement of the extremities. Theoretically, the Stagnara "wake-up test" (as the maneuver has come to be known) allows for prompt recognition of malpositioned hardware and its immediate removal in order to reverse or limit the degree of neurological injury. The wake-up test provides a fairly accurate assessment of gross motor changes resulting from surgical injury, however, it does very little to directly assess sensory or fine motor function.[16] Furthermore, this method of monitoring is not continuous and is inefficient. Other disadvantages include potential awareness under anesthesia and associated adverse events, such as self-extubation and self-removal of intravenous lines. The wake-up test has therefore become an adjunct to more progressive forms of spinal cord and nerve root monitoring, rather than a primary modality.

## Intraoperative Neurophysiological Monitoring

The disadvantages of the Stagnara wake-up test encouraged the development of safer and more continuous intraoperative neuromonitoring modalities. Somatosensory-evoked potential (SSEP) monitoring was the first neurophysiological modality to be developed, and it has been in clinical use since the 1980s.[17-18] SSEPs assess the functional integrity of the sensory pathways by following a response from a preselected peripheral nerve, through the dorsal column pathways, up to the sensory cortex. Stimulating electrodes are placed on the distal limbs (often over the posterior tibial or peroneal nerve), and receiving electrodes are inserted into the scalp over the sensory cortex. A small electric current is repeatedly applied to the distal peripheral nerve, and subsequent evoked potentials are then recorded over the sensory cortex to assess the response of the pathway to the sensory stimulus.[17,19] The amplitude and latency of each potential are analyzed and interpreted by a neurophysiologist, who compares the signals with baseline recordings obtained prior to surgical incision. An increase in SSEP latency equal to or greater than 10%, or a decrease in SSEP amplitude equal to or greater than 50%, serve as the generally accepted warning criteria for alerting the surgeon, anesthesiologist, and other perioperative team members of potential neurologic insult and the immediate need for corrective action.[17] SSEPs are, however, unreliable in detecting surgical trespass that is isolated to the motor pathways, as demonstrated by clinical experience.[17]

Transcranial motor-evoked potentials (TcMEPs) were therefore developed in response to cases of postoperative paralysis that occurred in the absence of intraoperative SSEP changes. An electrode inserted into the scalp region overlying the motor cortex initiates an electrical stimulus to a peripheral muscle (commonly abductor pollicis brevis, adductor hallucis brevis, or tibialis anterior), producing recordings whose amplitudes and latencies are then analyzed.[17,19] A decrease in TcMEP amplitude by 50% or more triggers a threshold alert for the perioperative team to immediately consider corrective actions. Compared to SSEPs, TcMEPS possess a major advantage in that the time required to conduct stimulation is very brief. Motor evoked potentials are averaged over a minute or less, thus detecting potentially significant changes in signal amplitude or latency in a very short period of time. In contrast, SSEPs are continuously averaged over a period of about 5 minutes and therefore require at least that much time to recognize meaningful compromise within the pathway.[20]

Spinal nerve roots are also at risk for surgical injury but cannot be reliably monitored via SSEPs or TcMEPs. Electromyography (EMG) is used to help ensure spinal nerve root integrity via two widely applied methods. Spontaneous EMG, also known as continuous EMG, records electrical activity within myotome(s) preselected to coordinate with the operative level(s) of interest (see Table 20.1). When surgical manipulation of a nerve root occurs (e.g., stretching, impingement, retraction), "burst" activity is emitted from the monitored muscle and the surgical team is informed. Additionally, triggered EMG is used to guide pedicle screw placement, on the basis that intact cortical bone electrically insulates a properly placed screw from the adjacent nerve root. Testing pedicle screws for triggered EMG involves

**Table 20.1** Frequently Used Vertebral Level–Specific Nerves and Muscles for Neuromonitoring

| Vertebral Level | Nerve | Muscle |
| --- | --- | --- |
| C3, C4 | CN XI (accessory) | Trapezius |
| C5 | Axillary | Deltoid |
| C5,C6 | Musculocutaneous | Biceps brachii |
| C6, C7 | Radial | Triceps |
| C8, T1 | Median | Abductor pollicis brevis |
| C8, T1 | Ulnar | Adductor pollicis |
| T7 – T12 | | External oblique |
| T7 – T12 | | Rectus abdominis |
| L2, L3 | Lumbar plexus | Iliacus |
| L3, L4 | Femoral | Vastus lateralis/medialis Rectus femoris |
| L4, L5 | Sciatic | Semitendinosus Semimembranosus |
| L4, L5 | Peroneal | Tibialis anterior |
| L5, S1 | Peroneal | Extensor hallicus |
| L5, S1 | Tibial | Gastrocnemius lateral |
| S1, S2 | Tibial | Gastrocnemius medial Abductor hallicus |
| S3, S4, S5 | Pudendal | External anal sphincter |

directly applying voltage to them one by one via an electrified probe. Requiring a high level of electrical stimulation in order to trigger EMG activity implies that the pedicle cortex is intact and the screw is appropriately placed. Concern is raised when relatively low stimulation is required to evoke muscle activity in the corresponding myotomes since it is likely that the pedicle screw is misplaced and in close proximity to the nerve root. In general, stimulus thresholds of less than 4–6 mA are suggestive of cortical bone perforation by pedicle instrumentation when the adjacent nerve root is healthy.[21]

The use of intraoperative neurophysiological monitoring has markedly improved the ability to detect neurological injury during spine surgery. Compared to the Stagnara wake-up test, neurophysiological monitoring modalities afford continuous, real-time feedback about the condition of spinal pathways and nerve roots. No modality is without limitations, however. In addition to surgical injury, other factors can adversely affect signal quality. Inhalational anesthesia can decrease amplitude and increase latency of TcMEPs and, to a lesser extent, SSEPs, thereby complicating signal interpretation. Intravenous anesthetics also affect SSEPs and TcMEPs, although to a much lesser degree. Therefore, when these monitoring modalities are employed, it is prudent to limit the amount of inhalational agent used and instead rely on total intravenous anesthesia (TIVA) techniques. It is also necessary to avoid muscle relaxants when TcMEPs and EMG are employed. Other variables that can affect signal strength include systemic hypotension, hypothermia, electrolyte derangement, and severe anemia.[17,19]

It is important to emphasize that the various monitoring modalities discussed (SSEPs, MEPs, and EMG) complement one another and that combining them increases the reliability in detecting neurologic compromise. Relying on a single modality alone is not recommended in most cases.[19] A review of 32 studies examining the evidence for intraoperative neuromonitoring concluded the following[17]:

Based on strong evidence that multimodality intraoperative neuromonitoring (MIOM) is sensitive and specific for detecting intraoperative neurologic injury during spine surgery, it is recommended that the use of MIOM be considered in spine surgery where the spinal cord or nerve roots are deemed to be at risk, including procedures involving deformity correction and procedures that require the placement of instrumentation. There is a need to develop evidence-based protocols to deal with intraoperative changes in MIOM and to validate these prospectively.

## NEUROPROTECTION STRATEGIES
### Physiologic Interventions

### Blood Pressure

The spinal cord is highly susceptible to ischemia due to a blood supply that includes watershed areas. The lack of adequate collateral flow, particularly in the thoracic cord, is apparent intraoperatively with multimodality intraoperative neuromonitoring (MIOM) as the amplitude of SSEPs decreases to less than 50–60% of baseline during the first 20 minutes of decreased cord perfusion.[22–23]

An understanding of the blood supply to the spinal cord underscores the importance of maintaining adequate intraoperative blood pressure, especially during procedures that include correction of malformation curves. The blood supply to the spinal cord is organized into central and peripheral vascular systems. The central system, which is derived from the anterior spinal artery, supplies the anterior two-thirds of the spinal cord (i.e., the anterior gray and white matter columns and the anterior portions of the posterior gray matter and white matter columns).[24] The peripheral system, supplied by the posterior spinal artery and pial arterial plexus, supplies the posterior one-third of the spinal cord (i.e., the posterior portions of the posterior gray matter and white matter posterior columns). There are no interconnections between the central and peripheral blood supplies, but their terminal branches marginally overlap, resulting in watershed areas. The blood flow of the central system intrinsically flows away from the center of the spinal cord, while that of the peripheral system flows toward the center, creating watershed areas within the spinal cord as well.[15] Therefore, areas within the cord that are susceptible to poor perfusion exist not only at the watershed areas where the anterior two-thirds overlaps with the posterior one-third, but also internally, where the central system overlaps with the peripheral system.

Recognition of the spinal cord regions most susceptible to injury permits the practitioner to manipulate physiologic parameters such as mean arterial blood pressure and intrathecal pressure perioperatively to improve blood supply to ischemic areas. Reliable and reproducible evoked potentials have been observed during deliberate hypotension with mean arterial pressures (MAP) as low as 60 to 70 mm Hg.[25–27] Not all patients, however, can tolerate perfusion pressures this low, and blood pressure augmentation is often the primary physiologic intervention used to avoid or reverse actual or impending ischemia.

Cord perfusion can be jeopardized by surgical dissection, vessel clipping, low perfusion pressure, retraction, and vasospasm. Wiedemayer et al. investigated spinal cord hypoperfusion within a cohort of 423 spine surgery patients, 11 of whom experienced a threshold change in monitoring potentials.[28] Of these 11 patients, only 2 had a systolic blood pressure below 90 mm Hg (target for response) at the time of the monitoring alert. All 11 patients were treated by augmentation of blood pressure, which resulted in recovery of evoked potentials in 9. This led the authors to conclude that perfusion to the spinal cord may be compromised even at normal systolic blood pressures when intraoperative mechanical stress is applied to the neural tissue.

Schwartz et al. reached similar conclusions based on a review of intraoperative neurophysiological monitoring records for 1,121 consecutive spine surgery patients treated for adolescent idiopathic scoliosis.[29] Changes in TcMEPs were observed in 38 patients. In nine of these patients, the TcMEP changes were due solely to hypotension. In each of these nine cases there was a greater than 75% decrease in TcMEP amplitude and no change in SSEPs. The average MAP during these monitoring changes was 59 mm Hg, and in response, the anesthesiologist raised the MAP to at least 90 mm Hg in each instance. As a result, the TcMEP amplitudes returned to normal or near baseline values within 5 minutes of intervention. The remaining 29 patients who experienced amplitude changes in TcMEPs also underwent blood pressure augmentation to a MAP of greater than 90 mm Hg, but without successful correction of the TcMEPs. Instead, TcMEP amplitudes returned to baseline only after surgical causes of signal change were identified and reversed (i.e., removing vessel clamps or reducing retraction).

Induction of controlled hypotension may seem counterintuitive, but this is a well-established method of reducing intraoperative bleeding. Limited intraoperative hypotension for hemorrhage control should occur in the presence of neuromonitoring and careful titration of blood pressure. Despite the safety seen with some medications, such as clevidipine and milrinone, the general consensus is to discontinue hypotensive medications should clinically significant evoked potential changes occur.[30-31]

## Anemia

Blood loss secondary to long operation times, large wound surfaces, and trauma to vascular-rich bone is a major concern in spine surgery. Perioperative techniques can reduce the risks of both blood loss and the need for allogenic blood transfusion. Controlled hypotension can limit blood loss simply by decreasing perfusion to exposed tissue areas. Acute normovolemic hemodilution is also widely used and has been shown to be safe and effective at reducing the need for allogenic blood transfusion.[32] At this time, other techniques such as maintenance of hypothermia and minimally invasive surgical approaches have not shown conclusive or sufficient evidence toward this goal.[33]

In addition to limiting blood loss with physiologic and mechanical techniques, certain medications have also proved beneficial in reducing perioperative anemia. A meta-analysis of 11 randomized control trials (RCT) that compared the effects of tranexamic acid (TXA) versus placebo on surgical bleeding during spine surgery found that TXA was associated with significantly less total perioperative blood loss and need for allogenic blood transfusion.[34] Although antifibrinolytic agents may theoretically increase the risk of thromboembolism, TXA did not significantly increase the incidence of pulmonary embolism, deep vein thrombosis, or myocardial infarction. Intrathecal morphine administered before lumbar spine operations has also been associated with reduction in intraoperative blood loss by as much as 50–65%, although the mechanism is not clear.[35–38]

## Hypothermia and Electrolyte Imbalances

Intraoperative hypothermia has been found to be linearly associated with decreased spinal cord blood flow and increased latency in MIOM potentials.[39] Hypothermia also strongly inhibits multiple steps of the coagulation cascade, disrupts synthesis of thrombin and fibrinogen, and inhibits platelet activation.[40–46] The incidence of perioperative hypothermia is very high, especially during long-duration procedures requiring large incisions. A 2014 retrospective review, however, found that hypothermia during lumbar spine surgery has no effect on perioperative blood loss when covariates such as operative time and surgery type were taken into account.[47] Another 2014 review examining the use of hypothermia during spinal tumor resection found no statistically significant difference between patients in the hypothermic versus normothermic cohorts in terms of rate of surgical, medical, neurological, or overall complications.[48] Despite the fact that hypothermia can contribute to coagulopathy, it is unlikely to significantly increase blood loss and the need for allogenic blood transfusion. Utilizing warmed saline irrigation, intravenous fluids, and external heating blankets can help prevent hypothermia and SCI.[49]

Another consequence of hypothermia is a leftward shift of the oxygen dissociation curve that impairs oxygen delivery to the tissues, including the spinal cord. It is possible that a critical reduction of neuronal tissue oxygenation by either reduced oxygen delivery or decreased inspired oxygen concentrations can inhibit TcMEPs by disturbing oxygen metabolism and cell homeostasis. Other theories for why hypothermia is associated with decreased or lost evoked potentials during spine surgery include accumulated extracellular potassium derived from local tissue damage, thereby acting as a strong axonal blocking agent.[50] To remove these irritating blood products and metabolites, it is common practice to irrigate the surgical field with a warm saline solution.

Changes in arterial carbon dioxide tension may also negatively affect evoked potentials. At a $PaCO_2$ range of 20–50 mm Hg, evoked potentials remain unchanged; however, extreme hyperventilation leading to $EtCO_2$ of less than 20 mm Hg can result in a small 2–4% increase in latency and decrease in amplitude of SSEPs.[51] These small changes are likely to be irrelevant clinically since much larger changes in evoked potentials are necessary to invoke a threshold alert for possible neuronal damage.

Intraoperative neuroprotective strategies during spine surgery involve maintaining physiologic stability throughout the procedure. This includes adjusting hemodynamic and physiologic parameters, minimizing bleeding, and promoting oxygen delivery to the spinal cord. Close communication among surgeon, anesthesiologist, and neurophysiologist plays an important role in avoiding, detecting, and reversing perioperative nerve injury.

## Pharmacologic Interventions

There is a large body of research investigating the efficacy of pharmacologic therapies in patients suffering from acute SCI, summarized in Table 20.2. Much of the

**Table 20.2** Research Summarizing the Efficacy of Pharmacologic Therapies in Patients Suffering from Acute Spinal Cord Injury (SCI)

| Pharmacologic agent studied | Reference | Type of Study | Study description | Conclusions and outcomes |
|---|---|---|---|---|
| Methylprednisolone | Bracken et al., *JAMA* 1984 (original publication)/ Bracken et al., *J Neurosurg* 1985 (1-year follow-up) | Randomized controlled trial (NASCIS I) | Compared MP 1,000 mg/d (high-dose) with 100 mg/d (low-dose) in 330 patients with SCI. Treatment effect was measured at 6 weeks, 6 months, and 1 year. | No significant difference noted at 6 weeks, 6 months or 1 year after injury. Incidence of wound infection was significantly higher in high-dose group and death within 14 days was more common in high dose group. |
| Methylprednisolone | Bracken et al., *N Engl J Med.* 1990 (original publication)/ Bracken et al., *J Neurosurg*, 1992 (1-year follow-up) | Randomized controlled trial (NASCIS II) | Compared outcomes of MP with the opioid antagonist naloxone and placebo in 487 patients | Post hoc analysis showed neurologic improvement at 6 months and 1 year in patients who were administered MP within 8 hours of injury. However, at 6-week and 6-month follow-up there was no difference between groups in the study's primary comparisons. All primary comparisons were negative at 1-year follow-up. Incidence of wound infections, GI bleed, and pulmonary embolus was increased in MP group. |
| Methylprednisolone | Bracken et al., *JAMA*, 1997 | Randomized controlled trial | Compared outcomes between 24- hour MP administration, 48-hour MP administration and 48-hour tirilazad mesylate administration in 499 patients with SCI | Post hoc analysis showed neurologic improvement at 6 weeks and 6 months in patients administered 48-hour MP compared to 24-hour MP. However, no difference was found in all primary comparisons. Rates of severe sepsis and severe pneumonia were highest in 48-hour MP group. |

*(continued)*

Table 20.2 Continued

| Pharmacologic agent studied | Reference | Type of Study | Study description | Conclusions and outcomes |
|---|---|---|---|---|
| Methylprednisolone | Pointillart et al., *Spinal Cord* 2000 | Randomized controlled trial | Compared neurologic outcomes in 106 patients with SCI randomized to four groups: MP, nimodipine, MP + nimodipine, and placebo | No difference in neurological outcome. Increased incidence of hyperglycemia infection and GI bleed in those patients treated with MP. |
| Methylprednisolone | Ito et. al, *Spine* 2009 | Prospective case series | Case series of 38 patients treated with MP compared with another series of 41 patients not treated with MP. Neurologic exam scores followed over 3 months. | No difference in neurological improvement outcome but significantly higher incidence of respiratory and wound infection. |
| GM-1 Ganglioside | Geisler et al., *NEJM* 1991 | Randomized controlled trial | Thirty-seven SCI patients randomized to receive either GM-1 ganglioside or placebo with recovery of neurological function compared between the two groups | Improvement in GM-1 ganglioside group was statistically significant. Study was underpowered due to small sample of patient questioning result validity. |
| GM-1 Ganglioside | Geisler et al., *Spine* 2001 | Randomized controlled trial | 760 SCI patients randomized to receive GM-1 ganglioside or placebo | No statistically significant differences in neurological outcome at 1 year. |

| Agent | Citation | Study Type | Description | Findings |
|---|---|---|---|---|
| GM-1 Ganglioside | Dayong et al., *Pak J Pharm Sci* 2015 | Randomized controlled trial | 53 SCI patients randomized to receive GM-1 ganglioside or MP | Found statistically significant improvement in neurologic function with administration of GM-1 ganglioside |
| Thyrotropin-Releasing Hormone (TRH) | Pitts et al., *J Neurotrauma* 1995 | Randomized controlled trial | 20 patients with SCI randomized to treatment with either TRH or placebo | TRH treatment was associated with significantly higher neurological improvement. Small sample size limits the validity of these results. |
| Thyrotropin-Releasing Hormone (TRH) | Vaidyanathan et al., *Ann Clin R* 1983 | Randomized controlled trial | 13 patients with bladder dysfunction following SCI randomized to treatment with either TRH or placebo (normal saline). | TRH treatment was associated with bladder function improvement. Validity is questionable due to small sample size. |
| Riluzole | Grossman et al., *J Neurotrauma* 2014 | Phase I matched-comparison group trial | 36 patients with SCI treated with riluzole and compared with other spinal cord injury registry patients | Statistically significant neurological improvement was noted in patients treated with riluzole. No serious adverse advents or deaths were reported. |

literature has focused on high-dose methylprednisolone and GM-1 ganglioside. Less-studied agents include thyrotropin-releasing hormone and riluzole. Although these studies have been conducted in patients suffering from acute SCI outside of the operating room, it is reasonable to extrapolate these findings to patients with neurologic injury resulting from spine surgery.

## Methylprednisolone

No single drug studied for neuroprotective benefits after SCI has received as much attention as methylprednisolone (MP). Three landmark RCTs, widely referred to as the National Acute Spinal Cord Injury Study (NASCIS) I, II, and III, respectively, investigated the neuroprotective effects of glucocorticoid administration after SCI.[52-57] While the NASCIS I trial showed no significant neurologic benefit with high-dose MP administered following acute SCI, the NASCIS II and III trials both showed that MP administration was associated with improved neurologic outcome after SCI. These findings provided much of the evidence base for MP administration following acute SCI in the two decades following the publication of NASCIS II and III.

The strength of the evidence supporting MP administration in the NASCIS II and III trials has been critically re-examined by Hurlbert and colleagues.[58] Weaknesses of NASCIS II include an arbitrary assignment of an 8-hour therapeutic window, the absence of functional outcome measures, and omission of data. Furthermore, the primary positive finding of improved motor function was inconsistent and apparent only in a post hoc analysis of a partial dataset. In NASCIS III, patients were randomized to one of three study arms: MP infusion for 24 hours versus MP infusion for 48 hours versus tirilazad mesylate infusion for 48 hours.[56] All primary comparisons were negative among the three groups, with post hoc analysis demonstrating improved motor scores of questionable significance in the 48-hour treatment arm compared to the 24-hour treatment arm among patients who started treatment between 3 and 8 hours after injury.[56-58] Additionally, all three NASCIS trials demonstrated high rates of complications, such as wound infection, gastrointestinal (GI) bleed, and respiratory compromise that may have had some relationship to glucocorticoid use.[52-57]

Subsequent studies have also called into question the reported benefits of MP following acute SCI. An RCT performed in 106 acute SCI patients compared outcomes following treatment with MP, nimodipine, MP + nimodipine, or no pharmacologic agent.[59] There was no difference in neurological outcomes at 1-year follow-up. Patients treated with MP did, however, have higher rates of infection, GI bleeding, and hyperglycemia necessitating treatment with insulin. Similarly, a consecutive cohort study investigating neurological outcomes in cervical SCI patients over 4 years found no difference in neurological outcomes with MP administration.[60] During the first 2 years of the study, all enrolled patients were treated with early spinal decompression and stabilization and high-dose MP administered within 8 hours of injury ($N = 38$). In the second 2 years of the study, all enrolled patients were treated with early surgery without MP ($N = 41$). Neurologic outcomes were similar in both groups. The incidence of pneumonia, however, was significantly increased with the use of high-dose MP.

In 2002, a committee selected and sponsored by the Joint Section on Spine and Peripheral Nerves of the American Association of Neurological Surgeons and Congress of Neurological Surgeons published the first evidence-based guidelines for the management of patients with acute cervical SCIs.[61] Recommendations regarding pharmacologic management at that time included the following for corticosteroids:

Treatment with methylprednisolone for either 24 or 48 h is recommended as an option in the treatment of patients with acute SCIs. It should be undertaken only with the knowledge that the evidence suggesting harmful side effects is more consistent than any suggestion of clinical benefit.

In 2013, the committee revised this recommendation as follows[62]:

Administration of methylprednisolone for the treatment of acute SCI is not recommended. Clinicians considering methylprednisolone therapy should bear in mind that the drug is not approved by the Food and Drug Administration for this application. There is no Class I or Class II medical evidence supporting the clinical benefit of methylprednisolone in the treatment of acute SCI. Scattered reports of Class III evidence claim inconsistent effects likely related to random chance or selection bias. However, Class I, II, and III evidence exists that high-dose steroids are associated with harmful side effects, including death.

Thus, current guidelines do not support use of glucocorticoids in the treatment of catastrophic perioperative SCI.

## GM-1 Ganglioside

GM-1 ganglioside is believed to promote neuronal plasticity, regrowth, and other repair mechanisms and therefore has also received considerable attention as a pharmacologic therapy for acute SCI. An RCT in which 37 patients with acute SCI received either intravenous GM-1 ganglioside or placebo found that the treatment group had superior recovery of neurologic function at 1-year follow-up without negative side effects.[63] In a follow-up multicenter RCT, in which 797 patients were randomized to receive either placebo, low-dose, or high-dose GM-1 ganglioside, there was no clinically significant difference in the percentage of patients with marked neurologic recovery among the three groups.[64] A third RCT in which 53 patients received either GM-1 ganglioside or MP following acute SCI found that GM-1 ganglioside was associated with neurological improvement (improved sphincter tone and motor function).[65] The small number of patients studied, however, limits interpretation of this finding.

Recommendations for the use of GM-1 ganglioside were included in the Joint Section on Spine and Peripheral Nerves of the American Association of Neurological Surgeons and Congress of Neurological Surgeons guidelines.[61] The 2002 recommendations read as follows: "Treatment of patients with acute SCIs with GM-1 ganglioside is recommended as an option without demonstrated clinical benefit." These recommendations were revised by the committee in 2013, stating that: "Administration of GM-1 ganglioside (Sygen™) for the treatment of acute SCI is not recommended."[62]

# IMPLICATIONS FOR CLINICAL PRACTICE

Spine surgery often provides excellent functional and anatomic results, but it carries a risk for neurologic injury. Awareness and prevention strategies can help alleviate these risks. Multiple controlled studies in animals have demonstrated that intervening after receiving an intraoperative neuromonitoring alert reduces the risk of neurologic injury. A 2012 meta-analysis conducted by a panel of neurophysiology experts sought to develop a set of evidence-based guidelines for the intraoperative use of somatosensory and transcranial electrical motor evoked potentials.[66] The studies reviewed demonstrated that all occurrences of postoperative paraparesis, paraplegia, or quadriplegia were associated with intraoperative evoked potential change. The panel therefore concluded that "IOM is established as effective to predict an increased risk of the adverse outcomes of paraparesis, paraplegia, and quadriplegia in spinal surgery."

Despite the seemingly obvious clinical benefits conferred by IOM in predicting neurologic injury, there is surprisingly little evidence to support this. Two recently published checklist protocols (see Table 20.3) outline suggested interventions when an intraoperative neurologic deficit is suspected and the respective role of each perioperative team member. Both were authored by panels of neurosurgery and orthopedic spine specialists and are quite similar.[67–68]

According to these protocols, in the event of a significant evoked potential change (defined as a decrease in SSEP amplitude by 50% or more or a decrease in TcMEP amplitude by more than 60%), the surgeon should (1) immediately stop the current manipulation, (2) assess the surgical field for possible causes of structural cord compression, and (3) review the events which occurred just prior to the alert for any potential etiology of the signal change. If spinal stenosis exists, then further decompression should be performed. Otherwise, decreasing traction and removing other corrective forces as well as rods and/or pedicle screws to inspect for possible neurologic trespass may be warranted. Intraoperative imaging to examine and evaluate implant placement should also be considered. During this time, the anesthesia care team should optimize blood pressure (augmentation to MAPs of 90–100 mm Hg). The anesthetic regimen should be checked for any recent changes that could affect monitoring, and any residual neuromuscular blockade should be reversed. Intraoperative assessments of hematocrit, arterial pH, and $PaCO_2$, as well as extremity positioning and body temperature are recommended.

The neurophysiologist's role in the intervention begins with repeating SSEPs and TcMEPs to rule out potential false positive readings. He or she should also check for any degree of neuromuscular blockade and check that monitoring leads are properly placed or evaluate the need for repositioning. An assessment of the pattern and timing of the signal changes should be performed and discussed with perioperative team members. Asymmetric changes, for example, would likely signify a cord or nerve root injury, whereas symmetric or global changes are more reliably associated with anesthetic-related changes or hypotension.

If the etiology of the signal changes is not discovered, then further measures need to be considered. These considerations include consulting colleagues, further blood pressure augmentation (MAPs >100 mm Hg), performing a wake-up test, and the option of performing the surgery in stages or aborting the surgery altogether.

The current literature does not support the use of pharmacologic therapy (i.e., glucocorticoid administration) in the management of acute SCI and argues against its routine use for neurological injury due to spinal surgery.[61–62]

**Table 20.3** Checklist for a Team-Based Response to an Intraoperative
Neuromonitoring Alert During Spine Surgery

*Gain control of operating room and call for senior and experienced team personnel*

| *Surgical Team* | *Anesthesiology Team* | *Neurophysiology Team* |
|---|---|---|
| • Stop current manipulation | • Ensure lack of neuromuscular blockade | • Communicate specific neuromonitoring signal changes |
| • Discuss events just prior to alert and consider reversing actions: | • Discuss any recent changes in administered anesthetic | • Repeat MEP and SSEP signals to rule out false positive |
|   • Remove or decrease traction | • Check and optimize mean arterial pressure | • Check all electrodes and connections |
|   • Remove rods | • (goal >90 mm Hg) | • Consider adding leads to proximal muscle groups |
|   • Remove screws and probe for breach | • Check and optimize hematocrit | • Assess pattern and timing of signal changes |
| • Evaluate surgical field for structural cord compression | • (goal >24%) |   • Asymmetric (cord or nerve root injury) |
| • Assess need for intraoperative fluoroscopy to evaluate hardware placement | • Check and optimize pH and electrolytes |   • Symmetric (hypotension or anesthetic issues) |
| | • Check extremity and neck positioning | • Check extremity and neck positioning |
| | • Check temperature, pursue normothermia | • Communicate and quantify any improvement in signals |
| | • Lighten depth of anesthesia | |
| |   • Reduce/eliminate inhaled agents | |
| |   • Consider reducing propofol dose | |
| |   • Consider adding ketamine (improves signals and allows reduction of suppressive agents) | |

**If NO Change**
• Increase mean arterial pressure >100 mm Hg
• Consult with colleagues
• Consider wake-up test
• Consider continuing or staging procedure

## FUTURE DIRECTIONS

There is a significant body of literature focusing on the etiology and detection of perioperative neurologic injury in spine surgery; however, there is very little in the way of management options once compromise has occurred. Current practice recommendations emphasize multimodal intraoperative neurophysiologic monitoring as the best means of detecting and reversing surgically induced injuries.

Adverse changes in physiologic parameters, such as blood pressure, temperature, electrolytes, and oxygen delivery, are all known to be reversible causes of neurologic injury. Irreversible causes of neurologic damage, such as surgical trauma and over-correction, have not received as much attention in the literature. MP has long been the cornerstone of pharmacologic management of acute SCI, but a strong base of evidence has refuted the administration of both MP and GM-1 ganglioside. The search for novel, effective, and safe therapeutic agents through additional research is needed.

Future efforts should focus on identifying surgical techniques that may further reduce the incidence of perioperative neurologic deficits related to spine surgery. Additionally, while checklists for interventions in response to neuromonitoring alerts exist, further investigation is necessary to validate their efficacy.

## REFERENCES

1. Vos T, Flaxman AD, Naghavi M, et al. Years lived with disability (YLDs) for 1160 sequelae of 289 diseases and injuries 1990-2010: a systematic analysis for the Global Burden of Disease Study 2010. *Lancet.* 2012;380(9859):2163–96.
2. Available from: www.hcup-us.ahrq.gov/nisoverview.jsp.
3. Cramer DE, Maher PC, Pettigrew DB, Kuntz C. Major neurologic deficit immediately after adult spinal surgery: incidence and etiology over 10 years at a single training institution. *J Spinal Disord Tech.* 2009;22(8):565–70.
4. Kamerlink JR, Errico T, Xavier S, et al. Major intraoperative neurologic monitoring deficits in consecutive pediatric and adult spinal deformity patients at one institution. *Spine.* 2010;35(2):240–45.
5. Diab M, Smith AR, Kuklo TR; Spinal Deformity Study Group. Neural complications in the surgical treatment of adolescent idiopathic scoliosis. *Spine.* 2007;32(24):2759–63.
6. Coe JD, Arlet V, Donaldson W, et al. Complications in spinal fusion for adolescent idiopathic scoliosis in the new millennium. A report of the Scoliosis Research Society Morbidity and Mortality Committee. *Spine.* 2006;31(3):345–9.
7. Garreau de Loubresse C. Neurological risks in scheduled spinal surgery. *Orthop Traumatol Surg Res.* 2014;100(1):S85–90.
8. Lykissas MG, Crawford AH, Jain VV. Complications of surgical treatment of pediatric spinal deformities. *Orthop Clin North Am.* 2013;44(3):357–70.
9. MacEwen GD, Bunnell WP, Sriram K. Acute neurological complications in the treatment of scoliosis. A report of the Scoliosis Research Society. *J Bone Jt Surg Am.* 1975;57(3):404–8.
10. Martirosyan NL, Feuerstein JS, Theodore N, Cavalcanti DD, Spetzler RF, Preul MC. Blood supply and vascular reactivity of the spinal cord under normal and pathological conditions: a review. *J Neurosurg Spine.* 2011;15(3):238–51.
11. Brallier JW, Deiner S. The elderly spine surgery patient: pre- and intraoperative management of drug therapy. *Drugs Aging.* 2015;32(8):601–9.
12. Gerstein NS, Schulman PM, Gerstein WH, Petersen TR, Tawil I. Should more patients continue aspirin therapy perioperatively?: Clinical impact of aspirin withdrawal syndrome. *Ann Surg.* 2012;255(5):811–9.
13. Devereaux PJ, Mrkobrada M, Sessler DI, et al. Aspirin in patients undergoing noncardiac surgery. *N Engl J Med.* 2014;370(16):1494–503.
14. Patel PA, Fleisher LA. Aspirin, clopidogrel, and the surgeon. *Adv Surg.* 2014;48(1):211–22.
15. Antithrombotic Trialists' (ATT) Collaboration, Baigent C, Blackwell L, Collins R, et al. Aspirin in the primary and secondary prevention of vascular disease: collaborative meta-analysis of individual participant data from randomised trials. *The Lancet.* 2009;373(9678):1849–60.

16. Vauzelle C, Stagnara P, Jouvinroux P. Functional monitoring of spinal cord activity during spinal surgery. *Clin Orthop*. 1973;(93):173–8.

17. Malhotra NR, Shaffrey CI. Intraoperative electrophysiological monitoring in spine surgery. *Spine*. 2010;35(25):2167–79.

18. Tamaki T, Kubota S. History of the development of intraoperative spinal cord monitoring. *Eur Spine J*. 2007;16(S2):140–6.

19. Gavaret M, Jouve JL, Péréon Y, et al. Intraoperative neurophysiologic monitoring in spine surgery. Developments and state of the art in France in 2011. *Orthop Traumatol Surg Res*. 2013;99(6):S319–27.

20. Pajewski TN, Arlet V, Phillips LH. Current approach on spinal cord monitoring: the point of view of the neurologist, the anesthesiologist and the spine surgeon. *Eur Spine J*. 2007;16 Suppl 2:S115–29.

21. Lall RR, Lall RR, Hauptman JS, et al. Intraoperative neurophysiological monitoring in spine surgery: indications, efficacy, and role of the preoperative checklist. *Neurosurg Focus*. 2012;33(5):E10.

22. Seyal M, Mull B. Mechanisms of signal change during intraoperative somatosensory evoked potential monitoring of the spinal cord. *J Clin Neurophysiol*. 2002;19(5):409–15.

23. Nielsen VK, Kardel T. Temporospatial effects on orthodromic sensory potential propagation during ischemia. *Ann Neurol*. 1981;9(6):597–604.

24. Turnbull IM. Chapter 5. Blood supply of the spinal cord: normal and pathological considerations. *Clin Neurosurg*. 1973;20:56–84.

25. Lotto ML, Banoub M, Schubert A. Effects of anesthetic agents and physiologic changes on intraoperative motor evoked potentials. *J Neurosurg Anesthesiol*. 2004;16(1):32–42.

26. Stephen JP, Sullivan MR, Hicks RG, Burke DJ, Woodforth IJ, Crawford MR. Cotrel-Dubousset instrumentation in children using simultaneous motor and somatosensory evoked potential monitoring. *Spine*. 1996;21(21):2450–7.

27. Lin BC, Chen IH. Modified transcranial electromagnetic motor evoked potential obtained with train-of-four monitor for scoliosis surgery. *Acta Anaesthesiol Sin*. 1998; 36(4):199–206.

28. Wiedemayer H, Fauser B, Sandalcioglu IE, Schäfer H, Stolke D. The impact of neurophysiological intraoperative monitoring on surgical decisions: a critical analysis of 423 cases. *J Neurosurg*. 2002;96(2):255–62.

29. Schwartz DM, Auerbach JD, Dormans JP, et al. Neurophysiological detection of impending spinal cord injury during scoliosis surgery. *J Bone Joint Surg Am*. 2007;89(11):2440–9.

30. Kako H, Gable A, Martin D, et al. A prospective, open-label trial of clevidipine for controlled hypotension during posterior spinal fusion. *J Pediatr Pharmacol*. 2015;20(1):54–60.

31. Hwang W, Kim E. The effect of milrinone on induced hypotension in elderly patients during spinal surgery: a randomized controlled trial. *Spine J*. 2014;14(8):1532–7.

32. Epstein NE. Bloodless spinal surgery: a review of the normovolemic hemodilution technique. *Surg Neurol*. 2008;70(6):614–8.

33. Tse EY, Cheung WY, Ng KF, Luk KD. Reducing perioperative blood loss and allogeneic blood transfusion in patients undergoing major spine surgery. *J Bone Joint Surg Am*. 2011;93(13):1268–77.

34. Cheriyan T, Maier SP, Bianco K, et al. Efficacy of tranexamic acid on surgical bleeding in spine surgery: a meta-analysis. *Spine J*. 2015;15(4):752–61.

35. Guay J. The effect of neuraxial blocks on surgical blood loss and blood transfusion requirements: a meta-analysis. *J Clin Anesth*. 2006;18(2):124–8.

36. Goodarzi M. The advantages of intrathecal opioids for spinal fusion in children. *Paediatr Anaesth.* 1998;8(2):131–4.

37. Gall O, Aubineau JV, Bernière J, Desjeux L, Murat I. Analgesic effect of low-dose intrathecal morphine after spinal fusion in children. *Anesthesiology.* 2001;94(3):447–52.

38. Eschertzhuber S, Hohlrieder M, Keller C, Oswald E, Kuehbacher G, Innerhofer P. Comparison of high- and low-dose intrathecal morphine for spinal fusion in children. *Br J Anaesth.* 2008;100(4):538–43.

39. Kano T, Sadanaga M, Sakamoto M, Higashi K, Matsumoto M. Effects of systemic cooling and rewarming on the evoked spinal cord potentials and local spinal cord blood flow in dogs. *Anesth Analg.* 1994;78(5):897–904.

40. Rohrer MJ, Natale AM. Effect of hypothermia on the coagulation cascade. *Crit Care Med.* 1992;20(10):1402–5.

41. Wolberg AS, Meng ZH, Monroe DM 3rd, Hoffman M. A systematic evaluation of the effect of temperature on coagulation enzyme activity and platelet function. *J Trauma Inj Infect.* 2004;56(6):1221–8.

42. Michelson AD, MacGregor H, Barnard MR, Kestin AS, Rohrer MJ, Valeri CR. Reversible inhibition of human platelet activation by hypothermia in vivo and in vitro. *Thromb Haemost.* 1994;71(5):633–40.

43. Martini WZ. Coagulopathy by hypothermia and acidosis: mechanisms of thrombin generation and fibrinogen availability. *J Trauma.* 2009;67(1):202–8; discussion 208–9.

44. Valeri CR, Feingold H, Cassidy G, Ragno G, Khuri S, Altschule MD. Hypothermia-induced reversible platelet dysfunction. *Ann Surg.* 1987;205(2):175–81.

45. Kermode JC, Zheng Q, Milner EP. Marked temperature dependence of the platelet calcium signal induced by human von Willebrand factor. *Blood.* 1999;94(1):199–207.

46. Reed RL 2nd, Bracey AW Jr, Hudson JD, Miller TA, Fischer RP. Hypothermia and blood coagulation: dissociation between enzyme activity and clotting factor levels. *Circ Shock.* 1990;32(2):141–52.

47. Tedesco NS, Korpi FP, Pazdernik VK, Cochran JM. Relationship between hypothermia and blood loss in adult patients undergoing open lumbar spine surgery. *J Am Osteopath Assoc.* 2014;114(11):828–38.

48. Johnson JN, Cummock MD, Levi AD, Green BA, Wang MY. Moderate hypothermia for intradural spinal tumor resection: a cohort comparison and feasibility study. *Ther Hypothermia Temp Manag.* 2014;4(3):137–44.

49. Sala F, Bricolo A, Faccioli F, Lanteri P, Gerosa M. Surgery for intramedullary spinal cord tumors: the role of intraoperative (neurophysiological) monitoring. *Eur Spine J.* 2007;16 Suppl 2:S130–9.

50. Park J-H, Hyun S-J. Intraoperative neurophysiological monitoring in spinal surgery. *World J Clin Cases.* 2015;3(9):765–73.

51. Kalkman CJ, Boezeman EH, Ribberink AA, Oosting J, Deen L, Bovill JG. Influence of changes in arterial carbon dioxide tension on the electroencephalogram and posterior tibial nerve somatosensory cortical evoked potentials during alfentanil/nitrous oxide anesthesia. *Anesthesiology.* 1991;75(1):68–74.

52. Bracken MB, Collins WF, Freeman DF, et al. Efficacy of methylprednisolone in acute spinal cord injury. *JAMA.* 1984;251(1):45–52.

53. Bracken MB, Shepard MJ, Hellenbrand KG, et al. Methylprednisolone and neurological function 1 year after spinal cord injury. Results of the National Acute Spinal Cord Injury Study. *J Neurosurg.* 1985;63(5):704–13.

54. Bracken MB, Shepard MJ, Collins WF, et al. A randomized, controlled trial of methyl-prednisolone or naloxone in the treatment of acute spinal-cord injury. *N Engl J Med.* 1990;322(20):1405–11.

55. Bracken MB, Shepard MJ, Collins WF, et al. Methylprednisolone or naloxone treatment after acute spinal cord injury: 1-year follow-up data. Results of the second National Acute Spinal Cord Injury Study. *J Neurosurg.* 1992;76(1):23–31.

56. Bracken MB, Shepard MJ, Holford TR, et al. Administration of methylpred-nisolone for 24 or 48 hours or tirilazad mesylate for 48 hours in the treatment of acute spinal cord injury. Results of the Third National Acute Spinal Cord Injury Randomized Controlled Trial. National Acute Spinal Cord Injury Study. *JAMA.* 1997;277(20):1597–604.

57. Bracken MB, Shepard MJ, Holford TR, et al. Methylprednisolone or tirilazad mesyl-ate administration after acute spinal cord injury: 1-year follow up. Results of the third National Acute Spinal Cord Injury randomized controlled trial. *J Neurosurg.* 1998;89(5):699–706.

58. Hurlbert RJ, Hadley MN, Walters BC, et al. Pharmacological therapy for acute spinal cord injury. *Neurosurgery.* 2015;76 Suppl 1:S71–83.

59. Pointillart V, Petitjean ME, Wiart L, et al. Pharmacological therapy of spinal cord injury during the acute phase. *Spinal Cord.* 2000;38(2):71–6.

60. Ito Y, Sugimoto Y, Tomioka M, Kai N, Tanaka M. Does high dose methylprednisolone sodium succinate really improve neurological status in patient with acute cervical cord injury?: a prospective study about neurological recovery and early complications. *Spine.* 2009;34(20):2121–4.

61. Chappell ET. Pharmacological therapy after acute cervical spinal cord injury. *Neurosurgery.* 2002;51(3):855–6.

62. Walters BC, Hadley MN, Hurlbert RJ, et al. Guidelines for the management of acute cer-vical spine and spinal cord injuries: 2013 update. *Neurosurgery.* 2013;60 Suppl 1:82–91.

63. Geisler FH, Dorsey FC, Coleman WP. Recovery of motor function after spinal-cord injury--a randomized, placebo-controlled trial with GM-1 ganglioside. *N Engl J Med.* 1991;324(26):1829–38.

64. Geisler FH, Coleman WP, Grieco G, Poonian D; Sygen Study Group. The Sygen multi-center acute spinal cord injury study. *Spine.* 2001;26(24 Suppl):S87–98.

65. Xu D, Yang L, Li Y, Sun Y. Clinical study of ganglioside (GM) combined with methylpred-nisolone (MP) for early acute spinal injury. *Pak J Pharm Sci.* 2015;28(2 Suppl):701–4.

66. Nuwer MR, Emerson RG, Galloway G, et al. Evidence-based guideline update: intraop-erative spinal monitoring with somatosensory and transcranial electrical motor evoked potentials. *J Clin Neurophysiol.* 2012;29(1):101–8.

67. Ziewacz JE, Berven SH, Mummaneni VP, et al. The design, development, and imple-mentation of a checklist for intraoperative neuromonitoring changes. *Neurosurg Focus.* 2012;33(5):E11.

68. Vitale MG, Skaggs DL, Pace GI, et al. Best practices in intraoperative neuromonitor-ing in spine deformity surgery: development of an intraoperative checklist to optimize response. *Spine Deform.* 2014;2(5):333–9.

# 21 Neuroprotection for General, Orthopedic, Peripheral Vascular, and ENT Surgery

Magdy Selim

## GENERAL CONSIDERATIONS

Stroke is an infrequent yet devastating complication of general; orthopedic; peripheral vascular; and ear, nose, and throat (ENT) surgery. It increases morbidity, length and cost of hospitalization, and mortality, and offsets the potential benefits of surgery. Stroke during and after these surgical procedures is relatively poorly investigated. The purpose of this chapter is to review the incidence, predisposing risk factors, and etiological mechanisms of stroke in these surgical procedures, and to provide preventive and management recommendations.

### Incidence and Burden of Perioperative Stroke

The occurrence of stroke in patients undergoing noncardiac and noncerebrovascular surgical procedures is uncommon. Data from the American College of Surgeons National Quality improvement Program (ACS-NSQIP) database indicate that approximately 0.1% of patients undergoing noncardiac, noncerebrovascular surgical procedures, including orthopedic, ENT, and peripheral vascular surgery, suffer a perioperative stroke.[1] The actual incidence of stroke, however, is likely higher than reported because the vast majority of published studies have been retrospective and lack detailed neurological and radiological assessments. Many patients with minor or rapidly resolving deficits due to stroke might be erroneously diagnosed with postoperative "confusion" or "residual effects of anesthesia." In a pilot multicenter prospective study of 70 patients undergoing general and orthopedic surgery, routine brain magnetic resonance imaging (MRI) between postoperative days 3 and 10 revealed a covert stroke in 11.4% of patients.[2]

The incidence of perioperative stroke likely varies with the type of surgery. It was thought that the incidence of perioperative stroke was particularly high in patients undergoing surgeries involving dissection of the neck, with an incidence estimate of 4.8% in a single-center case series study.[3] Subsequent studies, however, have reported much lower rates, varying from 0% to 0.2%.[1,4] Excluding cardiac, cerebro-vascular, and major vascular surgeries, it seems that the overall incidence of stroke is highest among patients undergoing peripheral vascular and orthopedic surgery. Data from the ACS-NSQIP database indicate that during the period from 2005 to 2009, the overall incidence of perioperative stroke was 0.6% in patients who underwent aortic procedures or elective peripheral vascular procedures such as lower extremity amputation or revascularization.[1] A nationwide Danish matched-cohort study found that patients undergoing hip replacement surgery had a 4.7 times increased risk of ischemic stroke (95% confidence interval [CI] 3.12–7.06) and 4.4 times increased risk of hemorrhagic stroke (95% CI 2.01–9.62) within 2 weeks post surgery.[5] A small case series has also suggested elevated stroke risk after shoulder arthroscopy in the beach chair position.[6]

Despite the low incidence of perioperative stroke in general, orthopedic, peripheral vascular, and ENT surgical patients, stroke is an important cause of morbidity and mortality.[7] It increases the length of surgical hospitalization, often requires intensive care and discharge to rehabilitation, and therefore increases the overall costs of care. In the ACS-NSQIP database, perioperative stroke after noncardiac, non-neurological surgery was associated with an eightfold increase in perioperative mortality within 30 days (95% CI, 4.6–12.6).[1]

## MECHANISMS OF AND RISKS FOR NEUROLOGICAL INJURY

An understanding of the risk factors and mechanisms for perioperative stroke is essential to determine the best strategies for prevention and management of stroke in general, orthopedic, peripheral vascular, and ENT surgery patients.

### Risk Factors

A case-control study of 61 patients with ischemic strokes after noncardiac surgical procedures (including orthopedic surgical procedures) and 122 age-, sex-, and procedure-matched controls showed that surgery and anesthesia themselves contribute to increased risk of stroke.[8] The length of the surgical procedure may influence the risk for perioperative stroke. In one study, the incidence of negative surgical outcome, defined as hospital stay of more than 10 days with a morbid condition including stroke or death, was 10.3% in operations lasting less than 220 minutes versus 38.2% in those lasting more than 220 minutes.[9]

Patient baseline comorbidities and cardiovascular risk factors play a predominant role. Advanced age (usually >70 years), preoperative history of stroke or transient ischemic attack (TIA), renal failure, and atrial fibrillation emerge as the most important risk factors for stroke in patients undergoing general surgery.[10–14] Other factors include female sex, history of myocardial infarction or congestive heart failure, diabetes mellitus, smoking, and chronic obstructive pulmonary disease.[15–16]

### Mechanisms of Neurological Injury

By far, most perioperative strokes are ischemic; only few are hemorrhagic.[10–12] The mechanisms of stroke in patients undergoing surgery are variable and depend on the nature of the surgical procedure, patient risk factors, and intra- and postoperative

**Table 21.1** Potential Mechanisms of Perioperative Stroke After General Surgery

| Hemorrhagic Stroke | Ischemic Stroke |
|---|---|
| • Perioperative anticoagulation | • Thromboembolism<br>  • Cardioembolism<br>  • Atrial fibrillation<br>  • Myocardial infarction<br>  • Heart failure<br> • Hypercoagulability<br>  • Surgery-induced<br>  • Perioperative cessation of antithrombotic therapy<br>  • Paradoxical embolism (with intra- or extra-cardiac left-to-right shunt)<br> • Artery-to-artery embolism (extracranial or intracranial arterial stenosis) |
| • Perioperative hypertension | • Hypoperfusion<br>  • Perioperative blood loss<br>  • Hypotension<br>  • Hemodynamic insufficiency<br>  • Extracranial or intracranial arterial stenosis<br> • OTHER<br>  • Fat, air, or fibrocartilaginous embolism<br>  • Arterial dissection during induction of anesthesia<br>  • Kinking of pre-existing extracranial arterial stenosis or rupture of pre-existing plaque during neck manipulations and induction of anesthesia |

course. Table 21.1 summarizes the potential etiological mechanisms of perioperative stroke in general, orthopedic, peripheral vascular, and ENT surgery patients. Several studies reported that the majority of perioperative strokes occur during the postoperative period.[10–14] Fewer than 6% of patients with perioperative stroke awaken from a general surgical procedure with stroke symptoms, suggesting that intraoperative mechanisms are rarely the immediate cause of perioperative stroke and that postoperative events are more important. In a case-control study of 24,241 patients who underwent noncardiac, non-neurological surgeries, the total duration that the mean blood pressure was decreased greater than 30% from baseline was associated with the occurrence of postoperative stroke.[17] Most studies, however, support little or no association between intraoperative hypotension and perioperative stroke risk in general surgery patients.[10,13] Hypotension during the postoperative period seems to be more important.

Most strokes after general surgery are related to thromboembolism that may be multifactorial. Cardiac embolism is most frequently due to postoperative atrial fibrillation or myocardial infarction as a result of supply–demand mismatch caused by hypertension, hypotension, or tachycardia during the perioperative period. Transient perioperative hypercoagulability may be caused by dehydration, bed rest, blood stasis, blood loss, and withholding of antithrombotic agents.[18–20] Fat, air, or fibrocartilaginous embolism during orthopedic procedures are other sources of embolization. In this regard, it is important to point out that spinal cord infarction might complicate orthopedic and spinal surgery as a result of significant and prolonged hypotension or embolization of fibrocartilaginous debris.[21–22]

## NEUROPROTECTION STRATEGIES
### Preoperative Strategies

Careful assessment to identify patients at high risk for perioperative stroke is essential for selection of appropriate surgical candidates. The individual risk factors listed in Box 21.1 should not be viewed in isolation during preoperative assessment of stroke risk. Some studies suggest that the incidence of stroke following general surgical procedures rises to 1.9% in patients with more than five of the mentioned risk factors.[1] Predictive models for preoperative estimation of stroke risk in patients undergoing general surgical procedures have not been fully studied or validated. A revised cardiac risk index (Box 21.1) has been proposed to predict cardiovascular complications including stroke in general surgery patients.[23–25] The $CHADS_2$ or $CHA_2DS_2$-VASc scores may be used to predict major perioperative events, including stroke, in patients with atrial fibrillation undergoing noncardiac procedures.[26–27]

A detailed neurological history for signs or symptoms of prior stroke or TIA is required in a comprehensive preoperative evaluation in patients with significant risk factors. A history suggestive of prior stroke or TIA should prompt neurological consultation and detailed neurological assessment with brain and vascular imaging to identify and treat the underlying etiology, particularly if these neurological events were not previously investigated or prior workup was incomplete. The timing of surgery in a patient who had a recent stroke should be carefully considered based on the urgency of surgery and its risks, the cause and size of the infarct, and stability of neurological deficits. Cerebrovascular reserve can be tenuous during the days to weeks following a stroke and may increase the risk of stroke recurrence during the perioperative period. A nationwide Danish cohort study of 481,183 patients who underwent noncardiac surgical procedures found that the risk of adverse neurological outcomes following surgery is particularly high if the time interval from previous stroke to surgery is less than 9 months.[28] It is therefore advisable to delay elective surgery in patients who had a recent stroke or TIA for as long as possible to

---

Box 21.1 The Revised Cardiac Risk Index

Independent predictors of perioperative complications:

1. High-risk type of surgery
2. History of ischemic heart disease
3. History of congestive heart failure
4. History of cerebrovascular disease
5. Preoperative treatment with insulin
6. Preoperative serum creatinine >2.0 mg/dL (176 μmol/L).

The presence of ≥2 of the preceding factors can aid with preoperative identification of patients undergoing nonurgent, noncardiac, surgery, as follows:

- Moderate perioperative complication rates (7%) in patients with 2 factors
- High perioperative complication rates (11%) in patients with >2 factors

allow the cerebral autoregulation to recover before encountering the hemodynamic stresses of surgery.

## Perioperative Strategies

Optimal management of the patient's risk factors in the perioperative period is essential to minimize the risk for stroke and to minimize the neurological deficits if a stroke occurs. Special considerations include serum glucose, blood pressure, atrial fibrillation, and antithrombotic agents.

## Serum Glucose

Preoperative hyperglycemia and impaired fasting glucose levels, independent of diabetes and other comorbidities, are associated with increased risk for perioperative stroke, myocardial infarction, and death.[29] Hyperglycemia is also associated with worse outcome after stroke.[30] Therefore, close attention should be paid to glucose monitoring and glycemic control during the perioperative period. The recommended target range for perioperative blood glucose is 60–180 mg/dL, despite the limitations of retrospective data analyses.[31]

## Blood Pressure

Optimal control of blood pressure preoperatively, coupled with careful monitoring of blood pressure intra- and postoperatively, is of critical importance to prevent hypertensive or hypotensive episodes and to maintain adequate cerebral perfusion. Therefore, antihypertensive agents should be continued up to the time of surgery to maintain a near-normal blood pressure.

Special caution should be considered with (1) abrupt preoperative discontinuation of some antihypertensive medications, such as clonidine, that may result in rebound hypertension; and (2) initiation of de novo therapy with β-blockers, particularly metoprolol, shortly before surgery, as this might be associated with increased risk of postoperative stroke.[32] A meta-analysis of 33 trials including 12,306 noncardiac surgery patients found that perioperative use of β-blockers was associated with an increase (odds ratio [OR] 2.01, 1.27–3.68) in nonfatal strokes. The use of β-blockers was not associated with any significant reduction in the risk of all-cause mortality, cardiovascular mortality, or heart failure, but it was associated with a high risk of perioperative bradycardia and hypotension requiring treatment.[33] In one study of noncardiac surgery patients, the use of intraoperative metoprolol, but not the shorter acting β-blockers esmolol or labetalol, was associated with a 3.3-fold increase in perioperative stroke, indicating that metoprolol should be used with caution or potentially avoided when perioperative β-blockade is required in patients at high risk of stroke.[34]

The optimal intraoperative target range for blood pressure is uncertain. Some recommend maintaining mean or systolic blood pressure within 20% of the preoperative baseline blood pressure.[35] Particular attention should be paid to patients undergoing shoulder surgery in the beach chair position. Case reports have linked this procedure to increased risk of perioperative stroke, presumably attributed to positional hypotension during the procedure or overestimation of cerebral perfusion pressure due to blood pressure determination from lower extremity cuffs (with failure to adjust for hydrostatic differences).[6] Indeed, some studies using near-infrared spectroscopy have documented a high incidence of desaturation in the beach chair position.[36] A recent consensus statement from the Society for Neuroscience in Anesthesiology and Critical Care recommends that induced hypotension for shoulder surgery in the beach chair position should be cautiously considered, particularly in patients at high risk for stroke, and that blood pressure measurements should be done using a cuff placed on the nonoperative arm as opposed to the lower extremity.[31]

## Management of Atrial Fibrillation

Patients with chronic atrial fibrillation should be closely monitored during the perioperative period. Antiarrhythmia and rate-controlling medications usually should be continued without interruption, and electrolytes and fluid status should be carefully monitored and corrected on an ongoing basis. The question always arises as to whether anticoagulation should be interrupted preoperatively or whether bridging therapy with heparin or heparinoids is required during the perioperative period. Results from the Perioperative Bridging Anticoagulation in Patients with Atrial Fibrillation (BRIDGE) trial suggest that foregoing bridging anticoagulation decreases the risk of bleeding complications and is not inferior to perioperative bridging with low-molecular-weight heparin for the prevention of arterial thromboembolic events including stroke and TIA.[37] In that study, 100 IU/kg of dalteparin was administered subcutaneously twice daily for 3 days before the procedure until 24 hours before surgery, and then for 5–10 days postoperatively, for the prevention of arterial thromboembolic events including stroke and TIA. Few patients in this trial, however, had a $CHADS_2$ score of greater than 4, and the majority of patients underwent low-risk ambulatory procedures. It is still likely that patients with $CHADS_2$ scores of greater than 4, those with significant history of thromboembolism, and/or those undergoing high-risk procedures should be considered for bridging therapy during the perioperative period to minimize ischemic stroke risk Table 21.2.

Patients who develop atrial fibrillation de novo postoperatively may have increased risk of subsequent stroke after both noncardiac and cardiac surgery.[38] Initiation of anticoagulation may be warranted, especially in high-risk patients, such as those with a history of stroke or TIA. Anticoagulation therapy should continue for 30 days after the return of normal sinus rhythm based on the recommendations of the American College of Chest Physicians and the American Association for Thoracic Surgery guidelines.[39-40]

## Management of Antithrombotic Agents

Temporary withholding of antithrombotics in anticipation of a surgical procedure may be associated with increased risk of thromboembolic events, either due to the indication for treatment itself, rebound hypercoagulability due to discontinuation of the antithrombotic agent, or a surgery-induced hypercoagulable state.[19-20,41-42] A Danish study including 66,358 patients who underwent total hip replacement and matched controls found that outpatient antiplatelet drug use lowered the 6-week postoperative hazard ratios for ischemic stroke by 70% while not affecting the risk of hemorrhagic stroke.[5] Although continuation of antiplatelet therapy

**Table 21.2** Thromboembolic Risk Categories for Patients Taking Antithrombotic Therapy

| Thromboembolism Risk category | Indication for Antithrombotic Therapy | | | Perioperative Bridging Therapy |
|---|---|---|---|---|
| | *Prosthetic Heart Valve* | *Atrial Fibrillation* | *Venous Embolism* | *Therapy* |
| HIGH/MODERATE | History of stroke/TIA | History of stroke/TIA | Recent venous embolism (within 3 months) | Recommended |
| | Any mitral valve | Rheumatic valvular heart disease | Thrombophilia | |
| | Caged ball or single leaflet aortic valve | CHADS$_2$ score >4 | Venous embolism within 3–12 months | |
| | Bi-leaflet aortic valve | ≥ 2 stroke risk factors | Active cancer | |
| | ≥ 1 stroke risk factor | CHADS$_2$ score 3-4 | Recurrent venous thromboembolism | |
| LOW | Bi-leaflet aortic valve | No history of stroke/TIA | Single venous embolic event >12 months ago | Optional—probably not required |
| | No stroke risk factors | CHADS$_2$ score <3 | None of the above | |

TIA, transient ischemic attack.

during the perioperative period might increase the risk of intraoperative bleeding during ENT or peripheral vascular procedures, there does not seem to be an associated increased risk for neurological or medical complications.[43-44] Therefore, continuation of antiplatelet therapy, in particular aspirin, seems to be acceptable in many procedures.[45]

The decision of when to stop or continue antithrombotics during the perioperative period should be individualized and should always involve weighing the risk of bleeding complications against the benefit of preventing thromboembolic events during the perioperative period. Given that bleeding is usually a treatable perioperative complication, the decision-making should place a high value on preventing thromboembolism in patients at high risk for thromboembolism and preventing bleeding in patients at low risk for thromboembolism.[46] Continuing clopidogrel and aspirin during the perioperative period has been advised in patients with a bare metal coronary stent who require surgery within 6 weeks of stent placement and in patients with a drug-eluting coronary stent who require surgery within 12 months of stent placement to prevent stent-related coronary thrombosis.[46] The period during which antithrombotic therapy is withheld should be minimized to decrease the risk of systemic thromboembolism and stroke during the perioperative period.

The American College of Chest Physicians Evidence-Based Clinical Practice Guidelines has made the following recommendations regarding perioperative management of anticoagulation.[46] (1) Bridging warfarin with therapeutic-dose subcutaneous low-molecular-weight heparin (SC LMWH), such as dalteparin 200 IU/kg once daily or enoxaparin 1.5 to 2 mg/kg once daily, or IV unfractionated heparin (UFH), is recommended preoperatively in patients with a mechanical heart valve, or atrial fibrillation, or venous thromboembolism, or clotting disorder at high or moderate risk for thromboembolism. The last preoperative dose of SC LMWH should approximate half the total daily dose instead of 100% and should be administered 24 hours before the procedure. If IV UFH is used as bridging anticoagulation, it should be stopped approximately 4 hours before surgery. (2) In patients with a mechanical heart valve, atrial fibrillation, or venous thromboembolism who are at low risk for future thromboembolism, low-dose SC LMWH, enoxaparin 30 mg twice daily or dalteparin 5000 IU once daily, or no bridging is recommended instead of bridging with therapeutic-dose SC LMWH or IV UFH.

Little is known about the perioperative management of newer anticoagulants such as direct thrombin or factor Xa inhibitors and their impact on perioperative bleeding risks. The duration for which these drugs need to be withheld prior to a procedure depends on baseline renal function and creatinine clearance.

## Intraoperative Strategies

To the extent that they can be avoided, reducing the intraoperative incidence of risk factors for perioperative stroke is a reasonable strategy. These risk factors include perioperative arrhythmias, respiratory compromise, extremes of hypotension or hypertension, cerebral hypoperfusion, and thromboembolism. Good surgical and anesthetic management is always tailored toward the goals of (1) appropriate selection of anesthetic technique and (2) maximizing homeostasis by use of techniques, medications, and intravenous fluid to normalize blood pressure, heart rate, and respiratory, fluid, and blood volume status during surgery.

When feasible, the use of local anesthesia and lesser degrees of sedation allows clinical monitoring of neurological function by assessing level of consciousness, speech, and strength of handgrip during surgical procedures, thus allowing timely detection of ischemia and the taking of necessary measures to correct inadequate cerebral perfusion. Neuraxial techniques are also associated with a lower incidence of perioperative stroke after orthopedic surgery. A large database study of more than 200,000 knee and hip arthroplasty patients found that neuraxial anesthesia was associated with a lower incidence of stroke (0.07%) compared to combined neur-axial and general anesthesia (0.12%) and general anesthesia (0.13%, $P = 0.006$).[47] Similarly, a single-center retrospective medical record review of 18,745 consecutive patients who underwent primary or revision total joint arthroplasty found that general anesthesia was an independent predictor of postoperative stroke within 30 days (OR 3.54, 95% CI 1.01–12.39).[48] As retrospective cohort investigations, these observations require confirmation in a prospective study. At present, there is no definitive evidence that choice of anesthetic technique is an effective strategy for reducing perioperative stroke.

## Postoperative Strategies

Continued and close monitoring of patients for postoperative arrhythmias, heart failure, neurological deterioration, vital signs, intravascular volume status, electrolytes, hemostasis, and blood sugar in the days after surgery is essential to implement prompt corrective actions to prevent conditions associated with stroke. It is also important to identify and treat causes of postoperative hypertension, such as pain, agitation, bladder distension, and hypoxia.

The personnel performing the monitoring should be educated about stroke warning symptoms and signs and trained to perform a thorough neurological assessment. They should be alerted that stroke symptoms in the postoperative phase can be misdiagnosed by incorrectly attributing them to "general deterioration" due to the effects of anesthesia or metabolic imbalances. Rapid identification of postoperative neurological complications, including focal neurological deficits, is essential and allows timely management to optimize the patient's recovery.

Early postoperative use of prophylactic strategies to minimize the risk of systemic thromboembolism is recommended to prevent potential paradoxical embolism and stroke. The incidence of thromboembolic complications, especially deep vein thrombosis (DVT), can be reduced by using graduated elastic compression stockings, intermittent pneumatic calf compression, early postoperative mobilization, maintenance of good cerebral perfusion (adequate hematocrit and normovolemia), and appropriate antiplatelet and anticoagulation protocols. A Cochrane database systematic review showed that the use of graduated compression stockings was effective in diminishing the risk of thromboembolic events in hospitalized patients after various surgeries and that using stockings with another method of DVT prophylaxis was more effective than using stockings alone.[49]

Rapid identification and correction of significant perioperative blood loss is also important yet often overlooked. In the Perioperative Ischemic Evaluation (POISE) trial, significant bleeding emerged as an independent predictor of postoperative stroke (adjusted OR 2.18, 95% CI 1.45–8.52) in the population of high-risk patients undergoing noncardiac surgery.[32] Similarly, patients with significant blood loss requiring more than 4 units of packed red blood cells had a 2.5-fold increased risk for stroke or myocardial infarction in a study of 651,775 patients undergoing general surgery.[50] Although highly controversial, it has been recommended that a hemoglobin level of less than 9.0 gm/dL should be avoided in order to minimize risk of stroke.[31]

## Management of Acute Stroke

Improved and early recognition of stroke by perioperative care teams and immediate consultation of the stroke team for suspected stroke are crucial to facilitate early treatment. Brain imaging should be performed as soon as possible to rule out intracranial hemorrhage or an undiagnosed brain lesion. Although many patients with ischemic stroke following general surgery may not be candidates for intravenous thrombolysis, which is often contraindicated during the first 2 weeks after a major procedure, they may be candidates for endovascular therapy. The use of endovascular revascularization strategies, especially thrombectomy, is a reasonable and safe alternative to IV thrombolysis for the management of hyperacute ischemic stroke in the perioperative setting.[51]

## IMPLICATIONS FOR CLINICAL PRACTICE

Stroke after orthopedic, ENT, peripheral vascular, and general surgical procedures usually occurs postoperatively, largely due to thromboembolism. Strategies to prevent perioperative stroke and to improve neurological outcomes are based on knowledge of the etiologies, pathophysiology, and risk factors for perioperative stroke. It is vital to use that knowledge to guide clinical approaches that are targeted to monitoring neurological status to guide early interventions.

A detailed neurological history and thorough evaluation of patients with prior stroke or TIA is mandatory before any elective surgical procedure. Both hyperglycemia and hypoglycemia should be avoided during the perioperative period. Although there are no randomized controlled trials to confirm the benefit of tight glycemic control in preventing or improving the outcome of perioperative stroke, there is consensus that blood glucose should be maintained in the 60–180 mg/dL range during the perioperative period.[31] Acute preoperative initiation of high doses of metoprolol should be avoided. Intraoperatively, techniques should be geared toward preventing excessive variability in blood pressure. In patients with atrial fibrillation, antiarrhythmia and rate-controlling medications should be continued without interruption, and electrolytes and fluid status should be carefully monitored and corrected during the perioperative period. Although recent data from the BRIDGE trial suggest that bridging warfarin with SC LMWH may not be necessary in patients with atrial fibrillation undergoing low-risk surgical procedures, the decision of whether to continue or withhold anticoagulation before surgery should be individualized and carefully discussed with each patient and his or her treating physicians.[37] Although antiplatelet drugs increase the risk of perioperative bleeding complications, temporary withholding of these agents, in particular aspirin, before general, orthopedic, and ENT procedures is unnecessary and could increase perioperative stroke risk. There is rising evidence to support the use of regional anesthetic techniques in appropriate settings.[47–48] In patients at high risk of stroke, there is a consensus statement recommending correction of postoperative blood loss to maintain a hemoglobin level of 9 gm/dL or greater, although this remains controversial.[31]

# FUTURE DIRECTIONS

The devastating effects of stroke after general surgical procedures, despite its uncommon occurrence, call for more research. Although the preceding recommendations can help to decrease the incidence of perioperative stroke, there is an unmet need to find novel and effective neuroprotective strategies that can be used pre- or intraoperatively to minimize the effects of stroke on brain tissue and resulting disability. Future studies should evaluate the potential usefulness of neuroprotective therapies or interventions, including various anesthetic agents that can be used prophylactically in the perioperative setting.

# REFERENCES

1. Mashour GA1, Shanks AM, Kheterpal S. Perioperative stroke and associated mortality after noncardiac, nonneurologic surgery. *Anesthesiology*. 2011;114(6):1289–96.

2. Mrkobrada M, Hill MD, Chan MT, et al. The Neurovision Pilot Study: non-cardiac surgery carries a significant risk of acute covert stroke. *Stroke*. 2013;44(2):ATMP9.

3. Nosan DK, Gomez CR, Maves MD. Perioperative stroke in patients undergoing head and neck surgery. *Ann Otol Rhinol Laryngol*. 1993;102(9):717–23.

4. MacNeil SD, Liu K, Garg AX, et al. A population-based study of 30-day incidence of ischemic stroke following surgical neck dissection. *Medicine (Baltimore)*. 2015;94(33):e1106.

5. Lalmohamed A, Vestergaard P, Cooper C, et al. Timing of stroke in patients undergoing total hip replacement and matched controls: a nationwide cohort study. *Stroke*. 2012;43(12):3225–9.

6. Pohl A, Cullen DJ. Cerebral ischemia during shoulder surgery in the upright position: a case series. *J Clin Anesth*. 2005;17(6):463–9.

7. Bateman BT, Schumacher HC, Wang S, Shaefi S, Berman MF. Perioperative acute ischemic stroke in non-cardiac and non-vascular surgery: incidence, risk factors, and outcomes. *Anaesthiology*. 2009;110:231–8.

8. Limburg M, Wijdicks EF, Li H. Ischemic stroke after surgical procedures: clinical features, neuroimaging, and stroke factors. *Neurology*. 1998;50:895–901.

9. Polanczyk CA, Marcantonio E, Goldman L, et al. Impact of age on perioperative complications and length of stay in patients undergoing noncardiac surgery. *Ann Intern Med*. 2001;134(8):637–43.

10. Hart R, Hindman B. Mechanisms of perioperative cerebral infarction. *Stroke*. 1982; 13:766–73.

11. Larsen SF, Zaric D, Bosen G. Postoperative cerebrovascular accidents in general surgery. *Acta Anaesthesiol Scand*. 1988;32:698–701.

12. Parikh S, Cohen JR. Postoperative stroke after general surgical procedures. *NY State J Med*. 1993;93:162–5.

13. Limburg M, Wijdicks EF, Li H. Ischemic stroke after surgical procedures: clinical features, neuroimaging, and stroke factors. *Neurology*. 1998;50:895–901.

14. Kikura M, Oikawa F, Yamamoto K, et al. Myocardial infarction and cerebrovascular accident following non-cardiac surgery: differences in postoperative temporal distribution and risk factors. *J Thromb Haemost*. 2008;6:742–8.

15. Bateman BT, Schumacher HC, Wang S, Shaefi S, Berman MF. Perioperative acute ischemic stroke in noncardiac and nonvascular surgery: incidence, risk factors, and outcomes. *Anesthesiology*. 2009;110(2):231–8.

16. Sharifpour M, Moore LE, Shanks AM, Didier TJ, Kheterpal S, Mashour GA. Incidence, predictors, and outcomes of perioperative stroke in noncarotid major vascular surgery. *Anesth Analg.* 2013;116(2):424–34.

17. Bijker JB, Persoon S, Peelen LM, et al. Intraoperative hypotension and perioperative ischemic stroke after general surgery: a nested case-control study. *Anesthesiology.* 2012;116(3):658–64.

18. Reich DL, Bennett-Guerrero E, Bodian CA, Hossain S, Winfree W, Krol M. Intraoperative tachycardia and hypertension are independently associated with adverse outcome in noncardiac surgery of long duration. *Anesth Analg.* 2002;95(2):273–7.

19. Hinterhuber G, Böhler K, Kittler H, Quehenberger P. Extended monitoring of hemostatic activation after varicose vein surgery under general anesthesia. *Dermatol Surg.* 2006;32(5):632–9.

20. Broderick JP, Bonomo JB, Kissela BM, et al. Withdrawal of antithrombotic agents and its impact on ischemic stroke occurrence. *Stroke.* 2011;42(9):2509–14.

21. Kim JS, Ko SB, Shin HE, Han SR, Lee KS. Perioperative stroke in the brain and spinal cord following an induced hypotension. *Yonsei Med J.* 2003;44(1):143–5.

22. Langmayr JJ, Ortler M, Obwegeser A, Felber S. Quadriplegia after lumbar disc surgery. A case report. *Spine.* 1996;21(16):1932–5.

23. Press MJ, Chassin MR, Wang J, Tuhrim S, Halm EA. Predicting medical and surgical complications of carotid endarterectomy: comparing the risk indexes. *Arch Intern Med.* 2006;166(8):914–20.

24. Lee TH, Marcantonio ER, Mangione CM, et al. Derivation and prospective validation of a simple index for prediction of cardiac risk of major noncardiac surgery. *Circulation.* 1999;100(10):1043–9.

25. Andersson C, Wissenberg M, Jørgensen ME, et al. Age-specific performance of the revised cardiac risk index for predicting cardiovascular risk in elective noncardiac surgery. *Circ Cardiovasc Qual Outcomes.* 2015;8(1):103–8.

26. McAlister FA, Jacka M, Graham M, et al. The prediction of postoperative stroke or death in patients with preoperative atrial fibrillation undergoing non-cardiac surgery: a VISION sub-study. *J Thromb Haemost.* 2015;13(10)1768–75.

27. van Diepen S, Youngson E, Ezekowitz JA, McAlister FA. Which risk score best predicts perioperative outcomes in nonvalvular atrial fibrillation patients undergoing noncardiac surgery? *Am Heart J.* 2014;168(1):60–7.e5.

28. Jorgensen ME, Torp-Pedersen C, Gislason GH, et al. Time elapsed after ischemic stroke and risk of adverse cardiovascular events and mortality following elective noncardiac surgery. *JAMA.* 2014;312(3):269–77.

29. Biteker M, Dayan A, Can MM, et al. Impaired fasting glucose is associated with increased perioperative cardiovascular event rates in patients undergoing major non-cardiothoracic surgery. *Cardiovasc Diabetol.* 2011;10:63.

30. Gentile NT, Seftchick MW, Huynh T, Kruus LK, Gaughan J. Decreased mortality by normalizing blood glucose after acute ischemic stroke. *Acad Emerg Med.* 2006;13(2):174–80.

31. Mashour GA, Moore LE, Lele AV, Robicsel SA, Gelb AW. Perioperative care of patients at high risk for stroke during or after non-cardiac, non-neurologic surgery: consensus statement from the Society for Neuroscience in Anesthesiology and Critical Care. *J Neuros Anesth.* 2014;26(4):273–85.

32. POISE Study Group, Devereaux PJ, Yang H, Yusuf S, et al. Effects of extended-release metoprolol succinate in patients undergoing non-cardiac surgery (POISE trial): a randomised controlled trial. *Lancet.* 2008;371(9627):1839–47.

33. Bangalore S, Wetterslev J, Pranesh S, Sawhney S, Gluud C, Messerli FH. Perioperative beta blockers in patients having non-cardiac surgery: a meta-analysis. *Lancet.* 2008; 372(9654):1962–76.

34. Mashour GA, Sharifpour M, Freundlich RE, et al. Perioperative metoprolol and risk of stroke after noncardiac surgery. *Anesthesiology.* 2013;119(6):1340–6.

35. Ng JL, Chan MT, Gelb AW. Perioperative stroke in noncardiac, nonneurosurgical surgery. *Anesthesiology.* 2011;115(4):879–90.

36. Pant S, Bokor DJ, Low AK. Cerebral oxygenation using near-infrared spectroscopy in the beach-chair position during shoulder arthroscopy under general anesthesia. *J Arthroscopic Related Surg.* 2014;30(11):1520–7.

37. Douketis JD, Spyropoulos AC, Kaatz S, et al. Perioperative bridging anticoagulation in patients with atrial fibrillation. *N Engl J Med.* 2015;373:823–33.

38. Gialdini G, Nearing K, Bhave PD, et al. Perioperative atrial fibrillation and the long-term risk of ischemic stroke. *JAMA.* 2014;312(6):616–22.

39. Epstein AE, Alexander JC, Gutterman DD, Maisel W, Wharton JM; American College of Chest Physicians. Anticoagulation: American college of chest physicians guidelines for the prevention and management of postoperative atrial fibrillation after cardiac surgery. *Chest.* 2005;128(2 Suppl):24S–27S.

40. Frendl G, Sodickson AC, Chung MK, et al.; American Association for Thoracic Surgery. 2014 AATS guidelines for the prevention and management of perioperative atrial fibrillation and flutter for thoracic surgical procedures. *J Thorac Cardiovasc Surg.* 2014;148(3):e153–93.

41. Maulaz AB, Bezerra DC, Michel P, Bogousslavsky J. Effect of discontinuing aspirin therapy on the risk of brain ischemic stroke. *Arch Neurol.* 2005;62(8):1217–20.

42. Genewein U, Haeberli A, Straub PW, Beer JH. Rebound after cessation of oral anticoagulant therapy: the biochemical evidence. *Br J Haematol.* 1996;92(2):479–85.

43. Knopf A, Freudelsperger L, Stark T, Scherer E. [ENT surgery in patients with anticoagulants and platelet aggregation inhibitors]. *HNO.* 2014;62(5):350–7.

44. Saadeh C, Sfeir J. Discontinuation of preoperative clopidogrel is unnecessary in peripheral arterial surgery. *J Vasc Surg.* 2013;58(6):1586–92.

45. Ferraris VA, Swanson E. Aspirin usage and perioperative blood loss in patients undergoing unexpected operations. *Surg Gynecol Obstet.* 1983;156(4):439–42.

46. Douketis JD, Spyropoulos AC, Spencer FA, et al.; American College of Chest Physicians. Perioperative management of antithrombotic therapy: Antithrombotic Therapy and Prevention of Thrombosis, 9th ed.: American College of Chest Physicians Evidence-Based Clinical Practice Guidelines. *Chest.* 2012;141(2 Suppl):e326S–50S. Erratum in: *Chest.* 2012;141(4):1129.

47. Memtsoudis SG, Sun X, Chiu YL, et al. Perioperative comparative effectiveness of anesthetic technique in orthopedic patients. *Anesthesiology.* 2013;118:1046–58.

48. Mortazavi SM, Kakli H, Bican O, et al. Perioperative stroke after total joint arthroplasty: prevalence, predictors, and outcome. *J Bone Joint Surg Am.* 2010;92:2095–101.

49. Amarigiri SV, Lees TA. Elastic compression stockings for prevention of deep vein thrombosis. *Cochrane Database Syst Rev.* 2000;CD001484.

50. Kamel H, Johnston SC, Kirkham JC, et al. Association between major perioperative hemorrhage and stroke or Q wave myocardial infarction. *Circulation.* 2012;126:207–12.

51. Chalela JA, Katzan I, Liebeskind DS, et al. Safety of intra-arterial thrombolysis in the postoperative period. *Stroke.* 2001;32(6):1365–9.

# Index